The Healing Forces of Harmonic Sounds and Vibrations

Healing Through the Power of the Voice and the Mind

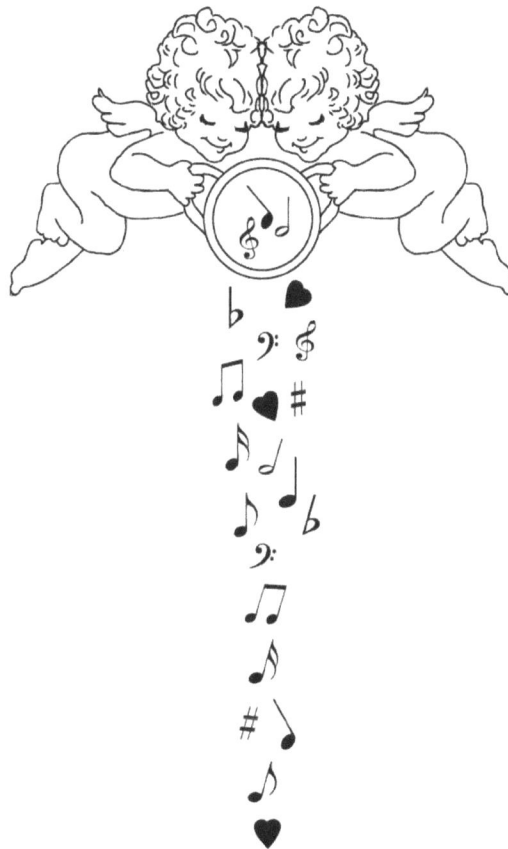

"The Healing Forces of Harmonic Sounds and Vibrations"

ISBN-13: 978-0-9916237-1-6
ISBN-10: 0-9916237-1-1

Published by: JEM Productions
Copyright © 2017 Jay Emmanuel Morales

All Rights Reserved

Technical Edition: Teodorico Enrique Ampudia
Editorial Review: Linda Russo
Production Management and Logistics: Teodorico Enrique Ampudia
Cover and Back Cover Design: Carlos Alberto Quintero
Photographs: Marco Antonio Olmos, Teodorico Enrique Ampudia

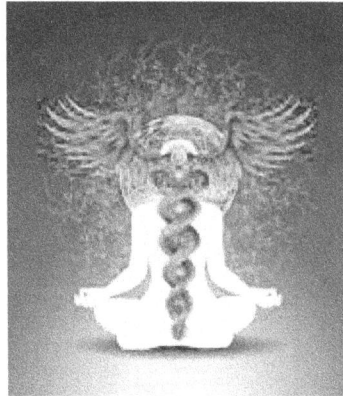

The Power of Harmony Organization, Health and Global Wellness Network:
Jay Emmanuel Morales, A.K., V.M.
P. O. Box 2618 New York, N.Y. 10108-2618
Tel: (212) 465-8163
E-mail: **powerofharmony1@gmail.com**
Web: **healingpowerofharmony.com**

Disclaimer: This book is for information, experimental research & self-education purposes only. No text in this book is used to treat disease.

Dedication

I dedicate this book "To the Universal Creative Intelligence" for granting me the gift of being able to sing, for being able to produce harmonic sounds through my voice, for giving me the blessing of being able to appreciate and enjoy the music created by great composers of classical music, Gregorian chants, Tibetan chants, Vedic chants, the melodious and inspiring voices of singers who sing with the strength of their hearts, and the musicians and composers who make music with the deepest sensitivity of their spirit, for giving me the opportunity to be of service, to inspire and assist humanity in a way that they can activate their natural healing process of the mind, body and spirit through "The Healing Forces of Harmonic Sounds and Vibrations and The Healing Power of the Voice and the Mind.

Because that healing power is latent within each of us through our mind and voice, when we generate creative harmonious thoughts and sounds and when we sharpen our perception capacities, the appreciation for music and the assimilation of those sounds, it manifests the atomic transformation that activates healing in all our systems.

I dedicate this book also to my beloved parents who humbly and with many sacrifices through life enriched me with the most powerful force in the universe, the love they gave me, the spiritual values, the compassion, the respect and consideration for humanity. To my beloved brother, to my political sister and to my dear nieces for all the love that they have given me. I dedicate this book to all the great masters, minds and scientists who have left legacies of wisdom that contribute and who will continue contributing through time, inspiring and awakening the consciousness and hearts of men and women in a way that we collectively can achieve to raise our vibrational frequency in the power of harmony, peace, unconditional love, goodwill, integrity, honesty, the wisdom of the highest spheres and primarily to create a better world where every man and woman values and protects our planet Earth's natural resources.

The Master of Teachers, Jesus Christ, Siddhartha Buddha, Ascended Masters, Tibetan Masters, Teachers of India, Egyptian Masters, Mayan Masters of Mexico and Guatemala, Chinese Buddhist Teachers, Sufis Teachers of Islam, Taoist and Shaolin Monks of China, Gregorian Monks, Rimpoche Tenzin Wangyal, Australian and Native Aborigines of North America, South America, Mexico, Central America, Geshi Lobsang Jamyang the Lama Thupten Kunkhyer, Pythagoras of Samos, Thoh (Hermes Trismegistus, The Atlante), Nicolas Tesla, Albert Einstein, George Lakhosky, Dr. Royal Raymond Rife, Dr. Alfred A. Tomatis, Leonardo Pisano Bigollo Fibonacci, Leonardo da Vinci, Guido de Arezzo, Dr. Daniel David Palmer, Edgard Cayce, Rudolf Steiner, Dr. Winfried Otto Shumann, Ernst Chladni, Dr. Hans Jenny, Dr. Josep Puleo, Dr. Leonard G. Horowitz, Dr. Lee Lorenze, Dr. Masaru Emoto, Maestro Pablo Casals, Maestro Jesus Maria Sanroman, Profesora Raquel Gandia, Dra. Valerie

V. Hunt, Dr. Robert O. Becker, Dr. Harold Saxton Burr, Dr. Reinhold Voll, Bruce Taino, Dr. Samuel Hahnemann, Dr. Herbertf Benson, Dr. Mitchell Gaynor, Dra. Pat Moffit Cook, Dr. Jeffrey Thompson, Professor Richard J. Saykally (UC), Dr. Steven Angel, Dr. Glen Rein, (NY), Victor Showell, John Stuart Reid, Thomas Aksness, Dr. Premala Brewster-Wilson, Dr. Leonel Eduardo Lechuga, Dra. Raquel Liberman, Dra. Estela Laufer, Dr. Jose Miguel Gonzalez, Dr. Bruno Casatelli, Dr. Ruben Ong, Dr. Edmund L. Gergerian, Dra. Gloria Godinez Leal, Dr. J.J. Hurtad, Dr. James Gimzewski, Dr. Paul T. Sprieser, Dr. June Leslie Wieder, Dr. John Beaulien, Dr. Herbert Berson, Dr. Neil Douglas Klotz, Manfred Clynes, Dr. Georgi Lozanov, Dr. Gordon Shaw, Dr. Francis Raucher and others.

Yogi-mahavatar Babaji, Paramahansa Yogananda, Maestre Serge Raynaud de la Ferriere, Maestro Rafael Elvira, Paquito Cordero, Nivea Solano, Sylvia de Grasse, Myrta Silva, Luis Vigoreaux, Nidiac Caro, Iris Chacon, Ednita Nasario, Emilio Cueto, Palmira Ubiñas, Pilar Alvear Farnsworth, Anita Velez Rieckehoff Mitchell, Marisol Carrere, Teodorico Enrique Ampudia, Marco Antonio Olmos, Carlos Quintero, Jesus Gutierrez, Laura Toapanta, William Jones (Lupito), Paul Utz (Crystal Tones), Susana Bastarrica, Antonio Kabral, Omar Cabrera, Miriam Cruz, María Rodríguez, Socorro García, Maria Guadalupe Doris Velez Marques, Dra. Maria Corbett, Dr. Bill Akpinar, Sonia Llanos, Linda Ruso, Nilda Tapia, Sigmund Jasinski, Thaddius Sadlowski, Yuli Zorov, Cely Carrillo Omrubia, Bonny Hughes, David Capurso, Michelangelo, Botticelli, Rafael, Pierre Seurat, Edward Bumes Jones, Salvador Dalí, John Hutchinson, Nancy Hutchinson, Lunartunar, John Lennon, Priscilla Spriesser and others.

"Our mind power is infinite and extraordinary as the whole universe and through it we create thoughts that generate vibrational frequencies of sounds that manifest and create our world."

- J.E.M.

Content

Prologue

In the infinite mystery of life and time, certain individuals incarnate into the world with a very specific talent and a unique and urgent mission engraved in the depths of their souls. This specific vocation is a call that in the evolutionary progress of human consciousness has been traveling through centuries and, in the sacred mystery of human redemption, requires a precise time for its realization. The American Indian tradition tells us we are now entering the Age of the Ear. This is a book of profound wisdom to impart a clarion call of awakening to all humanity at this critical time.

Jay Emmanuel Morales, born in Puerto Rico fewer than six decades ago, delivers in this book the entire legacy of his soul, with powerful ancient teachings and scientific evidence of the immense healing power of harmonic sounds, voice and mind. His informative text rekindles sacred fires dormant in our modern culture that are imperishable jewels of perennial wisdom to illumine our future.

The purpose of this book is to make people aware of the innate power that each of us possesses to manifest changes towards a more creative and more productive life, good health and spiritual growth.

Since age 18 when he came to the United States with a musical scholarship, Jay has been a great representative of Hispanic culture in New York City. In addition to music, he dedicated his life to the healing profession. The spine, that marvel of marvels in the sacred temple of our physical body first called him, so he studied applied kinesiology. He perceived the spine as a perfect cosmic musical instrument, that by the size, shape and weight of each vertebrae, held all the music of life. Performing arts, voice training, yoga, Qi Gong, esoteric and psychological studies and initiations, meditation, toning, chanting and mantra practice, plus the daily ubiquitous appreciation of music, coupled with extensive travel to ancient sacred sites on all continents, are among the ingredients that have come together to illumine this extraordinary work, the harvest of Jay's life. And yes also star charts, pyramid power and the modern magic of quartz crystal and Tibetan singing bowls…! His Puerto-Rican upbringing provided a very solid spiritual foundation.
In the pages of this great book, Jay walks us through many understandings of the Healing Forces of Harmonic Sounds and Vibrations with great care and patience.

Let us be grateful to receive the many soul promptings this book carries. Human beings are individualized aspects of the divine and are one humanity.

To each and to all of us God has given the voice, the divine legacy of sound and verb.
With our voice, let us consciously bless the world and heal our bodies.

Pilar Alvear Farnsworth,
Colombian writer, founder of a Movement for
Fully Conscious Natural Birth (Birth Movement)
http://www.farnsworthproductions.com/PilarDeLaLuz/

Preface

The extraordinary work performed by Jay Emmanuel Morales in this book exposes the use of innovative healing techniques through the power of harmonic sound, which he masterfully combines with the energies generated through the sounds of specific vowels of the Ancient Solfeggio codes, his melodious voice, the crystal quartz and Tibetan singing bowls. Jay Emmanuel studied singing and music at the Music Conservatory Pablo Casals of Puerto Rico.

More than a literary work, we could say that this is a didactic book, which describes a series of techniques where sound is the main element of his thesis, responsible for enhancing and awakening harmonic frequencies to create a perfect balance at the cellular level, resulting in the integration and self-healing of the body, mind and spirit.

We understand that today, modern medical science increasingly resorts to holistic healing techniques, as an alternative to make the treatments of traditional medicine more effective.

Jay Emmanuel is considered a great teacher in the healing areas of Vibrational Medicine, Kinesiology, Homeopathy, Ayurvedic Medicine, Nutrition and a great connoisseur of the ancient techniques from the Atlanteans, the Vedas of India, the Tibetans, the ancient wisdom schools of the Egyptians and other ancient civilizations that proved their effectiveness. All these therapeutic modalities have been scientifically corroborated and experimented with great success by the author in patients who have learned and who have managed to activate their natural healing process.

Congratulations, Jay, and I wish you many successes in your mission! A hug wrapped in divine light from my heart to yours…

Palmira Ubiñas
President and Founder: International Association of Hispanic Arts and Culture AIPEH
P. O. Box 720927, Orlando, FL 32872-0927, Tel: (407) 851-9191
Email: www.poetasyescritores@gmail.com

Scientific Testimonials

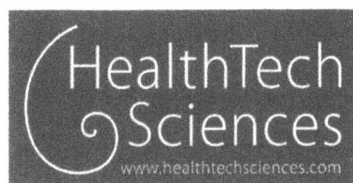

Sound therapy effective for chakra improvement

HealthTech Sciences is a research company focusing on health technologies, and is also behind the clinic franchise Health Optimizing, where the most effective health technologies for assessment and therapy within all categories are integrated.

We have tested Jay Emmanuel's chakra therapies on the CD "The Healing forces of Harmonic Sounds and Vibrations".

The tests have been performed with the "Voice Analysis" technology from Aquera, integrating all the different methodologies of analyzing emotional factors, chakras etc. from the voice.

Test subjects have been tested before and after listening 2 or 3 times to the chakra track specific for their weakest chakra according to the first test.

We have found Jay Emmanuel's sound therapy to be very effective, and in every test the treated chakra improved significantly.

Bergen, 27.12.13

Thomas Aksnes
Scientific Director
HealthTech Sciences AS

HealthTech Sciences AS
Org.nr: 892.976.562 MVA
www.healthtechsciences.com

Health-Optimizing Clinic
Daniel Hansens gate 9
5008 Bergen, Norway

Tel: (+47) 55 62 95 95
E-post: post@htsnorge.no
post@healthtechsciences.com

Institute of Preventive Medicine & Nutrition

1342 Atwood Road
Silver Spring, MD 20906
www.drbrewsterwilson.com
Tel: (301) 460-6600
Email: drpbwilson@gmail.com

Jay Emmanuel Morales, A.K., V.M.
Power of Harmony Organization, Health & Wellness Network
400 West 43rd Street, Suite 24-B
New York, N.Y. 10036

Ref: Sound Vibrational Therapy, excellent for stress management, wellness, prevention & longevity.

Since 1983 The Institute of Preventive Medicine and Nutrition has treated all diseases and all ages using only Natural "Wholistic" (Whole body) Therapies. For successful healing, we believe and depend heavily upon restoration of balance to the "Vital Force" energy, also referred to as the patient's immune system. Illness results when this Vital Force becomes untuned and re-tuning it back to harmonic balance is necessary in order to release the natural power of self healing.

We utilize a multidimensional comprehensive therapeutical approach which includes : Classical Homeopathy, Nutrition counseling, Herbs and Botanical Medicine, Energy Medicine.

To this end we are grateful and pleased to report the incredible benefit gained by our patients from listening to the CD Healing Forces of Harmonic Sounds and Vibrations, created by Jay Emmanuel Morales, for balancing of energy chakras. Since the year 2004 our patients have routinely been advised to listen to this CD as an important part of their health protocol. The results have been amazing and most user friendly. Some patients have even downloaded it on their computers to be able to listen to it as their schedule would permit "24/7"

My husband and I are personally the grateful recipients of the expert knowledge and intuitive treatments by Jay Emmanuel Morales, consisting of Applied Kinesiology, Sound Therapy with Crystal Bowls, Magnetic treatments, Exercise, and Nutrition advice.

Thank you Jay for giving of yourself, your touch, your voice, your heart, and spirit! May the Harmonic Sounds and Vibrations envelop the Planet bringing healing to all who choose to receive this gift and may the Creator of the Universe guide and bless your work.

Sincerely,

Premala E Brewster-Wilson

_____

Premala Brewster-Wilson, PhD. CCH. CNS. LN.
Founder & Director: Institute of Preventive Medicine and Nutrition

Gloria Godínez Leal, M.A.Sc., N.D., H.M.D., O.M.D
Founding President and Director of the
Institute of Energy Medicine and Biological S.C.
Autopista Escénica Tij-Ens # 12520-3 San Marino,
Tijuana B.C. México C.P. 22560
Tel. 52-664-6312725
www.papimimexico.com

February 5, 2014

"The Healing Forces of Harmonic Sounds and Vibrations and The Healing Power of the Voice and the Mind."

During the last two decades I have had the opportunity to conduct scientific and clinical research at the Institute of Energetic and Biological Medicine in Mexico. As an independent researcher I have traveled and known renowned scientists, physicians, researchers and inventors, who in essence were in the same search as me. It was there that Jay Emmanuel and I had a luminous meeting point: the resonance of a shared dream in developing a methodology that would be an adjunct to modern medicine, in order to ensure that human beings assume the integrative principles of Energy, Science and Life Spirit, and thereby regain the ability to heal themselves.

Vibrational Medicine or Quantum Medicine integrates the ancestral and natural wisdom of great scientific advances and nanotechnology, which allows us to evaluate and examine in detail the relationship between the physical body and the subtle bodies of light and the energy that contributes to the multidimensional nature of humans. It is becoming increasingly important to measure the therapeutic impact of the physical, emotional and subtle light body energy with the advanced bioelectro-diagnosis devices used in "Vibrational Medicine."

I have attended Jay Emmanuel Morales' workshops and have witnessed miraculous moments where harmonized mantralization, with peculiar crystals and Tibetan bowls open interdimensional portals, and create streams of light and harmony to recreate and manifest in nature. We ventured into historical, holy, and ceremonial sites and energy vortexes in the Basilica of Guadalupe, the Pyramid of the Sun at Teotihuacan, the Astronomical Chamber of the Acropolis in Morelos Xochicalco, Sedona Arizona, and the majestic Colorado Canyon.

I'm sure Jay Emmanuel's book will reveal important scientific and mystical aspects, due to his world view and as master custodian of therapeutic sound and the voice as an instrument of healing. He has been a faithful transmitter of ancient cultures and places, and understanding this ancient wisdom is now within our reach.

Jay Emmanuel, thank you for allowing us to participate as observers in the unveiling awareness of this great mystery!

Gloria Godínez Leal

M.A.Sc., N.D., H.M.D., O.M.D
Founding President and Director of the Institute of Energy Medicine and Biological S.C.
Autopista Escénica Tij-Ens # 12520-3 San Marino, Tijuana B.C. México C.P. 22560 Tel. 52-664-6312725
www.papimimexico.com

Dr. Leonel Eduardo Lechuga

Espacio Metatrón
Playa Mirador 427, CP 08830, México, D.F.
Tel: 011-52-55-5634-5969
Tel: 011-52-55-24-4848
Email: leo8888@prodigy.net.mx
Webpage: **metatron-galactron.com**

"The Healing Forces of Harmonic Sounds and Vibrations and The Healing Power of the Voice and the Mind."

What I particularly admire about Jay's healing system is the convergence of his profound knowledge, high technology and his heartfelt sincerity. Jay provides dedication and care with sensitivity and love to his patients, to help achieve an ultimate state of health and a near-perfect evolutionary life.

This result is due to a combination of Jay's disciplined lifestyle and his constant search for the latest scientific and spiritual advances. Jay's impressive and expressive treatments with healing sounds and Natural Ayurvédic Systems have a profound impact on the natural healing process of the body, mind and spirit. The body's healthy richness is due in part to Jay's generosity to humanity.

Therefore, the concepts noted in Jay's book are very beneficial for all people and for many alternative health professionals that are looking for holistic modalities that can help to stimulate the natural healing process of the body and mind.

February 3, 2014

Leonel Lechuga

Dr. Leonel Lechuga
Inventor, Arquitect, Teacher and Lecturer
Designer on people and spaces for harmonizing energy,
Director and Founder of Espacio Metatrón in Mexico City,
National Award of Science, 2006

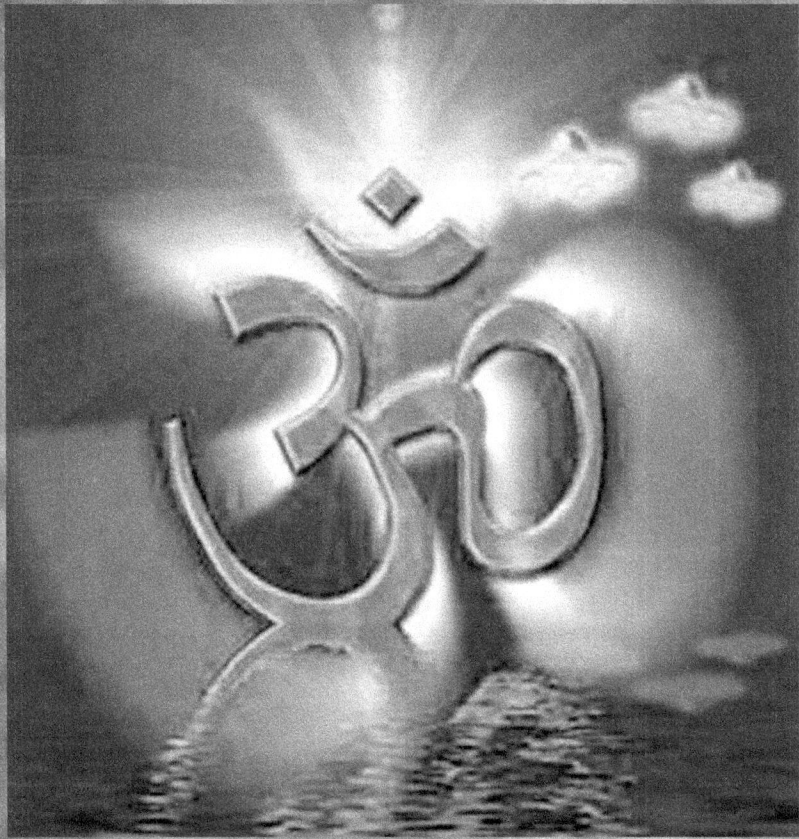

Introduction

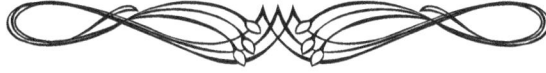

Since childhood I could see and feel the power of music and its impact on human beings. When I sang I observed that some people were filled with joy and laughed, while others were crying because on hearing the melody there was an activation of feelings and memories in their lives.

I once had a voice teacher who had several kittens. One day when I finished my vocal exercises, I burst into song and the kittens came to me and curled themselves around my feet. The kittens always stayed around me and near the piano while I sang. In the animal kingdom many species have a great sense of perception for harmonic sounds. I have noticed that in my apartment plants live for many years and I believe this is because I am usually singing and/or listening to classical music, mantras, Gregorian chants or New Age music. Plants are very receptive to the frequencies of sound and harmonic sounds which enhance their growth and development, and help to preserve their health.

I always loved good music, the arts and natural sciences. I am very fortunate that The Universal Creator gave me the gift of being able to sing. Music and singing inducted me on a life path where I was able to discover and truly understand the vast and mighty power of harmonic sounds and the vibrational frequencies generated by sound. I feel that I truly know how music and sound reach far beyond the world of matter into the highest spheres, and at quantum levels gave rise to the creation of the universe.

Later in life I would corroborate this information at metaphysical levels when I read the following excerpts in the Bible: In the first book of Moses in The Old Testament: "And God spoke and said Let there be Light and the light was revealed and the light was manifested," and in the New Testament, John 1: "In the beginning the Word was (the word is sound) and the Word was with God, and the Word was God." In the sacred books of India, the Vedas; "And in the beginning was Brahman which was the word and the word is Brahman."

The Power of the word gives rise to sounds, and sounds create vibrational frequencies that impact on all matter. Religions, spiritual trajectories and traditions of different cultures arrive at the same conclusion: that by a primordial sound, the paths were opened for the creation and manifestation for the existence of life on planet Earth.

Throughout my life I have been interested in knowing the music of different cultures. This led me to the study of sounds produced by the Vedic mantras of India, Egyptian, Tibetan and Hebrew mantras, and Latin and Gregorian chants. I have studied the impact of the harmonics produced by mantras and songs, and how they influence the natural healing process of the body and the mind through DNA repair.

Not only through the study of music produced by different cultures, but through life itself I have discovered and activated many feelings, in particular through my deep appreciation of the sounds of nature. This is the bottom line for me to get in touch with Mother Nature. I have achieved great states of communion with life when I walk in the woods, in parks surrounded by trees with lakes or rivers, or on the shore near the ocean surf. When I am in a natural environment my atoms, molecules and cells are revitalized, I feel energized, my senses of perception become sharpened and I rejoice with the sound of air, land, water, insects, birds, animals, and frogs - and when I am in Puerto Rico, with the sound of the coquí.

In fact, when I was studying at the University of Puerto Rico in the department of Ecology, I did a study of the sounds of the coqui (Eleutherodactylus Portoricensis - 16 species.) Those little frogs from the amphibian kingdom create a harmonic serenade with extraordinary vibrational frequencies that help establish the mental state of alpha 8 and 9-14 Hz, which is the most likely state to activate the natural healing process of the mind and body. In this mental state of alpha the process of learning, retention and assimilation of information is encouraged. In the CD recording companion to this book you will hear the sound of the coquí.

The power of sounds and harmonic vibrations and their effects on living things was greatly emphasized in ancient times. A great example was the Greek philosopher Pythagoras of Samos (560-480 BC.) He conceived the universe as a vast musical instrument and called the sacred sound of the universe and its vibrational energies **"The Music of the Spheres."** Long before him the great master Thoth the Atlantean "Father of Wisdom," also known as Hermes Trismegistus, who was deified in Egypt, reiterated that **music has the power to attract cosmic energy to planet Earth.**

According to the mythology of Atlantis and Ancient Egypt, Thoth spoke and the power of his words originated the sound that set in motion the plan that gave rise to the structure of the creation of the universe.

The universe is pure energy of vibrational frequencies. The sounds and vibrational frequencies are the fundamental building blocks of the macrocosmic universe, and also the basic structures that form our microcosmic universe, i.e. our energy body, the mind and the physical body. Without sound and vibrations nothing would exist in the third dimension.

Sound is vibration and vibration is energy. The human body functions using vibrational energy. Cells, tissues and organs respond to energy produced by sounds and vibrations. The sounds and vibrations have a direct effect on our DNA, our physiology and our consciousness. Sound can influence the body in many ways: slowing and accelerating the rhythmic process of our respiration, altering the temperature of the skin, reducing blood pressure, and most important, it can directly affect our brain waves, the five basic mental states: Beta, Alpha, Theta, Delta and Gamma. Sound, therefore, can be used to promote enhanced states of health.

Sound emerges from a non-manifest state. What I am hinting at is that it is in our brain where a mental process gives rise to the production of sound. In other words, the sounds we produce when we speak and when we sing contain mental messages that will be stored in the cellular memory of our DNA.

Thus, externalized mind messages through the word produce sounds that reflect the state of consciousness of the individual. Thus, you could say that consciousness is sound. If at deeper levels of consciousness we would positively change the messages generated by our mind, then we would be able to bring forth positive changes in our lives that would remain active in our being for a long time, and these changes would also be reflected around us and in the affairs of our daily lives.

Throughout history great minds and wise scientists have recognized the healing power of harmonic sounds and vibrations. An example is Nicolas Tesla (1856 -1943 Smiljan, Croatia) who said "if we want to find the secrets of the universe we must think in terms of energy, frequencies and vibrations."

We live in an ocean of energy, frequency and vibration. Albert Einstein (1879 - 1955 Ulm, Germany,) recognized harmonic music as one of the principal factors that inspired and helped him in carrying out his great scientific discoveries. Dr. Royal Raymond Rife, (1888 - 1971 Nebraska, USA), invented a machine that uses a unique combination of electromagnetic radio wave pulses of high and low frequencies that effectively inactivate and kill microorganisms that cause disease. Dr. Alfred A. Tomatis (1920 - 2001 Nice, France) researched, developed and tested his theory that the voice produces only what the ear hears.

Based on my studies of vibrational medicine I produced a CD entitled **The Healing Forces of Harmonic Sounds and Vibrations,** which has been programmed with specific vocal sound frequencies, music harmony and tones that resonate, balance and harmonize the chakras. The exquisite and synergistic harmonic sounds in this CD production has a balancing energy effect in the mental, emotional and entire physical body. It is a potent "Musical Therapy" recording that vitalize, harmonize and energize the organs, meridians and systems for each of the seven basic chakras, and also balance and activate peace and serenity in the environment where this CD is played.

The power that sound and vibration have on us is beyond our imagination. Our mental, emotional and physical development is directly affected by the sounds and frequencies that are generated in our atmosphere from the moment we entered existence in this third dimension inside our mother's womb, and also from the very moment of our first breath at birth and throughout our lives.

1

The Macrocosmic and Microcosmic Universe

The Macro and Microcosmic Universe is a huge musical instrument in a constant state of vibration.

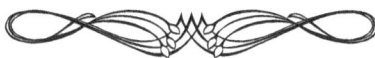

***

Modern science is recognizing what the ancient sages have been telling us over many centuries. Everything moves and vibrates, from the sub-atom, the atom to the molecule, producing sounds and vibrations. **All existing matter in the universe and in planet Earth is in a constant state of vibration and emits sound waves with specific frequencies.**

The most fundamental form of vibration in the creation of the universe is sound. On Planet Earth all beings of the plant kingdom and the animal kingdom are constantly breathing vibrational frequencies of sound and light signals which come from the sun, and from energy emitted by other celestial bodies in the universe.

The universe is a vast musical instrument that is in a constant state of vibration. Through vibrations and harmonic sounds new realities are created, sorted and organized.

Sound is vibration and vibration is energy. The human body is a **microcosmic universe** that operates by means of vibrational energy. The cells of the body respond to vibrations and energy that is produced by the sounds. The sounds and vibrations affect our DNA, our consciousness and our physiology. Sounds can influence the body in many ways: by slowing down the breathing rate, altering the skin temperature, reducing blood pressure and also by affecting the five brain wave states of Beta, Alpha, Theta, Delta and Gamma. Harmonic sound is used to produce homeostasis for the maintenance of good health in the entire biological system.

5

All our senses; what we see, hear, smell, taste, touch and perceive vibrates. Every sub-atom, atom, molecule, cell, tissue, organ, system and bone in our body vibrates. The vibrations generate sounds and light.

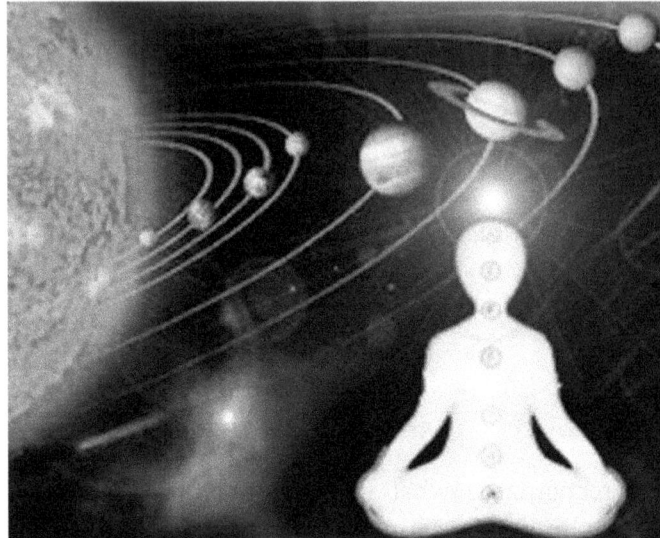

Our body is a microcosmic universe in a constant state of vibration producing sounds.

The macrocosmic and the microcosmic universes are constantly generating vibrations and sounds. **In conclusion, as we live and move, we continuously produce vibrations and sounds.**

The rotational and translation movement of the planets in their orbits around the sun generate electromagnetic energy which create sounds and vibrations of very high frequencies. The sun also emits a powerful electromagnetic energy with accompanying sounds and vibrations. It is like a majestic super symphony of high magnetic and vibrational energy that keeps the planets in their respective orbits.

Particulate matter and substances that vibrate and produce sounds at microcosmic and macrocosmic levels

- The motion of **electrons around the nucleus of the atom** emits sound (microcosmic level.)
- The movement of the **planets, solar systems and celestial bodies** in the galaxy produce high frequency sounds (macrocosmic level).
- The **cells, minerals and crystalline substances that travel in blood plasma through**

the arteries and veins of the body, emit sound waves and are in a constant state of vibration (microcosmic level).

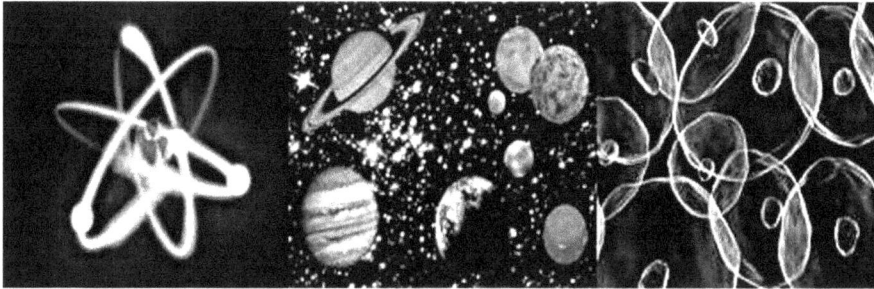

In conclusion, the motion of electrons around the atom, the movement of planets and celestial bodies in the galaxy, cell movement, minerals and crystalline substances inside our body, all emit sound waves and are in a constant state of vibration.

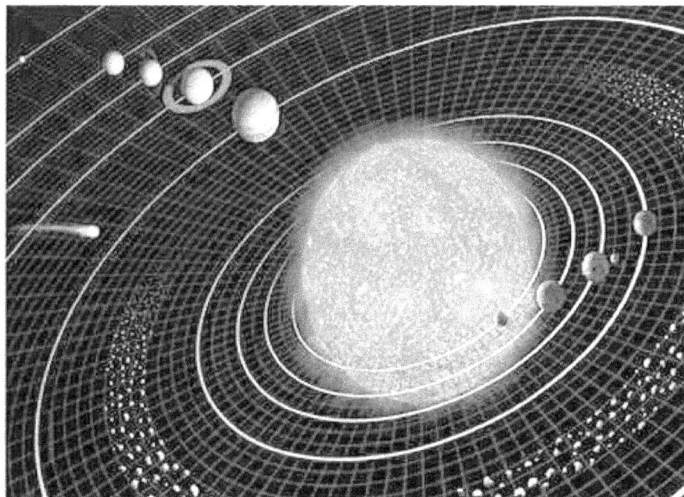

Effects of sound frequencies on the physiological systems of living beings both in their exterior and interior worlds

The exterior and interior worlds, including the creation of the universe through the famous Big Bang, allude to a unified theory of evolution which says there is but one cosmos in which everything that exists is in constant motion, expanding throughout space, and continuously generating vibrations at different frequencies.

What unifies the universe and cosmos is the existence of contiguous space infinitely expanding in such a way that the macrocosmic universe extends through contiguous space without interruption – from galaxies to stars, as well as through microcosmic particles such as neutrinos, sub-atoms and atoms. In the space of this macrocosmic universe exists the microcosmic universe of man, and within the physical body of man we find the same space. Therefore, the cosmos, the universe and humans are contained within a contiguous space of infinite extension.

There is evidence of the existence of additional universes in a third dimension within universes of different magnitudes of mass that simultaneously occupy the same space, and have the same internal axis. There is also evidence of the existence of a fourth spatial dimension occupying the same space.

The movement of the continuous expansion of space that gives birth to new galaxies, stars, solar systems, planets, as well as the simultaneous disintegration of other macrocosmic systems at a galactic level, is at all times in a constant state of vibration generating sound frequencies. Similarly, at a microcosmic level, the movement of blood through the arteries of the human body, the reproduction of the billions of cells as well as the daily disintegration of cells, is equally in a state of vibration which constantly produces sound frequencies.

According to numerous scientific studies and many mystical teachings of East and West, there is an inner universe (microcosm) and an external universe (macrocosm) and both universes emit a stream of sounds generating vibrational frequencies that permeate all creation.

Sound is constantly active all around us generating vibrational frequencies that affect every system in all living beings on Planet Earth. It could be defined as the sound waves of both macrophysics and microphysics cosmic symphonies that travel throughout all creation.

All the systems in the macrocosmic universe (galaxies, stars) and in the microcosmic universe (atoms, cells) generate frequency ranges of the Fundamental Harmonic Sounds that produce harmonic resonances that influence the creation of life, affecting the whole nature of our planet and most specifically the DNA of all living creatures.

Astrophysicist Don Jurtz says: "The stars broadcast sounds that are similar to the sound of gigantic bells or of immense musical instruments."

People who study the sounds of the stars are called astro-seismologists or asteroseismologists. It is closely related to helioseismology, the study of stellar oscillations specifically in the Sun.

You could say that the Greek philosopher and mathematician Pythagoras of Samos in the 6th century BC was the first to suggest the idea of "music of the spheres." Through current technology scientists have proven that it is indeed possible to hear the sounds of the stars and other celestial bodies in our universe.

Perseus sound waves present a fascinating way for defining the acoustic black hole. These sound waves may be the key to knowing how galaxies can converge and how the larger structures of the universe take form, expand and grow.

In modern quantum physics we know there is an average of 80 octaves to each side of the spectrum of sound produced by the macrocosmic universe, despite the fact that many of the combinations of cosmic vibrations are not perceived by our ears. However, we can connect to these vibrations through our subconscious and also through other internal body systems. According to the three gunas of the Sanskrit tradition, these inaudible vibrations come from higher, middle and lower resonance ranges of universal radiation.

The universe and our body is constantly generating sounds and vibrations. Everything is vibration -- hence, all emitted sounds and frequencies may be audible or inaudible. Researchers are experimenting with specific sounds that have measurable effects on atoms, molecules and body cells of humans and animals, and are studying how those sounds influence us and promote different states of consciousness. Through this new science that can be defined in many ways "Vibrational Therapy," "Vibrational Medicine, "Music Therapy," "Magnetic Harmonic Vibrational Therapy" and "The Healing Forces of Harmonic Sounds and Vibrations," we can stimulate and activate positive changes in psychological awareness and at physiological levels in most living beings.

Through specific low and high frequency sound waves we can stimulate the brain to tune the mind to different realities and multiple experiences. We understand that these vibrations have been expressed throughout all traditions in many sacred texts. Some examples include the OUM in Sanskrit books, AUM (or AM) in ancient Hebrew or Abba, and Amen in the Semitic languages and Christianity. The ancient Egyptians used the OM and AMON as a vibration of powerful qualities. Many invocations to Egyptian gods were preceded by the word Amon. Amen likewise, meaning "so be it," is a sacred word of Hebrew origin. The AUM from Hindu tradition is understood as the perfect reflection of the Absolute Reality, which is said to be "Adi Anadi," without beginning or end and encompasses all that exists.

The Bhagavad Gita states that the Universal Energy, or God, is the sound of OUM. The Bible states: "In the beginning was the Word, and the Word was with God, and the Word was God." Nada Yoga in the Sanskrit tradition sees everything in the macrocosmic and microcosmic world as composed of sound.

"OUM is the primordial heartbeat of the universe. It is the most rational form of consciousness (Atma) " Maitri Upanishad "Nadam" [Sanskrit] can be described as a stream of sound, the stream of life and consciousness, cosmic and supra-cosmic rhythmic vibration. We also have internal sounds (NADA BRAHMA) of worlds that are not heard. Sound manifests energy, all matter is composed of energy and therefore all living things generate different types of sound.

The great temples of the world, buildings, pyramids, churches, and the rocks and cave systems in nature produce specific sound patterns that relate to spectral stellar acoustics, and also to specific sounds generated by our biological systems. Our body is therefore a kind of temple of sound with geometric proportions relative to the pi and phi. Thus when our human bodies are unbalanced, they can be properly reprogrammed using biologically enhanced frequencies of sound.

If we look at the stars in the ancient Chinese maps, we can see the connection with "The Music of the Spheres." It reveals how the embryo, the human body and most patterns of the body are connected with the resonance to Major Stellar Systems. I am making reference here to the axiotonal lines described in the extraordinary book "The Keys of Enoch" by Dr. J.J. Hurtak. The axiotonal lines generate specific acoustic frequencies which are connected to the meridian system of the human body that resonate with the tubular pyramidal micro-structures found in our brain cells.

We humans are constantly emitting and receiving crystal radio waves; understanding this will help us realize how some sounds help reactivate the natural healing process of mind, body and spirit. Basically all beings are connected to the array of universal collective consciousness and can transmit frequencies of Sound and Light that directly affect our biological systems, our DNA, cells, organs and systems in our environment, our planet, and even in other planetary systems in the cosmos. We emit sounds and generate frequency waves that affect the atomic structures of the microcosmic and macrocosmic universe.

2

Pythagoras of Samos

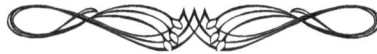

Pythagoras of Samos was a Greek philosopher and mathematician who lived from 580-495 BC. In a very real sense, he is considered the father of music therapy. In the Pythagorean Mystery School located on the island of Crete in Greece, he used the flute and the lyre as primary healing tools. He is considered one of the most significant pillars in the advancement of Greek mathematics, geometry and arithmetic.

Pythagoras conceived the universe as a vast musical instrument. He called the sacred sound of the Universe and its vibrational energy **The Music of the Spheres.**

The history of Western science begins with Pythagoras and the Pythagoreans. The school of Pythagoras was a Secret Mystery School and his teachings were transmitted only orally.

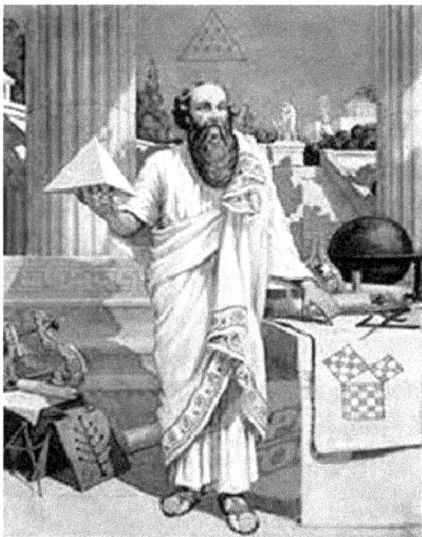

Pythagoras of Samos

In his school they used a musical instrument that dates back to ancient history called the monochord. It is believed that he was the inventor of that instrument. The monochord is a stringed musical instrument that uses a fixed weight to provide tension on the rope.

Pythagoras used the monochord to create the concepts of harmonic intervals of music, which were represented in integer ratios: 2:1 the octave, 3:03 the fifth, and the fourth 4:03. It is believed that this instrument also helped him describe his mathematical theory of natural phenomena and the numerical relationships.

According to the Greek writings, Pythagoras learned

geometry from the Egyptians and was influenced by the mathematicians of that mighty empire. He established that there was a relationship between numbers, music, geometry and astronomy. He founded the Pythagorean Brotherhood, which was a religious organization interested in philosophy, medicine, cosmology, ethics, politics and other disciplines.

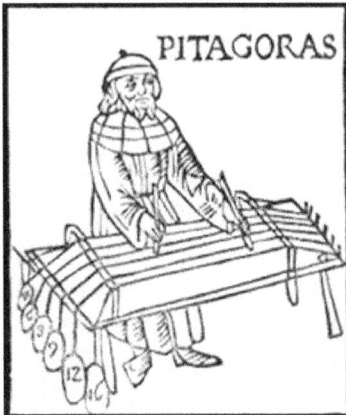

The monochord

Pythagoras considered that music contributed largely to health. He called his method **Musical Medicine.** Pythagoras and his followers would sing certain chants in unison during their meetings. Often his disciples employed music as medicine using composed melodies in order to help heal the psychic passions of anger and aggression.

Pythagoras discovered that there is an intrinsic arithmetic ratio between mathematics and the musical scale. The musical principles were equally as important to the Pythagorean system as the principles of mathematics. The phenomena taking place in the universe takes place in a mathematical sequence that can be expressed by numeric equations.

According to the Pythagorean scale, nature can be expressed in terms of mathematical proportions. Philosophers of that school concluded that musical harmony could also be expressed by means of numerical proportions.

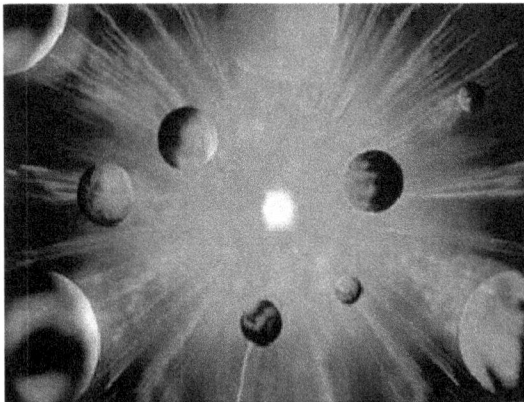

Pythagoras did research on the distance between the orbits of the Sun and the Moon, and of fixed stars. He concluded that these orbits correspond to the proportions of the octave, fifth and fourth of the seven planets and the fixed stars. The spaces between the orbits of the planets and heavenly bodies produce intervals that can be perfectly expressed through mathematical measurements and are also inherent in musical harmony.

Pythagoras had an intuitive gift that allowed him to sharpen his ears in perfect attunement to the music produced by the stars and other celestial bodies in the universe.

He said that many people cannot hear the music generated by the heavenly bodies in the universe. This is due to the fact that we are so used to constantly hearing these sounds that we have blocked the ability to consciously notice them. Another reason could be that the sound generated by the Celestial bodies is so subtle that it cannot be detected by our hearing capabilities. All of this inspired Pythagoras to call the sacred sound of the universe and its vibrational energy **The Music of the Spheres.**

By means of vibration, motion is manifested; by means of movement, color is expressed; and by means of color, tone is manifested. **Pythagoras was the first to say that the universe is governed by the laws of music.**

Sound and music have their origins in higher spheres

At the very precise instant when the first cosmic explosion happened in space that gave birth to the creation of the universe, galaxies, solar systems and celestial bodies, Sound originated. The universe is a vast musical instrument that is in a constant state of vibration and producing sounds.

The Pythagoreans used music to heal the body and elevate the soul and believed that the earthly music was but a weak echo of **"The Music of the Spheres" or "The universal harmony of the spheres".** In ancient cosmology, the planetary spheres ascended from Earth to the sky like the steps of a ladder. It is said that each sphere corresponded to a musical note different from the large musical scale. The particular tones emitted by the planets depended on the proportions of their respective orbits, just as the tone of a string of a lyre depended on its length. Another type of celestial scale related the planetary tones according to the numerical amount of the apparent time of its rotation around Earth.

Pythagoras discovered that the pitch of a musical note depends on the length of the string that produces it. This allowed him to correlate the intervals of the musical scale with simple numerical ratios. When a musician plays the string and stops exactly half way along its length, an octave occurs. The octave has the same sound quality as the note produced by the non-stop string, but as it vibrates at twice the frequency, it is heard at a higher pitch. The mathematical relationship between the musical note and its octave is expressed as a "frequency ratio" of 1: 2. In each type of musical scale, notes progress in a series of intervals from a note to the octave up or down. The notes separated by intervals of a perfect fifth (ratio 2: 3) and a perfect quarter (3: 4) have always been the most important tunes of Western music. **Recognizing these proportions, Pythagoras discovered the basis for mathematical foundations of musical harmony.**

Based on his discovery of the relationship between music and mathematics, **Pythagoras has also invented Western science.** By associating length measurements with musical tones, he made the first known reduction of the quality of a (sound) by an amount of (length and ratio). Understanding nature through mathematics remains a primary goal of today's science. **Pythagoras also recognized that the musical octave is the simplest and most profound expression of the relationship between spirit and matter.** The **"miracle of the octave"** is that it divides wholeness into two parts that can be audibly distinguished, but which remains recognizable as the same musical note, tangible manifestation of the hermetic maxim **"as above, so below." The short but deeply influential Brotherhood of Pythagoras sought to unite "religion and science, mathematics and music, medicine and cosmology, body, mind and spirit in an inspired and luminous synthesis."**

"In The Beginning"

The infinite Universal Intelligence Sound,
Birthing the First Explosion of Cosmic Light,
Rays of Love Frequencies, Sound and Light,
Expanding beyond dimensions, space and time,
Materializing Universes, Galaxies and Stars
In the endless evolutive journey of cosmic light,
Morphing matter, antimatter, energy,
atoms, molecules and cells,
Into the perfect creation,
giving formation to all cosmic life.

J. E. M.

3

Sounds in Space and Auditory Perception of Humans and Other Mammals

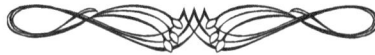

Sounds in Space

The Pythagorean tenet of conceiving **the universe as a vast musical instrument** by the great Greek philosopher Pythagoras of Samos, rose 495 years before Christ with its sublime concept of **The Music of The Spheres,** and has been scientifically endorsed in modern times.

From the mid-20th century and on, scientists have been collecting sounds from space by astronomical instruments such as the radio telescope.

Radio astronomy through telescopes, and especially through one of the largest in the world located in the center of the Caribbean islands, in Arecibo, Puerto Rico, receives signals from radio waves emitted by celestial bodies in space, and other cosmic phenomena.

A total vacuum exists in outer space where sound is not propagated; however, emissions of polar discharges like the auroras borealis, solar wind emissions, and emissions of planets like Jupiter can be audibly detected.

In exterior space, sound propagation is only possible where there is no vacuum. Multiple sounds from the atmosphere of celestial bodies can be detected through microphones. Scientists have been able to capture and classify the sounds of many different celestial bodies in our solar system. Among them are sounds emitted by Jupiter, solar storms, the magnetic field of Earth and other places where there is atmosphere. The atmosphere of celestial bodies such as "Titan," a natural satellite of Saturn, and the surface of Mars, have been detected by the radio telescope.

The sounds of radio and television are transported through the atmosphere via radio waves with short wavelengths that are less than a meter in diameter. These waves are modulated to broadcast frequencies that activate the sounds on the radio and video television. Radio waves are also produced by stars in distant galaxies, and can be detected by astronomers using specialized telescopes like the one located in Arecibo, Puerto Rico. Very large longitudinal waves have been detected radiating toward Earth and coming from several millions of miles long from the depths of space. Because these signals are very weak, the radio telescope is equipped with many different sets of antennas with parallel receivers to record radio waves and sounds from distant celestial bodies.

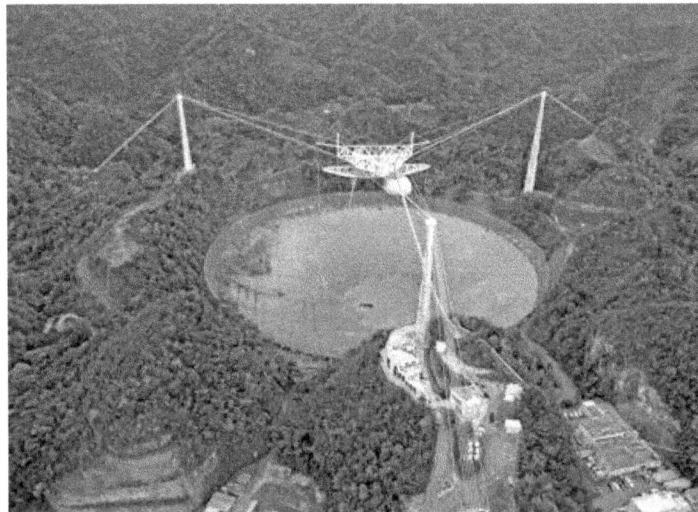

The world's largest radio telescope, located in Arecibo, Puerto Rico.

On August 15, 2006 the California Institute for Human Science's Neuro-Acoustic Research Center published an article about recordings from outer space supplied by NASA. These recordings from outer space are remarkably similar to the sounds of the ocean, choirs of voices singing, dolphins, birds and crickets.

They also observed that the sounds produced by the rings of Uranus are quite similar to the sounds produced by Tibetan Bowls. The sound of Tibetan Bowls and choir chants have healing effects on living beings. Does this point to the Collective Unconscious? or perhaps a Collective Library containing all the knowledge of the universe?

Astronomers using instruments such as the **radio telescope** have collected sounds from space, and therefore scientifically confirmed that **all existing matter in the universe (including Earth) is in a constant state of vibration and emitting sound wave frequencies.** Thus, it has also been scientifically confirmed that the understandings of the great Greek philosopher Pythagoras (who conceived the Universe as an immense vast Sacred Musical Instrument,) and the concept of the **Music of the Spheres** are accurate.

Ability for auditory perception in humans, dolphins, whales and other mammals

Our ears cannot detect many of the sounds that are generated around us, but this does not mean that the sounds do not exist. The human ear has the ability to hear only from 16 to 20 Hz up to 16,000 to 20,000 Hz or cycles per second, which is considered a limited hearing range.

Dolphins and whales have a greater ability to hear sounds and can sense from 75 to 150,000 Hz and some up to 200,000 Hz or cycles per second. Marine biologists have found that whales and dolphins communicate with members of the same species through a language of sound waves that they emit at distances covering hundreds and thousands of miles. These intelligent animals, besides having a great perceptive sound capacity up to 200,000 Hz per second, also have at their favor the milieu they inhabit, as sound produced inside of water travels 4 to 5 times faster than in the air.

Most dolphins have a large repertoire of sounds. They emit sounds in the form of two types of pulses : sounds used for eco localization and sounds that define their emotional state. Dolphins also emit pure tone sounds called whistles. Each dolphin emits its own whistle that identifies and distinguishes it from all other dolphins.

The language of the dolphins is being decoded with new technology

A new artificial intelligence software technology called Gavagai AB that was successfully used to analyze 40 different human dialects, and has been lately used in analyzing Swedish for unlocking dolphin's language.

Researchers at the KTH Royal Institute of Technology have compiled numerous data on the sounds produced by dolphins with the aim of decoding the language of these intelligent creatures.

According to Digital Trends, research suggests that dolphins communicate in a language that shares similarities with ours. It is based on sentences made from individual words whose order is relevant to determine the meaning; The dolphins even pause to let themselves talk. As such, the decoding of its language implies mainly to link a certain sound to a specific meaning.

Given that dolphins are one of the most intelligent species on Earth, what we might expect in the future could go beyond our imagination. This type of data will allow us to communicate directly with the dolphins translating our messages to the corresponding sounds that they used in their language.

Dolphins also have more developed hearing senses than humans; They can hear a wider range of frequencies. Dolphins when compared to whales, usually communicate using high frequencies while whales often use low frequencies. However, the whales can communicate at farther distances (several hundred or kilometers away) than dolphins can.

Our bodies have the ability to absorb and detect sounds beyond the hearing ability of our ears. We not only hear and perceive sounds and vibrations through the ears, but also by our bodies, through our bones, epidermal tissue and crystalline substances in our bloodstreams. Ducts, arteries, veins and capillaries are particularly large sound drivers and receivers of vibrations. The famous Dr. Alfred A. Tomatis (1920 -2001) demonstrated scientifically that epidermal tissue (skin), bone mass and bone have the ability to perceive sounds that are not perceived by the ear. In conclusion we also perceive the vibrations of sound through our bodies.

The capacity of auditory perception of humans compared to the hearing ability of other living beings on planet Earth

Elephants--------------= 5-16 Hz to 12,000 Hz
Humans---------------= 20-30 Hz to 16,000-20,000 Hz
Dogs------------------= 40-50 Hz to 46,000 Hz
Cats-------------------= 45-100 Hz to 32,000-65,000 Hz
Mice-------------------= 70 Hz to 150,000 Hz
Bats--------------------= 1,000-2,000 Hz to 150,000 Hz
Beluga Whales---------= 1,000 Hz to120,000 Hz
Dolphins---------------= 8-100 Hz to 150,000-200,000 Hz

The ability of auditory perception in humans is very limited compared with other beings that inhabit Earth. However, humans have a greater ability to perceive frequencies of sounds through tissue, bone structure, and epidermal tissue (skin), and also through crystalline mineral substances that travel in the bloodstream through arteries and veins.

The healing power of the sounds produced by dolphins and whales

Dolphins emit sounds that generate vibrational frequencies of 8 Hz per second. Those sounds are inaudible to the human ear, but naturally lead the brain and the whole bio-molecular system of the body to its natural vibrational state of 8 Hz.

Scientific studies have shown that 8 Hz sounds produced by dolphins activate a mental and physical balance in humans when they are exposed to these sounds. These sounds are also effective for releasing stress and activating a broad sense of calm and tranquility. This is because 8 Hz frequencies are naturally present in the harmonic field of Earth and effectively stimulate the mental state of Alpha and Theta in humans.

It has also been scientifically proven that dolphins emit sound frequencies of 8 Hz as well as frequency waves from 20 Hz to 20,000 Hz, which trigger physiological changes in tissue and blood chemistry. This contributes to an acceleration of the natural healing process of the body. Some experts believe that dolphins are able to concentrate their sonar capacity to the affected area of a person. These exceptional animals can locate tumors and problems in a person that is swimming with them, and intuitively send curative healing frequencies to the individual's affected area.

Communication exchanges between whales produce very low sound frequencies that travel thousands of miles inside of sea water. Scientific studies have shown that when listening to the sounds of whales, our brain rhythms tend to slow down to match and harmonize with the frequency of the musical sound produced by these wonderful cetaceans which helps to produce deep delta states for restful sleep. It has been proven that the sound emitted by whales helps us sleep very soundly.

8 Hz sound frequencies are recognized by the brain and activate a perfect vibrational wave flow through the neurons of our nervous systems, which promote balance in all body systems.

In my CD, **The Healing Forces of Harmonic Sounds and Vibrations,** I include the sound of dolphins and whales, because the 8 Hz sounds that these intelligent animals emit generate frequencies which produce therapeutic effects in humans, plants and all other living things. Similarly, when those sounds are combined with the harmonic vocal sounds emitted by the human voice and the sounds of pure quartz crystals bowls, we are able to effectively induce mental states of alpha and theta. It has been scientifically proven that sounds emitted by dolphins, whales, birds and harmonic vocal sounds emitted by humans are beneficial and help to activate the natural healing process of mind, body and spirit.

Scientific researchers found that when people meditate properly with their eyes closed, the alpha state of mind is stimulated which leads to the synchronization of the right and left cerebral hemispheres of the brain. This process begins from 8 Hz cycles per second, and on.

Albert Einstein said that his theory of relativity had been formulated thanks to the synchronization of the two hemispheres of his brain that allowed him a further expansion of his brain power. The synchronization of the two hemispheres of the brain increases endorphin production and fosters the release of endogenous substances that act like painkillers.

In the sixties, Dr. Puharich and Dr. John Taylor found that the vibrational frequency of 8 Hz cycles per second activated extrasensory abilities such as telepathy, remote viewing, telekinesis and many other capabilities that are present only in a latent state in most of us.

Thanks to the scientific background of Dr. Puharich, he was able to observe that specific frequencies have a powerful effect on the human mind. For example, 8 Hz frequency cycles per second are able to increase a predisposition to learning, leading the person to the Theta brain state. The frequencies of 8 Hz cycles per second also stimulate an attitude of creativity and activate profound intuitions of a mystical and scientific nature.

If the two hemispheres of our brain are synchronized at 8 Hz cycles per second, they work more harmoniously and with a maximum flow of information. In other words, the frequency of 8 Hz seems to be essential for the activation of the full and sovereign potential of our brain.

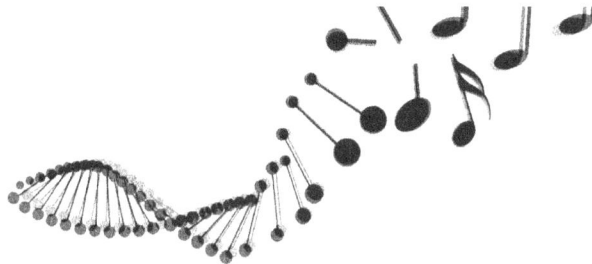

8 Hz frequency is the harmonic sound of the DNA double helix in its replicating state.

The frequency of 8 Hz per second is also the frequency of the double helix of DNA replication. Melatonin and Pinolina work in DNA, inducing an 8 Hz signal to enable replication of DNA and mitosis. This process activates a form of superconductivity that has effects on the temperature generated by the human body.

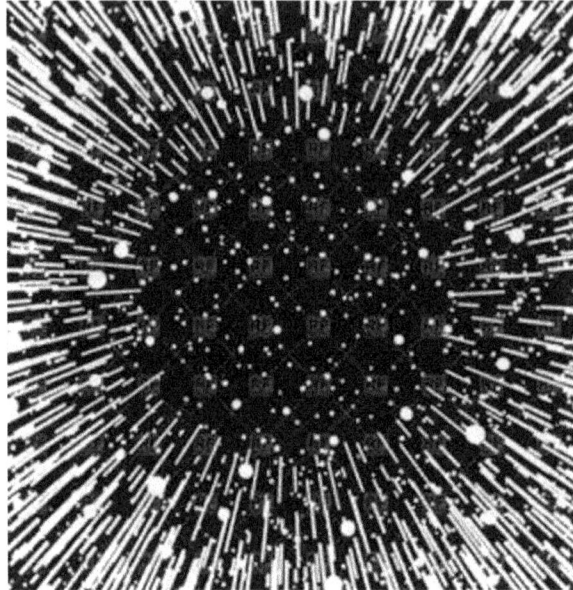

A sound from the Infinite Consciousness,

Giving birth to the cosmic light,

Expanding beyond space and time,

Materializing Universes, galaxies and stars,

In the endless evolutive journey,

Turning Infinite Consciousness into life.   -J.E.M.

4

Healing Effects From Animal and Nature Sounds

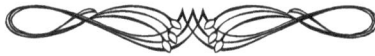

Animal Sounds That Have Healing Effects

Elizabeth Von Muggenthaler, a scientific researcher and specialist in bio-acoustics, has delved into an area that has never before been researched. She has studied the mysterious realm of the healing power of purring cats, whale songs, and sounds of the Sumatran Rhino. She also investigates sounds that we can feel and yet never hear. She is president of the Fauna Communication Research Institute.

Sumatran Rhinos expel air through their nostrils and produce sounds that are very similar to whale sounds. Elizabeth observed that the whistle of the rhino produces a vibrational frequency which is similar to that produced by whales and often travels for miles.

In nature, these rhinos are supposedly solitary and are rarely seen together. It is curious that a solitary creature has developed such a wide repertoire of sounds. These creatures enjoy being in their mud wallows and like to sing. Elizabeth thinks it is a type of meditation.

There are only about 200 rhinos worldwide, whales are also diminishing and not much is being done for their preservation. These wonderful creatures may eventually become extinct, and if so, we will lose the benefits of their therapeutic sounds.

The Chirping of Birds

Birdsong and the sound produced by many species of birds creates relaxing effects all around the world. The vibrational frequency generated by the sound of a singing bird is 5 Hz to 7 Hz which is the same frequency of theta brainwaves. Besides producing deep relaxation, listening to bird sounds can help individuals focus and resolve their problems with greater ease.

Bird sounds also generate vibrational frequencies that stimulate the growth of grass and vegetation. This was published in the journal NATURE over twenty years ago. The prevailing note of a bird song differs a few decibels from our F sharp (F#) note. The Chinese call this central note of nature, which is prevalent in bird songs, Yellow Bell. In India it is called Ma.

The Frog Sounds

The sounds that tree frogs emit coincide with theta brain wave frequencies which are associated with creativity. These sounds are in the lower end of the theta range of 3 Hz to 7 Hz, and therefore activate deep into our subconscious minds, and connect to our creative sides.

The Healing Sound of Purring Cats

Purring cats produce a vibrational frequency in the anabolic range of 20 to 50 Hz, and can extend up to 140 Hz. The purring sound is created from a cat's diaphragm and larynx. All members of the cat family, except leopards, have a strong harmonic resonance of 50 Hz.

About two years ago, scientists discovered that the vibrations between 20 and 140 Hz help heal bone fractures, repair muscle and ligament tears, and reduce inflammation and pain. Three species of cats fall exactly on or within 2 points of 120 Hz, which is a frequency that has been found to repair tendons and help heal bone fractures.

The Fauna Communications Institute located in North Carolina (USA), has found that a cat's purr matches vibrations of 20 to 140 Hz. The dominant frequencies produced by a purring cat are from 25 to 50 Hz. These are the optimal frequencies that stimulate growth in bone mass and also stimulate the healing of fractures.

All cats, including pumas, ocelots and lions, have additional sets of strong harmonics ranging from 25 to 50 Hertz to help them generate muscle strength, increase joint mobility and relieve pain. Notably, it was recently discovered that when cats purr, it helps them eliminate the excess of carbon dioxide from their bodies.

The frequency that is produced by a purring cat is good for healing muscle, tendon and ligament injuries, as well as for strength and muscle toning. It is also good for any type of joint injury, wound healing, reduction of infections and inflammation and for pain relief. The purring sound also helps soothe chronic lung disease in cats.

The authors of a manual about veterinary surgery note that cats do not develop health problems such as lung diseases, muscle injuries, and tendon and bone diseases as often as dogs and other animals.

The sound of a purring cat begins in the brain when neurons in the central nervous system fire a rhythmic, repetitive message. This type of message is called a neural oscillator; an electric pulse is sent to the muscles of the larynx which cause them to contract at a rate of 25 to 150 vibrations per second in a consistent and constant pattern.

Scientific studies have shown that all cats purr at the same frequency. The vibrational frequency of a purring cat is similar to the one created when the sound of OUM is vocalized in a deep tone at low volume during meditation. It is a guttural sound in a very deep tone that comes from deep in the throat and the chest area. The sound is similar to the sound of the purr of an engine, but with a very low frequency at a very low tone, soft and pleasant to the ear.

Humans can mimic this sound, but it is important when making this sound to also think about the meaning of the OUM. First, the lips stay together with the mouth almost closed and filled with air. Then the air is expelled from the diaphragm slowly and it feels as if the sound vibrates the vocal cords with a deep tone at a low volume. We visualize and feel the sound emerging from the area between the chest cavity above the thymus gland area and near the lower base of the throat. When we produce this sound, the powerful frequency that is internally generated stimulates the natural healing process of the body.

When the sound we make approximates the purring of a cat, we can obtain great health benefits. Studies have shown that the sound of a purring cat can relieve stress, lower blood pressure, and induce tranquility, peace and calm in humans.

We have much to learn from the intuitive power of animals, from the sounds they emit and how their sounds can stimulate a natural healing process in our bodies. If we would make an effort to imitate at least some sounds that animals produce, we would begin to experience the benefits and would be on our way toward good health.

Sounds of Planet Earth

"Our Planet Mother Earth (Gaia)
is like a gigantic symphony orchestra,
incessantly in concert, generating
sounds and vibrations naturally."
- J.E.M.

Mother Nature takes care of balancing all planetary systems. All systems on Earth are in a constant state of vibration and producing vibrational frequencies of Sound. There are the external surface sounds of air, wind, and water, as well as the Earth's internal sounds. Myriad sounds – volcanoes, trees, insects, animals, birds, and sounds produced by Earth's magnetic field – all these sounds have a direct effect on the ecosystem and on the biophysical and mental systems of our bodies.

The natural ecosystem of our planet is directly linked to sound frequencies produced by birds, insects (i.e. bees, butterflies, crickets,) amphibians (i.e. frogs,) reptiles (i.e. snakes) and many other sound sources, which help to maintain balance in the natural production of seeds, flowers and fruit. Crops that are exposed to natural sounds produced by birds, insects, amphibians, reptiles and the five natural elements, grow healthier and faster. In botanical science we refer to this as the Agro Bio Sonic effect.

Studies demonstrate that plants that were exposed to Mozart's music, grew 50% to 100% faster than normal. Sound permanently interacts with the physiology of plants, animals and humans. If we can learn to harness and focus these different sound frequencies we could achieve specific effects for the benefit of all living beings on Earth.

The sounds and vibrational frequencies produced by air, wind, rain, thunder and lightning have powerful effects on Earth's ecosystems. For example, thunderstorms trigger ozone production which increases oxygen levels and helps reduce pollution caused by carbon monoxide and other noxious gases in the atmosphere.

Water is the most abundant element on Earth and covers three fourths of the planet's surface. Oceans, rivers and lakes are constantly moving and producing sound frequencies. The animal and plant life in the bodies of water generate sounds that impact the natural ecosystems of water and land. The dolphins and whales in their extraordinary interspecies communications produce powerful sounds that travel thousands of miles through the ocean.

Humpback whales sing in intervals of seven-eighths (similar to the range of the piano keyboard). Like humans, whales remember their songs and repeat them from season to season. These intelligent creatures have a sophisticated form of communication by which they produce extraordinary low tones that can travel for hundreds of miles.

Whales are knowledgeable about the thermal layers of the ocean. They take advantage of thermal currents of the ocean when the water is warm, because intuitively they know that sound frequencies travel more efficiently in warmer water. Marine biologists estimate that humpback whales use songs to communicate with other members of their species at distances of over hundreds or even thousands of miles.

Marine biologists have discovered, through scientific studies, that the sounds produced by whales and dolphins can deliver therapeutic effects to humans.

In the forest, nature creates innumerable and delightful harmonic frequencies. In the evenings in forest regions of Puerto Rico, extremely tiny frogs produce enchanting continuous harmonized sound frequencies that can activate the mental state of Alpha relaxation.

These tiny frogs are known as the **coqui** (eleutherodactylus portoricensis - 16 species). The first syllable of sound they produce "co" reached a record pitch of 1,160 Hertz and is intended by that tiny frog to warn other males of its species to stay away from its particular territory. The second syllable "kii", which hits a record sound of 2,090 Hertz, is used to invite the females of the species to mate and reproduce.

Although both sexes vocalize aggressively against intruders entering their territory, only males call during courtship at 1 and 2 meters above the ground, usually while sitting on the leaf of a plant. The females travel long distances to answer the calls of the males.

The experience of the sounds produced by the coquii, "co-kii, kii co-co-kii" is indigenous to Puerto Rico. The musical serenade and frequencies of sound produced by coquís have powerful effects that activate the alpha state of mind and relaxation in humans and therefore can produce healing effects.

My friend Pilar, told me she first encountered the sound of the Coqui in Hawaii when she attended a seminar in Kalani, a holistic retreat center near Pele, in the Big Island. On the evening she arrived, there was a presentation about the center in an open pavilion outside that included the magical background sound of the Coqui. She was fascinated. She was so entranced by the spectacular sound, that when the presentation was finished she asked the presenter if she could buy the CD of the beautiful frog songs. The presenter laughed and explained to her that it had not been a CD, but the actual sound of the Puerto Rican Coqui that someone had probably brought to Hawaii (likely in a clandestine way) and were now thriving there.

I explained to Pilar that Hawaii and Puerto Rico have nearly identical tropical, topographical and ecological conditions and when Puerto Rico's sugar industry was devastated by two hurricanes in 1899. The devastation caused a worldwide shortage in sugar production and a huge demand for the product from Hawaii. Hawaiian sugar plantation owners began to recruit the jobless, but experienced, laborers from Puerto Rico. On November 22, 1900, the first group of Puerto Ricans consisting of 56 men began their long journey to Maui, Hawaii. The trip was long and unpleasant. They first set sail from San Juan, Puerto Rico harbor, to New Orleans, Louisiana. Once in New Orleans, they were boarded on a railroad train and sent to Port Los Angeles, California. From there they set sail aboard the Rio de Janeiro to Hawaii and by the year 2000 the Puerto Rican population was over 30,005 and by 2015 it surpasses that amount many times.

During the late 20th century, the **"coquí,"** a thumbnail-sized tree frog endemic to Puerto Rico, became established in Hawaii, most likely as stowaways in shipments of potted plants. While its loud and magical sound, was considered "music to the ears" by the Puerto Rican people in Puerto Rico and Hawaii, it was considered an annoyance by some Hawaiians. However, this invasive species reached much higher population densities through the years. They made many efforts to exterminate the **"Coquí's"** fast growing population but they were not able to exterminate them and the **"Coquí"** population continue expanding every day through the many island of Hawaii. There is a saying that "The Puerto Ricans that immigrated to Hawaii took along with them their music, their typical instruments, the Cuatro, the Guitar, the Guiro, the Maracas, the Palitos and of course they took with them the nice **"Coquí"** healing music serenade.

A brief historical account about the music receptivity of Puerto Ricans and their connection with the "Coqui"

The natives of Puerto Rico known as **"Taíno Indians"** that migrated to the island from the Northern Coast of South America and settled in Puerto Rico around 900 A.D., played a percussion instrument called **"mayohavau"** that was played during religious rituals. According to Fray Ramon Pane who arrived in **Borinquen** (as the natives used to call Puerto Rico) in 1508 after Juan Ponce de Leon, the **"mayohavau"** was a percussion instrument made of thin wood, shaped like an elongate gourd, and measured up to one meter long and a half meter wide. The sound of the **"mayohavau"** could be heard from 2.4 to 4.6 miles, or 3,862 to 7,403 meters. Fray R. Pane reported that this instrument was played by the tribe leader as an accompaniment to songs and dances which were used to pass on customs and laws to younger generations.

The **Taino Indians** also played "güiros", made from higüeros (gourds) which varied in size from quite small to about a meter in length. Another musical instrument they commonly used was a flute made from conch shells or reeds. The Taínos also used maracas, although the design was different from the modern version; using a single large ball instead of many small ones.

Puerto Ricans were influenced by music hundreds of years prior to 1492 when Christopher Columbus arrived. Puerto Ricans' love for music is encoded in their DNA, deep in their roots, from the **"Taino Indians,"** to the 1508 Spaniard Colonization (who brought with them the Flamenco and Arabic music) and Africans that came to Puerto Rico with Spaniards. From the moment Puerto Ricans are born, they are exposed to the Coqui's beautiful healing tropical sounds and musical serenade.

I have been intrigued with the Greek philosopher Plato's writings, and by a recent underwater archaeological discovery that most of the Caribbean Islands and Puerto Rico are the remains of an ancient civilization from more than 11,600 years ago. Written documents exist that claim crystals and harmonic sounds were used to treat and heal the people of Atlantis and to perform other advanced technological functions. It is not mere chance that my passion and love for singing, nature and music has led me to dedicate my life to researching and writing my thesis about **"The Healing Forces of Harmonic Sounds and Vibrations and Healing Through the Power of the Voice and the Mind."** I believe this goes back thousands of years to my ancestors, and is encoded in my DNA, since I was born in beautiful Puerto Rico.

5

The Nature of Sound and Electromagnetic Energy

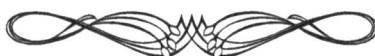

The Nature of Sound, Electromagnetic Energy and Vibrational Frequencies

Sounds are composed of different frequencies. Hertz is the scientific measurement used to measure the frequencies of sounds. Sounds below 30 Hz are not heard or perceived by the human ear. However, sounds above 20 Hz can be perceived by the human ear. Brainwave patterns usually range from 40 Hz and in many cases up to 100 Hz or more. Brain waves of 40 Hz can be recorded by an electroencephalogram ("EEG") and are referred to as Gamma brainwaves. We refer to frequencies that are significantly higher than 40Hz as Hyper-Gamma brainwaves. Such frequencies have the enormous potential to boost the lower and higher ranges.

Recently, research reports have been obtained through EEG investigations during ecstatic states of consciousness associated with brainwave frequencies of up to 200 Hz. These frequencies have been labeled **Lambda** brainwaves.

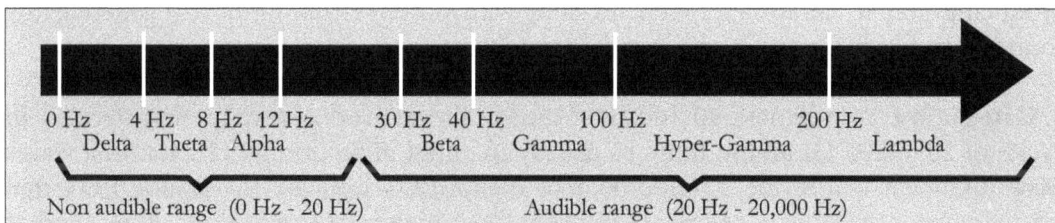

0 Hz	4 Hz	8 Hz	12 Hz	30 Hz	40 Hz	100 Hz	200 Hz
Delta	Theta	Alpha		Beta	Gamma	Hyper-Gamma	Lambda

Non audible range (0 Hz - 20 Hz)   Audible range (20 Hz - 20,000 Hz)

0 Hz a 20 Hz = Frequencies NOT PERCEIVED by the human ear.
20 Hz a 20,000 Hz = Frequencies PERCEIVED by the human ear.

Delta waves: fluctuate between 1/3 and 4 Hz
Theta waves: fluctuate between 4 and 7 Hz
Alpha waves: fluctuate between 8 and 14 Hz
Beta waves: fluctuate between 14 and 40 Hz
Gamma waves: fluctuate between 40Hz and 100Hz

The electroencephalogram (EEG) is the method used to measure and record the electrical activity of neurons in the brain. Neurons are specialized cells of the nervous system. By using an EEG doctors can record and identify abnormalities in the brain, such as coma, brain death, tumor, or stroke. An EEG is performed by placing electrodes and wires on different areas of the head. This procedure is painless.

The role of different waves and vibrational frequencies generated by the human brain

The discovery of various waves and vibrational frequencies generated by the human brain occurred after World War II by the German psychiatrist Hans Berger. His studies revealed that there was an electrical potential in the human brain, and by an instrument he called an encephalograph, he was able to measure vibrational frequency waves in the brain.

The brain is an electrochemical organ and it has been scientifically proven that when the brain is in full operation it can generate up to 10 watts of electrical potential or electricity. Conservative scientists estimate that if the 86 billion cells that compose the human nervous system were to be interconnected at a given time, and were to discharge their electric charge in a single electrode placed on the scalp, it would record between 5 million and 50 million volts. Although this electric power is rather limited, it takes a very specific form in the human brain. The electrical activity that emanates from the brain is shown as brainwaves. It is through this electrical activity that our minds operate.

There are five basic categories of brainwaves, ranging from the highest to the lowest brain activity. The categories are gamma, beta, alpha, theta and delta. These different brain states are classified according to the speed of the predominant neurological brain wave signals from one point to another during a given time. The speed and vibrational frequency are measured in Hertz, and the figures are obtained using an EEG. Brain neurons are constantly producing electric vibratory frequencies along with powerful vibrations that generate tiny sounds. The five brain waves are described as follows:

1. Gamma Waves (alertness, 40-100 Hz) Gama brainwaves are generally characterized in cycles of 25 to 100 Hz and in humans usually manifest at around 40 Hz. Gamma waves were unknown before the development of digital-EEG because the analog-EEG that existed previously could not measure waves at those higher frequencies. Its upper limit of measurement was around 25 Hz. However, neuroscientists are now beginning to discover the wonderful properties of the brain when gamma frequency waves occur.

A gamma brainwave is the fastest brainwave frequency with the smallest amplitude. Gamma brainwaves have been reported in EEGs of experienced meditators like monks and nuns. These waves are associated with the "feeling of the ecstasy of blessings." In this state there is a maximum level of mental concentration and cognitive functioning.

Neuroscientists believe that gamma waves are able to link and connect information from all parts of the brain. Gamma waves originate in the thalamus and move from the back of the brain toward the front of the brain, at about 40 times per second, and the entire brain is influenced by these waves. The quick action of gamma waves causes the brain to achieve peak physical and mental performance. In this condition a person has the feeling that he or she has arrived in a powerful zone where he or she can achieve whatever is desired.

All human beings generate gamma brain waves, but the amount of gamma waves varies with each person. Low amounts of gamma brainwaves have been linked to learning disabilities, poor memory and impaired mental processing. In a low level gamma (30-40 Hz/Sec.) a person can become very excited and anxious and can fall into a state of panic and hysteria. This state is manifested oftentimes when a person faces an extremely tense situation or receives bad news that causes the adrenal glands to secrete adrenaline that is out of control. In these cases other hormonal substances also become activated, such as somatotropic hormones and corticosteroids.

People in the high ranges of gamma activity are exceptionally intelligent, compassionate and ususaly very happy. They usually have excellent memories and self-control of all their senses. People with high levels of gamma activity are also known to have high Intelectual Coefficient (IQ). Athletes, musicians, teachers, lecturers, scientists, artists and intellectuals who achieve success in their work generate high levels of gamma activity.

The frequency of 40 Hz regulates and accelerates memory processing. People with high gamma brain activity are exceptionally vibrant and may have photographic memories. In other words, they get the information from the memory bank of the brain almost instantly or in fractions of seconds. This is because 40 Hz gamma sharpens sensory perception. The brain becomes much more sensitive to sensory stimuli; therefore, food tastes better and the senses of sight, hearing and smell are heightened. A sense of true living and better perception is activated.

One of the most remarkable properties of the gamma state is the acceleration of brain information and a heightening of the senses, which results in enhanced focus and attention. The brain is able to process extraordinary amounts of sensory information quickly, and can easily retrieve the information at a later time. People with high gamma activity are naturally happier, calmer and radiate a harmonious state of peace. Gamma is the best antidepressant and is activated naturally. People with depression typically have low gamma activity.

How Can We Produce Gamma Brain Waves?

The answer is simple. When we meditate and sense the power of love and compassion deep within ourselves, we produce gamma brainwaves. Thus, we achieve a state of harmony, happiness, high awareness of mental focus and self-control where our senses are heightened, and perception and coordination of neurovascular brain processes in our nervous systems are increased.

Love is the most powerful energy in the universe which creates, regenerates, heals and transforms. When love is coupled with compassion - generated when we meditate, pray, practice mantras, intone vowel sounds, sing harmonies in the diatonic scale, and listen to the music of **"The Healing Forces of Harmonic Sounds and Vibrations,"** we create in ourselves heightened states of sensory perception and divine order.

Gamma waves are also present during sleep and creative visualization. Compassion comes from a feeling of oneness with all creation. This is the "feeling of the ecstasy of blessings" that accompanies high levels of gamma brain wave activity.

Many studies and experiments have been performed with meditators, especially Tibetan Buddhist monks and Celestine nuns. Both groups demonstrated the ability to produce gamma waves during meditation. The studies showed a significant increase in brain activity in the left prefrontal cortex, which is associated with self-control, happiness and compassion.

When you meditate with the help of music and sounds (including **"The Healing Forces of Harmonic Sounds and Vibrations,"** flutes, classical music, Tibetan bowls and pure quartz crystal singing bowls, Gregorian chants in Latin, Tibetan mantras, and nature and animal sounds like the coqui, birds, dolphins, whales, insects, and crickets) and through prayer, affirmations, mantras, creative visualization and the powerful energy of love coupled with a sense of compassion, you begin to activate the sense of oneness with Universal Consciousness and achieve successful brainwave activity that triggers high levels of gamma waves.

2. Beta Waves. Our minds usually operate at this frequency in everyday life. In this state we are in a full conscious state and can pay attention to everything around us, and usually only one side of the brain is functioning. In this state we experience logical reasoning and common conversations. Beta is generally characterized by brainwave cycles of **15 to 40 Hz** (cycles per second). Higher cycles of beta frequency usually generate tension and anxiety, and make a person think too much which can cause confusion, wrong decisions and negative reactions. The high vibrational frequencies of beta brain waves also generate hypertension, increased heart rate, increased blood flow, cortisone production and glucose consumption. Generally, we do not wish to experience a state of high frequency beta because it can negatively affect our health.

3. Alpha Waves. Here we are between sleep and wakefulness in a state of mild sleep or a state of light relaxation. When we meditate, alpha waves are usually activated. The person is in a state of mental and muscular relaxation and fluctuates between conscious and unconscious access. Creative insight and imagination become active. Suggestions and behaviors can be induced in this state. This state is achieved when we meditate, pray and recite mantras. We may also go into alpha state when we travel in a car and observe a beautiful landscape, when relaxed on a cruise, or while reading a good book. We lose track of what is happening around us. The brain works in cycles of between **8 to 9 Hz and 14 Hz.** Alpha state is characterized by the partial state of the conscious mind and the partial state of the subconscious mind being activated simultaneously. It is a favorable state to absorb information, and to study and assimilate new concepts. Alpha state promotes more left brain use in the assimilation and processing of information. In alpha state, information is amplified, either positively or negatively. Thus, it is important to ensure that we are positive and have constructive thoughts during alpha state. It has been scientifically proven that alpha brain waves create the most effective mental state for the activation of the natural healing process of the body, mind and spirit.

4. Theta Waves. Here we are in a state of deep relaxation, mentally and physically. The conscious mind is mostly **off** and the subconscious mind ceases to flourish. The theta state is generally invoked when we are sleeping, dreaming or in a state of deep relaxation. This state is also achieved when we meditate deeply, repeat mantras, listen to **"The Healing Forces of Harmonic Sounds and Vibrations"** and the sounds produced by quartz crystal singing bowls, Tibetan bowls and the flute. This is the state where hypnotists aim to take clients to enable them to enter into a deep state of hypnosis. In the theta state brainwave cycles range from **5 Hz to 8 Hz.** Theta is where ideas, visualizations and suggestions are more likely to enter the subconscious mind and we are less aware of what is happening around us.

5. Delta Waves. This is an extremely deep state of sleep and relaxation with full operation of the subconscious. Delta is a frequency we do not yet fully comprehend, as it is experienced during our deepest sleep for about 90 minutes each night. It has been proven that during this time in particular, the physical and mental body is reconditioned and begins to recover from wear and fatigue. We enter delta in the waking state when we are in advanced states of meditation. This state is associated with Kundalini meditation. It is interesting to note that delta, characterized by slow brain waves from **1 Hz to 4 Hz,** is the state that a skilled hypnotist wishes to lead his patients into, as a substitute for anesthesia during medical surgery. This procedure has been scientifically documented on numerous occasions and confirmed by many surgeons.

Harmonic sounds that stimulate brain states of alpha and theta

Scientific research has confirmed that harmonic sounds can induce mental and physical relaxation that stimulates alpha and theta brain states. Sounds such as those produced by "The Healing Power of Harmonic Sounds and Vibrations," pure quartz crystals bowls, Tibetan bowls, flutes, mantras, chants of Tibetan monks, and Gregorian chants help stimulate brain frequencies conductive to positive molecular responses. These responses induce physical and mental changes which improve the human state of consciousness and stimulate the natural healing process of the body, mind and spirit.

Frequencies and sounds that are not perceived by human ears

An example of the frequencies of sounds that we cannot perceive through our ears but are perceived through our skin (epidermal tissue), bones or nervous system are **electromagnetic microwave** emissions. Such emissions are produced by mobile phones, radio waves, radar, and radiation from microwave ovens. It has been scientifically proven that microwave frequencies emitted by mobile phones and radar have a negative effect on the brain, nervous system, immune system and endocrine system, and produce imbalances in the neurovascular system. Wireless routers that activate Internet access in computers also produce **electromagnetic microwave** emissions that generate vibrational frequencies that negatively impact our health.

The sound waves of microwave frequencies which are generated by mobile phones are intensified when a person is moving while talking in the phone, (i.e. when walking or riding in a car.) The stepped-up ultrasonic waves produced when we are moving augment the negative effects on our health. These tiny sound frequencies are not perceived by our ears, but are perceived by other systems in our bodies, including the neuro-vascular system (brain), epidermal tissue (skin), bone tissue and crystalline substances in the plasma in our blood. In conclusion, our bones, brain and skin have the ability to easily absorb sound frequencies **not** perceived by our ears.

Scientific studies have shown that sound frequencies, specifically sounds that are not detected by our ears, can produce changes in the endocrine system, immunological system, autonomic system, nervous system and other body systems. Indeed, the human body has a high capacity to absorb extremely tiny vibrational sound frequencies that are not perceived by the ear, but are perceived by the brain, skin, bones, and mineral and crystalline substances that travel in the bloodstream, through the arteries, veins and capillaries.

The Nature of Energy

Science has proven that all energy is electromagnetic in nature and is in a constant state of vibration and creating sound. Our bodies, organs and the billions of cells that make up our biophysical composition radiate their own electromagnetic fields where vibrations and sound occur.

The energy that is generated in our physical universe produces radiation, and this radiation emits energy: thermal energy (heat and cold), light and electricity, and sound frequencies. The Sun emits or radiates light, and sounds, and also electromagnetic frequencies. Earth emits electricity, magnetic energy and sounds. In quantum terms we speak of a certain particular kind of energy that Earth produces, and that we define as telluric energy. The energies emitted by the Sun and Earth come from substances that are different in nature, but all of them produce radiation, electromagnetic energy and sound frequencies.

Electromagnetism is a form of radiation that originates naturally and can also be produced artificially. Electromagnetism is the fundamental energy that is generated by the physical universe. Atoms, molecules, solids and liquids that are formed by sub-atomic reactions generate electromagnetic energy and vibrational frequencies which in turn also produce sound.

Electromagnetism is an electric charge balanced with magnetic energy that sustains the trajectory of orbits in subatomic particles that created matter, from atoms to galaxies, in all the celestial bodies of the universe. Quantum mechanics recognizes that the very nature of the physical universe is precisely electromagnetism and vibrational energy which generate sound frequencies.

Science has also recognized that at micro-cosmic levels, living organisms carry out their biological functions generating electrical currents and magnetism, issuing thermal energy (heat and cold) and therefore, generate sound frequencies.

The disruption of electromagnetic energy in cells generates frequencies and vibrations which damage the natural metabolism of the cells and leads to disease.

Electromagnetic energy and vibrational frequencies not of natural origin

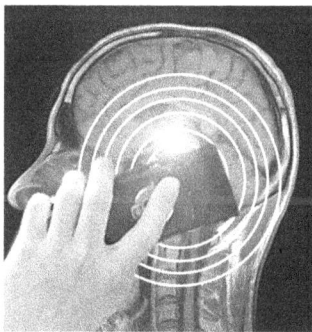

We are surrounded by power lines, radar and other systems that generate electromagnetic energy and vibrational frequencies that are not natural. This type of electromagnetic energy can be defined as abnormal energy because it is created by man. The vast majority of electromagnetic energy that is generated by radar, cell phones, microwaves, high-voltage electric lines and other electronic systems generates artificial electromagnetic energy fields with subtle energy, producing pollution and tiny vibrational sound frequencies. The human ear is not capable of perceiving such sound frequencies, but the frequencies are perceived by our epidermal tissue, bones, nervous system, and crystalline substances in our blood plasma.

All living things have their own energy fields that surround the physical body. The fields of artificial electromagnetic energy created by man can alter the energy of the subtle body which is around the physical body, producing changes that interfere with the energy balance of human beings and affect their health.

The human body is composed of trillions of cells and is one of the biophysical systems most endowed with a great capacity to perceive energy. The cell membrane has an extraordinary capacity for registering vibrational power through itself. Exposure to weak signals (low frequency signals) generated by cell phones creates electromagnetic energy which causes cells to release much of their vital energy. This creates a breakdown in the communication between cells and can cause uncontrollable reproduction thereof.

Power lines, radar, television signals, computer monitors, cell phones and systems that generate electromagnetic energy produce ionizing energy that is not naturally occurring. All these technologies generate extremely low vibrational sound frequencies.

Non-ionizing radiation is different from ionizing radiation because when it penetrates matter it does not break the nuclei of atoms, yet it alters the original position of the electrons, and thus alters the natural composition of the substance.

When the ionizing radiation that is not naturally occurring makes contact with atoms in the human body, the natural composition of atoms is altered by adding or removing electrons. All of this activates the process of cell oxidation and gives rise to the production of free radicals that contributes to the origin of many diseases.

Due to modern technology, artificial ionizing radiation is creating enormous health problems for humanity and for many other living organisms on Earth.

Ionizing radiation of natural origin comes to us from the Sun, through its rays. There are also natural materials such as Uranium, Radium, Cobalt, Selenium, Plutonium and Radon gas which produce ionizing radiation of a natural origin. It is imperative to consider that all of these elements are constantly in a state of vibration and producing sounds.

6

The Emission of Frequencies

**Sound frequencies produced by our solar system, and
sounds that can cause harm to human beings**

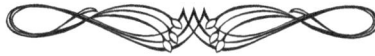

The Sun Produces Ionic Energy and Sounds That Make the Earth Dance

The Sun generates the most powerful energy that gives rise to life and creation on Earth. The Sun is like a giant burning ball of gas that is maintained by active thermonuclear reactions and reactions using fusion. The fusion process occurs when hydrogen atoms join together to form a larger chemical compound, giving rise to helium, a new element.

The temperature on the Sun's surface is about 4000 C to 6000 C. The Sun burns four million tons of its chemical composition every second. Powerful sunspots and solar waves are produced and they create interference with radio waves. Earth is eight light minutes away from the Sun. The energy generated by the Sun produces natural ionizing energy that is in a constant state of vibration and in turn generates sound frequencies.

David Thomson and Louis Lanzerotti are members of the experimental team HISCALE aboard Ulysses. Along with their colleagues Frank Vernon, Marc Lessard and Lindsay Smith, they have shown that sounds generated inside the Sun cause vibrations that produce tremors and movements on Earth. These sounds make Earth ground vibrate in solidarity with the Sun. The team also demonstrated that distinct isolated tones generated by pressure waves and the gravity in the Sun are present in a wide variety of terrestrial systems.

Different tones emitted by the Sun have been recorded by geological instruments and seismic data on Earth. It has been discovered that the Earth's magnetic field, the atmosphere and even the voltage induced in ocean cables are part of **"the cosmic symphony of sounds."**

The **"cosmic symphony of sounds"** is active around us but our ears cannot detect all the sounds. This is because some sounds have a pitch that is too low to be perceived by the human ear. Sound frequencies typically generate from 100-5000 micro Hertz (1 micro Hertz corresponds to 1 vibration every 278 hours). This is equivalent to 12 octaves below the lowest audible note on the musical scale that humans can hear. In comparison, the note that symphony orchestras use to tune their instruments is LA (A) above the central DO (C) that is located in the middle of the piano keyboard and corresponds to 440 Hertz.

Low-frequency sounds produced by the Sun have been recorded by the Spaceship ESA / NASA SOHO. Videos exist that demonstrate how atmospheric circulation inside the Sun causes **very low frequency sounds.**

Solar oscillations have been observed from Earth, both optically using SOHO instruments, and by networks of radio telescopes. Solar oscillations are caused by pressure waves in the Sun, and are known as g modes. The deepest sounds associated with the Sun's gravitational waves (g modes) are difficult to reach.

Scientists have examined a wide range of data covering natural phenomena and technological systems in fields as diverse as telecommunications and seismology, and continue to find new evidence of discrete tones related to solar oscillations among sounds that had been previously considered **"background noise."** This has added to the enigma posed by the findings of Ulysses.

According to the observations of David Thomson these sounds and background noises are related to the magnetic field. He suggests that g vibration modes occur within the magnetic field at the Sun's surface. Part of this magnetic field got carried from the Sun into interplanetary space by the solar winds, where it was detected by the space detectors in Ulysses.

Frequencies of the Universe, the Sun, Plants and Humans

All beings on our planet Earth are constantly receiving sound frequencies and sun flares. We breathe sounds, vibrations and light signals coming from the Sun. The energy of electrons from the Sun activates plant plasma and chlorophyll, and this energy is transformed into the oxygen that is used by all beings on Planet Earth.

There is a cycle of nine perfect frequency sounds in the universe. NASA has recordings of the Sun's tonal central frequency which indicates that the Sun is radiating in the key of 528 Hz. The 528 Hz tone is one among the nine fundamental creative frequencies of the primordial musical scale. Earth's botanicals are also vibrating at the tonal frequency of 528 Hz. The original western musical scale (solfeggio) consists of 6 notes C (DO), D (RE), E (MI), F (FA), G (SOL), A (LA), and E (MI) the third note (528 Hz) is defined as the miraculous note. The universe and the Sun are vibrating at the frequency of that miraculous sound.

The universe is organized into mathematical patterns; some believe this to be the language of the Creative Universal Intelligence, or God. The way in which the entire universe is constructed, including people, is through a mathematical matrix of 9 simple musical chords. In other words the universe is created by a mathematical matrix of sound frequencies.

Math geniuses and physics experts have concluded that the universe was created and is maintained by a mathematical matrix and sound frequencies that are extremelly powerful and sacred.

Sounds That Can Cause Serious Mental and Physical Harm To Humans

Military institutions in many countries have used **ultrasonic weapons** in their military exercises. Ultrasonic weapons technology uses powerful speakers to generate intense frequencies of sound, similar to explosions. These weapons are called **sound grenades or sound cannons.** The sound frequencies generated by ultrasonic weapons can cause serious harm to anyone who is exposed to them. Another technique used by military institutions is a series of recorded sounds projected through loudspeakers in battles to confuse the enemy, called **Psychological Warfare.** The high frequency sound waves generated by the ultrasonic weapons produce vibrational frequencies that can destroy the ear nerves and subsequently can also damage the nervous system and organs in the human body.

Ultrasonic weapons technology generates 7 Hz sounds. The sounds are sent through tubes into open space. These sound frequencies are so powerful that they can penetrate walls, as well as many other construction materials. Walls and other materials used to create divisions inside buildings offer little protection against these intense sound frequencies which are non-harmonic in nature and can cause serious damage to individuals.

Due to technological advances, there is now an instrument that produces **infrasound** frequencies from 0.3 Hz up to 18.9 Hz. This technology, confirmed by the engineer Vic Tandy, generates intense sound frequencies that can distort the vision field in the human eye, which can create an imbalance and may cause dizziness. Another example of infrasound causing a physical problem in individuals is car sickness. Car sickness is not always caused because the car is in motion; sometimes car sickness is caused by the sound vibration produced by a car's engine, which generates a frequency between 4-7 Hz.

The frequencies of 7 Hz can cause osteoporosis. Low frequencies such as 18 Hz can cause dizziness, fainting, and feelings of terror. There is a theory that some ghostly apparitions in some places are caused by low-frequency vibrations of about 18 Hz.

A tiger's roar is around 18 Hz and can cause temporary paralysis, the weakening of muscles, feelings of terror, cold, fainting, headache and other symptoms (not just from fright!)

The loud music played in modern dance clubs generates intense wave frequencies that can have negative psychological and physical effects on the young patrons. Many of the sounds of modern dance music activate hostile attitudes, psychological imbalances and negative emotions in young people.

Individuals who frequently expose themselves to loud nightclubs and rock concerts find it difficult to hear sounds below 30 to 40 Hz. As time passes, they usually suffer ear problems that limit their sense of hearing.

Ultrasonic technology weapons, infrasound, loud nightclubs, loud rock concerts and the roar of a tiger are examples of the sound wave frequencies that can produce adverse effects in humans, unlike **The Healing Forces of Harmonic Sounds and Vibrations, which generates frequencies that balance the chakras, activate a positive mind state and stimulate the natural healing process of the biological systems in the body.**

7

The Human Body, Matter and Frequencies

The human body, with its systems, cells and four elements, produces sounds that have specific resonance frequencies

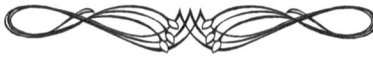

The Human Body and Its Organs, Cells and Systems

Every atom, molecule, macromolecule, organelle, cell, tissue, organ, gland and system in our body absorbs frequencies of sound, emits sound and has a frequency of resonance.

The cell is the smallest unit of life in the human body. Approximately 50 million cells die each second in the human body and simultaneously reproduce and become replaced by the same number of new cells. During that cycle of life, the trillions of cells that make up our bodies work in close collaboration, communicating with each other, absorbing sounds, producing sounds, and registering resonance frequencies.

The human body is composed of different chemical elements from Earth. There are over 90 elements that occur naturally on Earth and about 25 of them can be found in the human body. The four most important elements that constitute 9.2% of a human's body weight are: oxygen (65%), carbon (18.5%), hydrogen (9.5%), and nitrogen (3.2%). The elements that represent 3.7% of a human's body weight are: calcium 1.5%, phosphate 1.0%, potassium 0.4%, sulfur 0.3%, sodium 0.2%, chlorine 0.2% and magnesium 0.1%. The chemical ratio in the human body changes as we age, and during this process the elements vibrate, generate frequencies and behave in specific rhythms, like Earth.

Every person, animal, microorganism, planet, and celestial body; and each element, atom, cell, tissue, organ, bone and gland in the human body produces sounds and is in a constant state of vibration.

Everything that exists in the physical plane generates sounds, has its own vibrational frequency and projects its own specific resonance that differentiates it from other bodies.

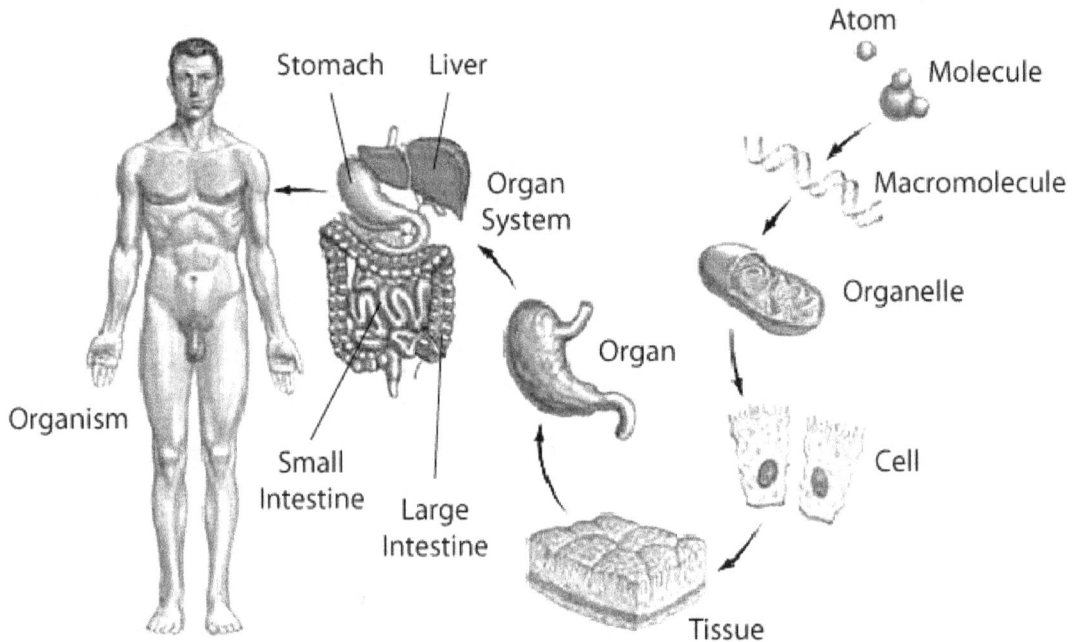

The human body's organizational systems, from the simplest (atom, molecule, macromolecule, organelle and cell) to the most complex (tissues, organs and systems.)

The human body consists of 10 core systems essential for life: the systems of bones and muscles, and the circulatory, digestive, urinary, nervous, reproductive, lymphatic, endocrine and respiratory systems. All of these systems produce sounds, absorb sounds and frequencies and have a specific resonance frequency.

Everything we see, hear, smell, taste, touch and perceive vibrates. Each sub-atom, atom, molecule, cell, tissue, organ, bone and body system produces sounds and vibrates. Vibrations produce sounds and sounds at high frequencies produce light.

The **macrocosmic and microcosmic universe** are constantly in a vibrational state, humans are constantly producing sounds and vibrations, and all elements on Earth are constantly producing sounds and vibrations.

Skeletal system	Muscular system	Circulatory system	Digestive system	Urinary system

Nervous system	Reproductive system	Lymphatic system	Endocrine system	Respiratory system

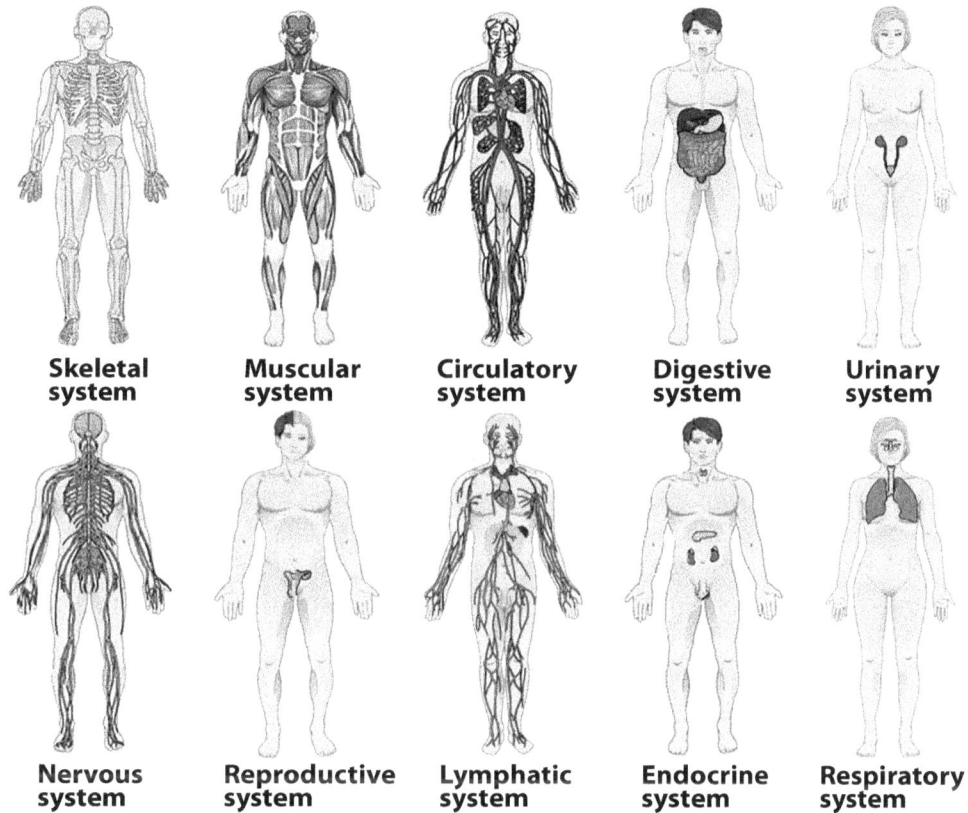

Diagram of the 10 essential systems of the human body.

It has been purported that humans were created by the power of sound and thus can produce sound using breath. Breath and air are the active forces of life and spirit. Breath and air is the prana, chi or qi energy of life.

The mind and heart's powerful energy, move oxygen through the lungs, and throat, which creates movement of the vocal cords and tongue, and the power of words is expressed: sounds have the power to alter the atomic structure of matter.

Earth, Water, Air and Fire

The four elements that give form and life to our planet, and which nurture and protect our bodies, survival and expression, are **Earth, Water, Air and Fire**. These elements are in a constant state of vibration and are continuously producing sound frequencies. They shape all life energy on Earth and nothing can exist without these elements, nor could anything exist without producing sound frequencies.

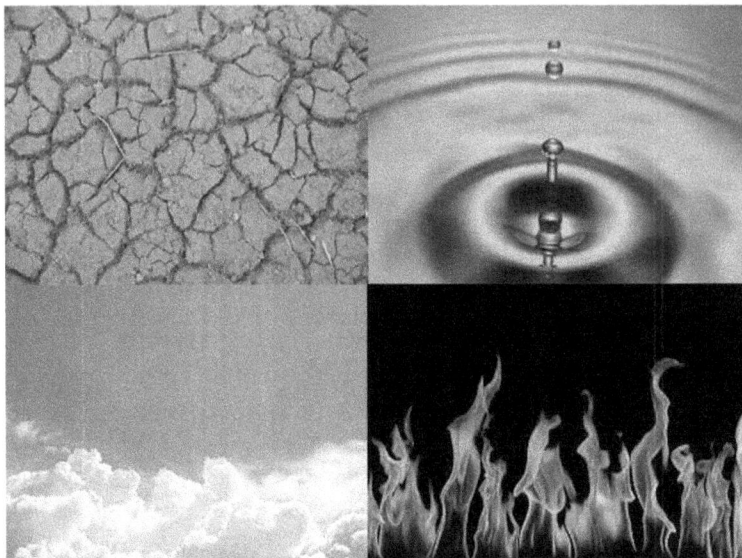

The four basic elements that give form and life.

Earth is anchored and tuned to a person's **physical body.**

Water receives, tunes and affects a person's **emotional body.** The emotional body fuels energy that is in motion. The throat and solar plexus are areas of the physical body that are stimulated by the emotional body.

We know that sound frequencies travel 4 to 5 times faster through water than air. Water is a liquid crystal superconductor of light and sound, and has the capacity to store memory. Water can be compared to a tape that records vibrational frequencies of sounds and videos. We can talk to water before drinking it and impregnate it with frequencies of creative love, gratitude, perfect health and divine order. When you drink water that has been programmed with powerful words, the opening of the heart chakra is stimulated and diffuses positive frequencies throughout the body's trillions of cells to activate the human capacity to achieve good health and spiritual transformation.

Air/Ether receives, tunes and affects a person's **mental body.** The mental body contains the seeds that give rise to thought.

Fire or Cosmic Fire receives, tunes and affects a person's **ethereal body**; the person's

being and soul.

Every sub-atom, atom, molecule and cell within the human body is a capacitor that stores memory, personal remembrances and vibrational energy patterns. Every feeling and thought stimulates the endocrine glands to secrete biochemical substances; the glands then emit vibratory frequencies and generate sounds that reflect the state of consciousness of the person, which will then manifest in health or disease.

The four elements are an integral part of the human body and promote self-realization and the evolutionary rise of human consciousness from a material plane to a spiritual plane. The four elements give rise to the creation of matter, because they originate from a creative power or universal intelligence, and are in a constant state of vibration, producing sounds.

8
Thoth

Thoth, the creation of the Universe, the mythological secret of the pyramid and its resonant tones

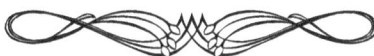

Thoth and the Creation of the Universe

In Egyptian mythology Thoth means **Father of Wisdom.** His Egyptian name is Tehuti or Djehuti. Thoth is the **Great Master of the Mysteries of Atlantis,** Guardian of the Records, Mighty King, and Wizard, who has lived from generation to generation; creator of the **Halls of Amenti** and keeper of the mighty wisdom of the **great continent of Atlantis.** His famous literary work is known as the **"Emerald Tablets of Thoth - The Atlantean."** In his writings, Thoth presents his mythological conception of the origin of the **"Creation of the Universe."**

According to the mythology of Atlantis and Egypt, Thoth designed and created the universe through the power of the word. Thoth spoke and thus, by the verb, began the sound that put a plan into motion, which led to the creation and structure of the universe. The powerful frequency echoed through time and space in the universe, and gave rise to all that exists. The great plan of creation was developed in the essence and mind of God. **The power of the verb, the word, and sound preceded light and is what truly led to the creation of the universe.**

According to ancient mythology Thoth worked directly with the creation of the universe and the creation of Earth. This was part of the great plan that took place under Ma'at as the presiding deity.

The universe was conceived as a holographic frequency. We understand the concept of frequency bands from radio waves and other communication technology systems. Other levels of existence can penetrate into our dimension easily through physical mechanisms that are created by frequency waves.

Although we cannot measure the essence of spirit, life, emotions and mind, such essences are present and can be recorded by multiple vibrational wave frequencies that generate sounds. Scientists do not attempt to explain this, but psychologists, theologians and mystics believe that there is something that goes beyond what is physically accessible through our senses.

This all coincides with the mythological context of creation as described by Thoth. The configuration of creation is symbolized by four elements and these elements represent various forms of behavior and levels of mind, of being and other mystical and religious aspects.

In essence, Nut-Nut represents the first element, the **physical plane**. Nut's body is the vehicle that created the physical universe. Hehut and Hehu represents the element of **fire** or cause, the plane by which an idea is first visualized and is manifested through the power of intention or disposition. Kekiu and Kekiut represent the element of **water** which is what we call the etheric plane or astral plane, where emotions and spirit meet and move through our being. Finally Kerh and Kerhet represent the element of **air** or thought, through which things are decreed and enabled. Through these elements, which are also part of our own being, each one of us is involved in the development, expansion and creation of the universe.

Egyptian legends mention Thoth as the father of wisdom and teacher of masters in the Atlantic continent and Egypt. He is known today in the hermetic philosophy as Hermes Trismegistus. He is thought to have been an instructor of ancient prophets. All religions and philosophies have their origins in basic scientific principles and historical facts.

The Hermetic schools that originated in Atlantis and Egypt under the principles of Hermes Trismagistus, teach us that everything is based upon the principles of vibration. The universe is governed by the laws of vibration, frequencies and sound; and at all times the sounds and movement of the heavenly bodies across the galaxy generate the **"Music of the Spheres."** Each star (i.e., suns, planets, moons and celestial bodies) in the galaxy has its own vibratory frequency and generates a specific sound at a macro cosmic level. At the microcosmic level, every living being on Earth has its own vibratory frequency and generates sound.

The mythological secret of the vibratory frequency generated by the pyramid and its relationship to the five elements

It was believed by some that on the continent of Atlantis, and later on in the Egyptian empire, architects and engineers incorporated sacred geometry to construct pyramids, temples, buildings and palaces. One of the most powerful buildings in our world is **The Great Pyramid of Cheops,** which was built in direct alignment with the stars of the cosmos. Its builders incorporated the principles by which the natural elements shape life on Earth, using the proportional sacred formula of Phi.

The secret of the pyramid is related to the four corners at the base and the fifth point at the top, which is the center of the pyramid and is known in Egypt as the **"Center of Creation."** The five points of the pyramid are related to the elements. These are:

First Element = **Earth (Ta)** = Symbolized by the color Green
Second Element = **Water (Mu)** = Symbolized by the color Blue
Third Element = **Air (Nefu)** = Symbolized by the color Yellow
Fourth Element = **Fire (Set)** = Symbolized by the color Red
Fifth Element = **(Hu)** = Creative Power of Being
The Fifth Element is **The Supreme Being**. It comes from Atum, which means **life.**

In the initiation within the Great Pyramid of Giza the combination of the four words represent the four elements plus the fifth element. When pronounced in the ancient Egyptian language, the words create **TA-MU-NEFU-SET-HU.**

TA-MU-NEFU-SET-HU that was and is the **powerful mantra** given to the pharaohs and those beings who were and are chosen to be initiated into the Great Pyramid of Cheops under the brotherhood of Tehuti or Thoth. This initiation activated great powers and enlightenment to the initiates. The vibrational frequency that is produced by this mantra creates a powerful sound that activates the power of the 5 elements, elevating a higher mental state of consciousness, activating powers beyond the 5 senses, and activating the powers of mind over matter.

The top of the pyramid (the capstone) emits energy that creates a vertical column of double helix frequency waves in spiral form. These waves are generated by the four sides of the pyramid and create a vortex of high frequency vibrational energy. This high frequency vibrational energy is the energy that powers the universe and is known as **Tachyon energy** and is defined as **NEH-EH** in ancient Egyptian language, meaning **eternity.**

Tachyon energy is the process by which the pyramid refocuses light into subatomic particles. **Tachyon energy** is defined in the American Heritage dictionary hypothetically as a **subatomic particle that travels faster than the speed of light.** The word Tachyon is derived from the root "tachy" meaning fast or accelerated. Tachymeter: comes from the Greek Takbu and Takbus.

When the pyramid is aligned with one side facing due North and the opposite side facing due South, the high amplitude of the piezoelectric limestone of the great pyramid creates an electromagnetic field around the structure. This electromagnetic field organizes the movement of the electrons as a **rotating toroid (doughnut).**

The length of the base of the great pyramid replicates the fundamental resonant tone created by its structure. Each side of the base of the pyramid has been calculated as approximately 748 feet (228 m), which creates a fundamental vibrational frequency of about 1.5 Hz when the pyramid is stimulated at a high amplitude.

The periodic pulsation of pyramids through resonance levels, creates a Fibonacci set of standing waves centered around a wavelength of 748 feet (228 m), delimited by the base of the pyramid. The angles of the standing waves which correspond exactly with the inclination of the faces of the pyramid are designed using the **Phi** of 51.85 degrees.

This base frequency of 1.5 Hz is defined as **tritalamic entrainment frequency.** This frequency pulsation attunes, unifies and synchronizes the functioning of the hypothalamus, pineal and pituitary glands. This frequency is the lowest frequency of Schumann resonance; therefore, the function of the pyramids can be, in fact, to change the terrestrial frequency, fluctuating around 7.3 Hz, to the 1.5 Hz tritalamic frequency.

In the center, or heart, of the Great Pyramid of Giza are openings or channels with 21 cm waves emanating from the pyramid's chambers, which point directly to the Belt of Orion in space. These openings are of great importance.

The great pyramid is a transmitting station for vibrational frequencies. We have obtained data to prove that the resonance frequency of the cavity opening into outer space is 1,420 GHz and this frequency coincides with the resonance frequency of hydrogen. The resonance frequency is amplified by a sophisticated technology inside the pyramid, and radiates great power by waves going across Earth's atmosphere to connect with the Belt of Orion.

The power of pyramids is activated when one side is aligned directly towards the

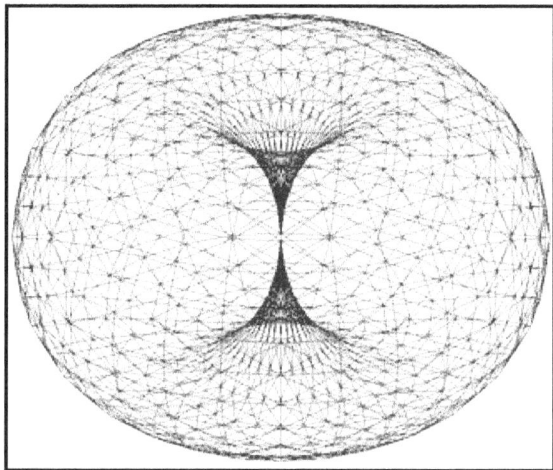

The motion of electrons in a toroid shape.

exact **Polar North** and the face at the opposite side to the **exact Polar South.** This activates **Tachyon energy** which is faster than the speed of light. Simultaneously, a high vibrational ionic frequency is activated, which influences the preservation of matter, prevents the breakdown of organic elements, balances the right and left hemispheres of the brain, energizes the pineal and pituitary glands, and calibrates the chakras. This process helps to stimulate the natural healing process of the body and mind, and occurs when a person is at rest or meditating within the powerful sacred geometric structure of the pyramid.

The high concentration of neutrinos and ionic energy which is generated by a pyramid's powerful energy field stimulates the natural process of healing in the human being at the cellular level. Energy waves are activated which decrease the colloidal precipitation of the cytoplasm of cells, thus preventing the oxidation and aging of the body. The system of energy waves generated by the pyramid activates high resonance pyramidal ions that resonate with biological and energetic systems in the body.

In the intercellular space where energetic transmission between cells takes place, permeability and exchange of sodium / potassium is activated. The molecules of water are activated with high vibrational pyramid frequencies resulting in the proper functioning of the cells and good health. This contributes to an increase in the cell's zeta potential and hence the body's natural healing process is activated.

The Resonant Tones of the Great Pyramid of Giza

Christopher Dunn has written a fascinating book called **"The Giza Power Plant."** The book is about Mr. Dunn's research on ancient Egyptian technologies that are hidden among the mysteries of the Great Pyramid of Giza. The book includes discoveries, studies and current research by Mr. Dunn. Mr. Dunn's acoustic analysis inside the king's chamber is fascinating and truly enlightening.

Subsequent experiments conducted by Tom Danley in the king's chamber of the Great

Pyramid of Giza, and in chambers above the king's chamber suggest that **the pyramid was built following an acoustic sound pattern.**

Danley identifies four frequencies inside the pyramid. He points out that certain notes are enhanced by the structure of the pyramid, and by the materials used in its construction. The sustained chord of F#, according to ancient Egyptian texts, forms part of the harmony of our planet. Danley's tests show that this note is present in the king's chamber even when no sound is produced.

The frequencies in the **king's chamber** range from **16 Hertz to 0.5 Hz.** However, these sounds cannot be perceived because they are well below the range of human hearing. According to Danley, these vibrations are caused by wind blowing across the ends of the shafts and openings of the pyramid, similar to when one blows across the top of a bottle.

It seems that the Great Pyramid of Giza was built with the principles of harmonic alignment in mind! The frequencies are sub-conical and go up to 0.5 Hz. Therefore, it follows that this harmoniously links the pyramid with the universe and Earth. However, this does not mean that all celestial bodies in the universe are tuned to **F#**. Each celestial body has its own specific frequency. Only the beginning – the first step of harmonic alignment – is absolute in the universe. **F#** is the chord resonance of Earth, and this is a fact inherent in the ancient wisdom of several cultures.

Mr. Sahi Hawass produced a video documentary about the Giza Plateau and the **theory of "Harmonic Creation"** which was used to construct the Great Pyramid of Giza. This video also addresses the four fundamental frequencies capable of generating **harmonic alignment.**

I have researched sound effects that stimulate the natural process of healing, and have noticed that when I tone vowel sounds such as AUM, EUM, IUM, OUM, in UUM diatonic harmony chords inside a pyramid, or with a pyramid placed on my head, I achieve a high sense of relaxation mentally and physically. This makes it possible and easier for me to arrive at the mental state of Alpha (8 Hz to 14 Hz).

When I am using the pyramid I feel that some areas in my brain are stimulated and trigger and enhance higher mental powers of perception, focus and concentration. The high power of perception that is achieved using the pyramid also produces an effect that creates an internal amplification of the volume of the sounds being vocalized and an amplification of perception in all the senses.

I experience similar effects using the pyramid when I vocalize Tibetan or Vedic Sanskrit mantras, and Latin prayers, and when I pray and make statements aloud while using different chords in the diatonic harmony.

I have experimented with vowel sounds and Vedic Sanskrit mantras along with pyramids when I have had stress, muscle tension or strain in the central nervous system. My success in eliminating tension, stress and pain through this practice is fascinating.

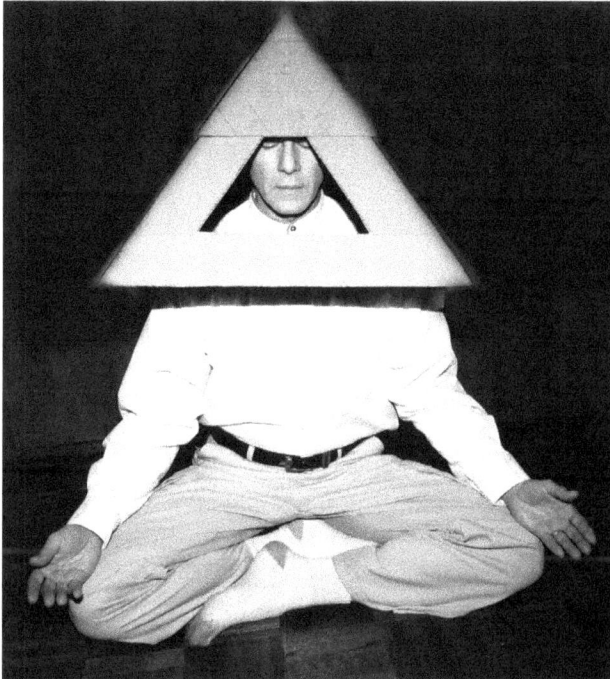

The therapeutic effects of the harmonic vowel sounds and of Vedic and Sanskrit mantras inside the pyramid.

The sacred geometry pyramid power, in combination with the power of vowel sounds and Sanskrit Vedic mantras, generates a powerful electromagnetic energy. This energy can balance and regenerate a particular area by amplifying the resonance of the harmonic sounds and vibrations, which releases energy blockages from the central nervous system, organs, tissues and meridians of the body.

Using a pyramid generates a vibrational frequency which synchronizes pulses from the hypothalamus, the pineal gland and pituitary gland, and triggers a unified functioning. By using powerful vowel sounds in diatonic harmonies, Vedic Sanskrit mantras, and a pyramid, the mind and body can fully regenerate and heal.

9

Books of Antiquity and Spiritual Beliefs in the Power of Sound

Ancient books which deal with the power of sound, harmonic sounds and the principle of resonance

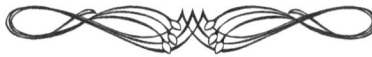

What are the spiritual beliefs that have been written in the ancient books about sound?

The Bible (Genesis): The first book of Moses. The Old Testament. God spoke and said, "Let there be light!" and light was manifested.

The Bible (New Testament): John 1: In the beginning was the Word (Word is sound) and the Word was with God, and the Word was God.

The Vedas (sacred book of India): In the beginning was Brahman which was the word and the word is Brahman.

The Tradition of the Hopi (old Native American Culture): The spider woman singing the song of creation gave life to all inanimate things on the planet.

The Popul Vuh (Sacred book of the Maya): The first real man and woman were created, absolutely, through the power of sound.

Ancient Egypt: The history of Thoth (Father of the wisdom of Egyptian mythology,) who gave names to objects and turned them into living beings. Thoth by speaking the verb, through the sound, began to put in motion the plan that would give rise to the creation and the structure of the universe.

In Polynesia: The gods blew the conch, the sound came and life was created.

China and Eastern Cultures: divine beings sounded the giant gong and life originated.

The religions, spiritual paths and traditions of different cultures came to the same conclusion that **the creation and manifestation of the existence of life on Earth came through a primordial sound.**

The light was created with seven basic colors from which thousands of combinations were further created. The stunning beauty of the energy of light was preceded by sound. The seven musical notes are the basic numbers that compose musical harmony, and the number seven appears in many evolutionary processes of this dimension.

Scientific studies have shown that frequencies of waves created by sound have direct effects on the human body, and may produce changes at the physical level in the autonomic, immune, endocrine and nervous systems.

The vibrations of harmonic sounds have the power to alter the atomic structure of matter and also contribute to stimulate the acceleration of the natural process of healing of body, mind and spirit.

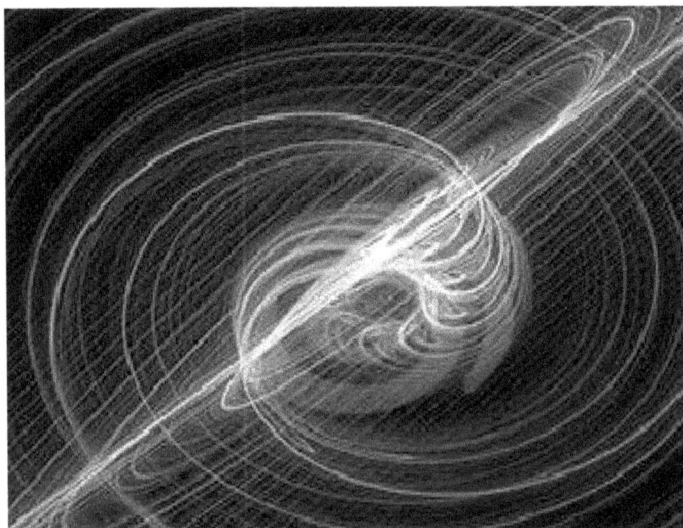

Illustration of vibrational waves of sounds.

Conversely, non-harmonic sound vibrations have negative effects on our body, creating imbalances in the nervous, endocrine and immune systems as well as in other body systems, at a cellular level.

The noise that occurs in cities produces negative sound frequencies which may induce stress and affect the body's health at the cellular level. This includes the sounds and sirens of police cars, and fire department vehicles, car alarms and loudspeakers, etc

Sound is Vibration and Vibration is Energy

The human body operates using vibrational energy. The body's cells respond to the vibrational energy produced by sound. The sounds and vibrations affect DNA and, therefore, the physiological structure of our bodies and consciousness. Sound can influence the body's respiration rate, skin temperature, and blood pressure. It also has a direct effect over the five mental states of Beta, Alpha, Theta, Delta and Gamma brainwaves. Harmonic sound is used to promote homeostasis, that is, to encourage good health.

The Principle of Resonance

Matter is organized in the form of waves and frequencies. For example, if we have two sound instruments like tuning forks, or two crystal bowls vibrating at the same musical note, when one begins to vibrate the other is automatically stimulated and starts to vibrate. This natural effect occurs because the two instruments have the same musical tone and frequency. This is defined as the principle of the law of resonance.

Resonance may be the most important principle in healing through sound. In the context of healing humans or animals, we can direct a specific frequency of vibration that is most natural to any of the body's systems (i.e., the heart, liver, lungs and other organs.) The specific and innate frequency of each organ system is targeted as its main resonant frequency.

All cells emit sounds as a result of metabolic processes. There is an interaction between the sounds of each cell, the sounds emitted by the environment, and the sounds produced by the instruments of healing. The principle of resonance refers to the cellular uptake of harmonic sounds that activate the healing process.

In curing by sound, resonance principles are used for the reharmonizing of cells that have been (hypothetically) imprinted with disturbing frequencies. The damage to cells that have been affected by disharmonic frequencies may be due to toxic substances, emotional trauma, pathogens, and/or long term exposure to noise pollution produced by ambulances, police cars, the low frequency sounds produced by cell phones, radars, microwave ovens and other utensils, etc.

Resonance is a basic principle that has an effect on matter and humans. The use of this principle applies to those who need physical healing, emotional and mental transformation. The correct frequency allows the organ or system of the body to recall its original existence, so that it may return to its proper energy field and gene code, and lead to a harmonization of its proper function.

Another example of the effect of the law of resonance may occur in the presence of people expressing joy. Their energy can make us resonate together with them on the same frequency of joy and happiness. This principle is true in positive moments and negative moments.

10

Sacred Geometry and Sounds

Sacred geometry, the healing of the cells in the human body systems through sound and resonance

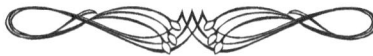

The relationship of sacred geometry and frequencies of sounds

The energy that is produced by the frequencies of sounds is based on **Sacred Geometry** and is encoded in minerals, vitamins, herbs, rare gases, amino acids, hormones, etc. These frequencies harmonize and calibrate physical, emotional, mental and spiritual bodies.

Example: All herbal supplements, vitamins and pharmaceutical drugs have particular given frequencies, a frequency signature. When we swallow an herbal tincture, vitamin, or pharmaceutical drug, the frequency encoded in the capsule or pill stimulates the area of the body that needs to be healed. Therefore, the original frequency of the tissue or organ is stimulated as it was when it was healthy. The frequency broadcasted in the pill or capsule stimulates the activation of the healing process.

How is sound capable of activating the healing process in the cells?

Ionic channels are located within cell membranes, through which the cell receives nourishment and communicates with neighboring cells. Cells become dysfunctional if some of their vital ion channels become closed, which causes cell aging or cell inactivation. The cell is literally dormant, or asleep. In theory, the vibrational frequencies produced by harmonic sounds stimulate the closed channels of cell membranes and these channels re-open, helping the cell to wake up, so that the normal operation and reproduction of the cell can resume.

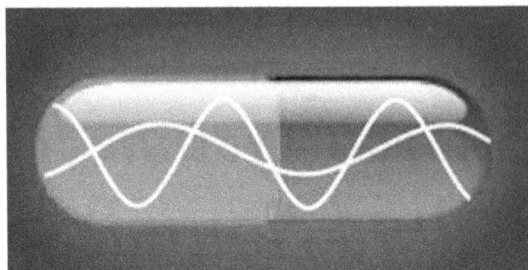

Illustration of a capsule with frequency waves inside.

Dr. James Gimzewski, from The University of California, (UCLA) adopted a revolutionary approach for the study of cellular function. He uses an atomic force microscope and a kind of high-sensitivity microphone to hear the sounds emitted or produced by the cells.

The focus of this new science called "Sonocytology" uses a method that can detect pulsations of the cell's outer membrane, and thus, the "song" or sound produced by the cell is identified. The work of Dr. Gimzewski has revealed that every cell in our body has a unique acoustic signature and sings to its neighboring cells.

Sonocytology is a potentially powerful diagnostic tool that can be used to identify the sound signatures produced by healthy cells, and also the sounds produced by diseased cells.

Dr. Gimzewski introduces an even more interesting prospective: the possibility of using the destructive sounds of diseased cells to implode and destroy diseased cells. In this scenario, no collateral damage to the surrounding tissue would happen, because healthy cells do not resonate with the frequencies produced by diseased cells.

Dr. Gimzewski won the Nobel Prize. His innovative mind led him to accomplish extraordinary work, where he shares a vision of creating new modalities through audible sound, which opens great potential for helping heal the body with noninvasive methods.

In the coming years we will probably see different types of diagnostic and therapeutic methods by means of harmonic sounds and vibrational frequencies that resemble scenes from the infirmary of the futuristic television series Star Trek. No doubt we will see a proliferation of healing modalities of harmonic sound frequencies that will lay the foundation for a new science that will be known as Vibrational Medicine. All this may be due to the Laws of Creation, where harmonic sound has the power to heal naturally.

The spine, bones, and biological systems of the human body are capable of resonance.

The spine, bones, organs and biological systems of the human body are constantly working, vibrating, producing sound frequencies and can resonate to different musical tones in the diatonic harmony (C, D, E, F, G, A, B.)

In Vibrational Medicine the human spine is compared to a xylophone, in view of the fact that each vertebra (and each organ) has the ability to resonate to a different musical note in the diatonic harmony.

Our spine, like our bones, has the ability to convert the vibrational energy in a way that generates an electromagnetic field. Dr. Valerie V. Hunt, pioneer in studies of bioenergy, emeritus research professor of physiological sciences and human energy fields at the Los Angeles University of California (UCLA), has found that all cells and even sub-atomic particles, contain small electrical elements.

Our bone structure has piezoelectric properties, which means that an electromagnetic pulse can be created in the surrounding field. Bones are capable of converting vibrational energy, such as light and sound, to electromagnetic energy and can create a link between cells, organs and bones to the periphery of our electromagnetic field.

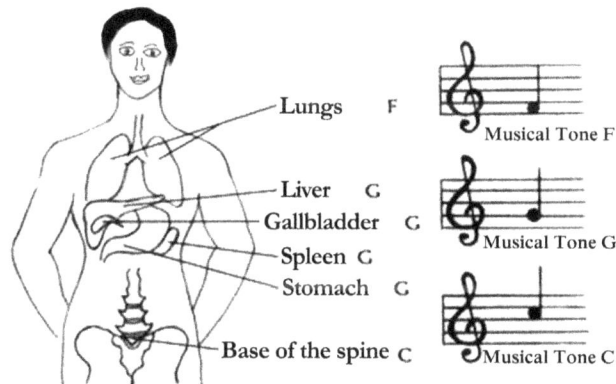

Lungs F — Musical Tone F
Liver G
Gallbladder G — Musical Tone G
Spleen G
Stomach G
Base of the spine C — Musical Tone C

The spine is like a living xylophone. The xylophone is a musical percussion instrument.

The heart, thymus and lungs are capable of resonance with the musical tone F.

The stomach, gallbladder, liver and spleen are capable of resonance with the musical tone G.

The base of the spine is capable of resonance with the musical tone C.

Sacred Geometry and Synchronization with Brain Waves

Sacred geometry is supposed to allow humans to explore new modes of perception, providing information on scientific, psychological, philosophical and mystical aspects of the universe. The physical world is made of sub-atoms, atoms and molecules which vibrate, make sounds and are governed by designs having geometric relationships. Ancient civilizations used universal principles in the design of temples and religious monuments, and incorporated sacred geometry in their buildings. Sacred geometry is related to the vibrations of atoms, its frequency and its motion in space.

Thoughts, feelings and emotions of humans correspond to brainwave patterns, and sacred geometry provides the means to develop methods to help orchestrate these brainwaves. The astrophysical parameters of Earth correspond to the alpha brainwave frequencies, and to frequencies and wavelengths of sound and light.

Modern science has revealed that geometric rhythms are present in the center of atomic structures. For example: Cymatics, the science of how sound waves physically create geometric patterns, has enabled the production of impressive sacred geometric shapes. Some of those geometric shapes are the flower of life, binaural rhythms, monoaural and isochronous tones that are implanted in the brain waves to produce different states and to generate a vibratory resonance in the body and mind.

Effects of Architecture that Incorporate Sacred Geometric Principles

Shape and symmetry influence the thoughts and feelings of human beings. Some examples are seen in the architecture of pyramids, shrines, temples, and cathedrals, along with yoga positions (asanas.) The sacred geometric shapes transmit frequencies that resonate with the genetic code of the original DNA of humans. An example is The Great Pyramid of Giza, whose inclination of about 51.49° refers to an unusual heptagon that is associated with sound, wisdom and the unknown, and is known as The Geometry of the Soul.

Platonic Solids, Sacred Geometry and the relationship with the universe, music and the human body

Plato discovered the **"platonic solids."** He believed that music has a powerful influence on the lives of all beings. In his treatise Temaeus, he describes the numerical creation of the physical universe, its relation to music with vibrations, and its effect on living beings. He urged his students to activate the ancient temples and sacred shrines of the land with sacred chants, using **"perpetual choruses"** to make these songs echo with the harmonies of the Celestial Choirs.

The term **"sacred geometry"** is used by archeologists, anthropologists and geometers to encompass the religious, philosophical and spiritual beliefs that have arisen around geometry in various cultures during the course of human history. Sacred geometry implies sacred universal patterns used in the design of sacred architecture and sacred art. The basic belief is that there is a harmonious relationship between geometry and mathematics, in proportion to musical chords, with light and cosmology. Sacred geometry is present in prehistory and physically in the elements, animals, plants and minerals.

Sacred Geometry was used by masters, architects and engineers of ancient civilizations about four-thousand five-hundred years ago; Their masterpieces were captured in the Pyramids and Temples in Egypt, buildings and monuments of the Sumerians, the mausoleums and Pyramids of Xi'an in China, and the Mayan Pyramids Chichen Itza, Uxmal, Teotihuacan, Ek Balam and others in Mexico. Other examples, included the Petén Pyramid (El Mirador) in Guatemala, and old European megalithic structures. Sacred Geometry continues to be used in modern buildings in the 21st century.

The Greeks also taught that five solids were the central patterns of physical creation. They associated four solids with the archetype of the elements earth, water, air and fire, and the fifth element was associated with ether which represented the vital force. Similar to the Egyptians in their initiation ceremonies of Pharaohs and Priests in the Great Pyramid of Cheops, they associated the four elements **(Ta)** Earth, **(Mu)** Water, **(Nefu)** Air, **(Set)** Fire and the fifth element **(Hu)** Ether, the creative and vital force of being. The four corners that form the square of the base of a pyramid are represented by the four elements Earth, Water, Fire, Air, and the top of the pyramid is represented by Ether. In their sacred initiations, they used a powerful mantra that was associated with the 5 elements **(Ta-Mu-Nefu-Set-Hu)**. In Scotland, there are also prehistoric Petrohilos or icons carved with platonic solids, that are estimated to go back more than a thousand years before the Greeks. Scientists have analyzed the five solids, the proton and neutron arrangements and the possible relationship with the elements of the periodic table.

The theory of **"The Music of the Spheres or Harmony of the Spheres"** was proposed by Plato 347 AD, and was followed by Pythagoras. Both shared the idea and belief that the secrets of the universe are expressed through numbers, mathematics and their close relationship with the **Five Platonic Solids.** They imagined the five perfect solids through **"Imaginary Spheres"** each placed inside the other. They proposed that each of the spheres surrounding each of the solids represented the distance from the sun and the planets and that they produce unique vibrations and sounds which they called **"The Music of the Spheres or Harmony of the Spheres."** Modern science has shown that Plato's and Pythagoras's proposition is true and scientifically valid.

The five Platonic solids comprise the alchemical elements and the Creation. They are represented as follows: (1) Tetrahedron **(Fire)**, (2) Cube **(Earth)**, (3) Octahedron **(Air)**, (4) Dodecahedron **(Ether)**, (5) Icosahedron **(Water)**.

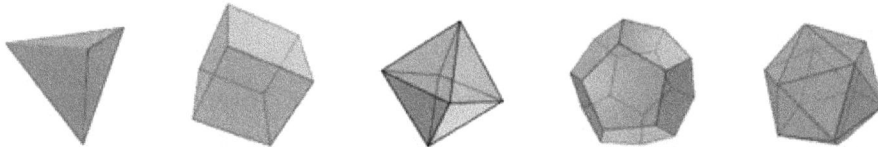

The five Platonic solids: tetrahedron, hexahedron, octahedron, dodecahedron and icosahedron

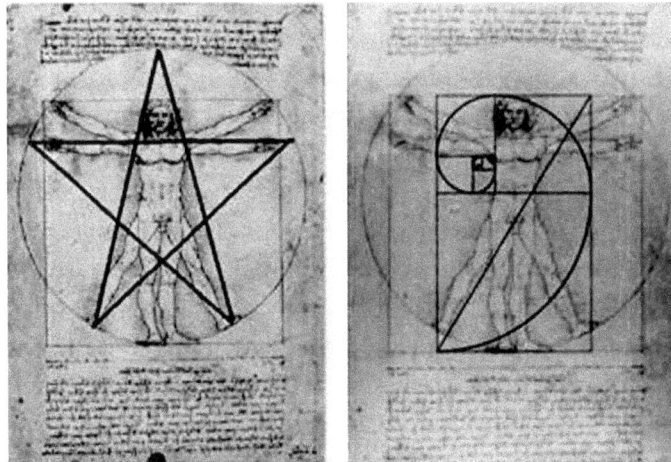

Pentagonal Human Body's Proportion & Human Body Golden Ratio Proportion

In addition to the five platonic solids and **five basic elements corresponding to solids and life;** the human race may be united in the same basic sacred proportions. In Leonardo da Vinci's drawings the physical body is presented with arms and legs extended forming a pentagonal figure, the fifth point is in the upper part of the head, and the reproductive organs correspond to the exact center. Each of these points refers to the number five:

five fingers on the hands of each arm, five toes on the foot of each leg, and five openings on the face. In addition, each of us possesses five senses of physical perception.

The proportions of the **"Golden Ratio"** of the cosmos and our bodies are closely aligned with **"The Music Harmony of Fifth."** The divine proportion of the Macrocosmic Universe of the stars and planets, and of the Microcosmic universe of the human body are vibrating in a harmonious perfection in the same frequencies and geometric proportions.

The chords or intervals of 5 notes (fifth) found in most sacred music and in **Gregorian chants** have a powerful harmonizing effect on the human energy system. They are also used in new age music and I use some of these chords in the music CD **"The Healing Forces of Harmonic Sounds and Vibrations."**

The famous German poet, playwright, novelist, scientist, theater director and artist Wolfgang von Goethe said **"Music is liquid architecture and architecture is frozen music".** He could see the connection and effect between music, geometry, architecture of buildings and the relationship with the natural architecture of the physiognomy of the human body. **Pythagoras** was the first to describe the **5-note chord interval (fifth)**, which is recognized worldwide for its harmonic beauty and because it demonstrates the relationship of the microcosms with the macrocosms and how the universe works.

I made a recording in the **Queen and the King Chambers of the Great Pyramid of Cheops in Egypt.** I have also experimented making sounds and harmonic songs in other grand places including the temple of the **Hathors in Denedera, the Isis Temple in Philea, Aswan and the Sekhmet Temple in Karnak in Egypt.** I have experienced and observed how the frequencies of sounds amplify, and through majestic echoes expand and spread within those spaces, travel and return to penetrate inside the body. The effect that it produces within the body is wonderful, activating a state of peace and serenity as if one were floating inside the building space but in another dimension. Each body fiber vibrates in harmony with the frequency that is encoded on the walls, columns and roofs of the temples and buildings. In some photographs of me, plasma circumferences have appeared floating in the air within the space of the buildings.

11

Vibrational Medicine and the Origin of Diseases

Vibrational medicine, the origin of diseases, and the six bodies of human beings

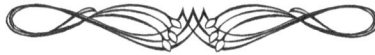

Vibrational medicine and the origin of diseases

Vibrational medicine is based on the theory that diseases are the result of blockages in the meridians, tissues, organs and body systems that do not allow life energy Chi, Prana or Vital Force to flow freely and efficiently. When an organ of the body is sick, the organ no longer vibrates in its original resonance and frequency.

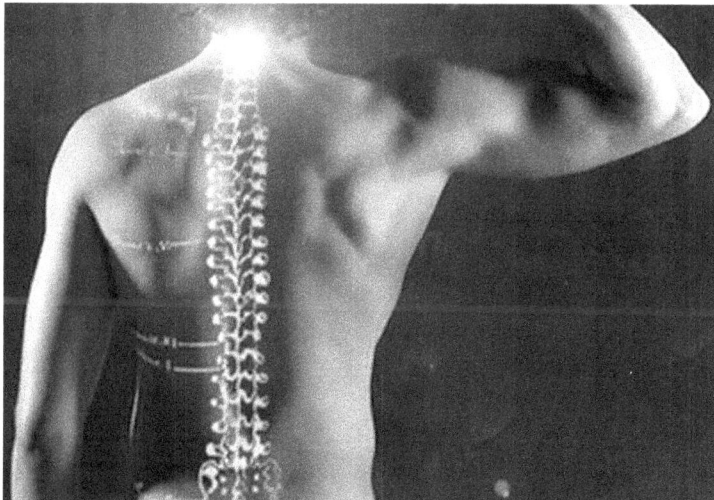

A Blockage in the central nervous system at the cervical area, which interrupts the flow of chi energy to the meridians of the human body.

When blockages exist in the meridians and the central nervous system, organs do not receive efficient vibrational frequencies. This can cause an imbalance in the rotating energy centers of the body, known as chakras and can cause disease.

Instead of using pharmaceuticals, chemicals or surgically removing organs, **the use of specific harmonic sound frequencies can stimulate the affected tissues and organs,** which can return them to their original, healthy frequencies.

The Healing Forces of Harmonic Sounds and Vibrations is a therapy that helps to stimulate the natural healing process of the body, mind and spirit. The use of sounds, musical tones and frequencies, produces specific vibrations that restore harmony to the chakras. Each energy center of the body, better known as the chakras, vibrates in its particular musical tone. **The Healing Forces of Harmonic Sounds and Vibration**s helps to harmonize the life force energy of the etheric body, the aura and the physical body.

We are not just physical beings, we are electromagnetic beings

We have to think that we are not just physical beings but that we are electromagnetic beings, with an electromagnetic vibrational energy field that is in constant interaction with our environment, in a way that goes beyond the perception of our five senses.

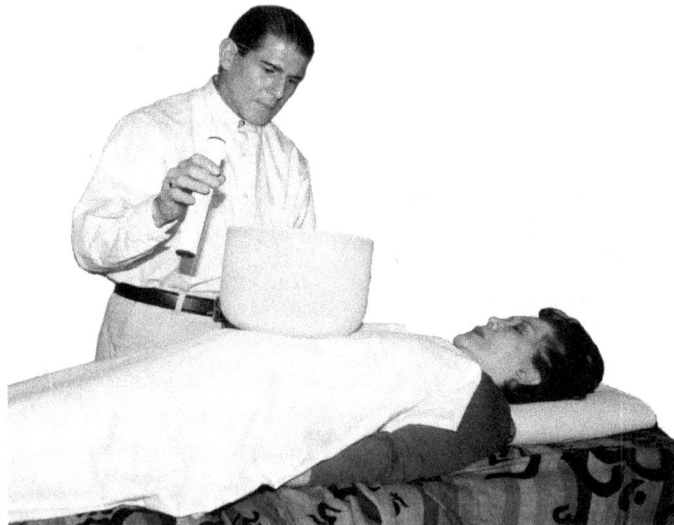

The bodies of living beings are surrounded by electromagnetic energy fields (holographic body and auric body.) The energy is produced through biochemical reactions that are metabolized by internal systems, and those vibrational frequencies have an emotional origin.

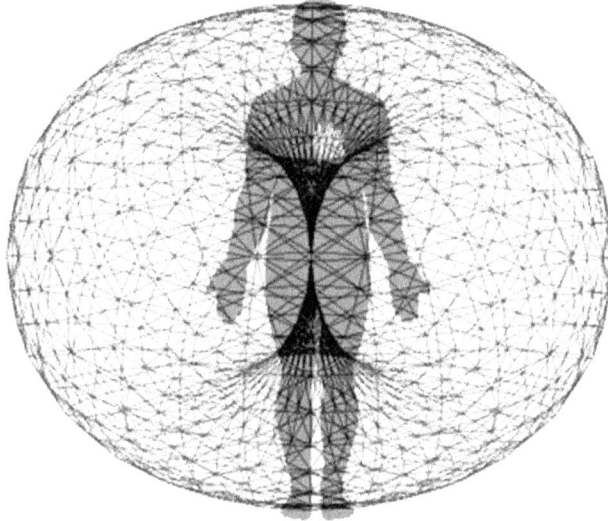

Illustration of the electromagnetic and energetic body of human beings and the human body to-roidal energy field generated by the heart.

Science has not elucidated with certainty the origin of life, but it has been able to conclude that the physical, mental and emotional state of living beings directly influences the electromagnetic energy fields (holographic body and auric body) that are generated around the body.

Human beings have basically six (6) bodies: The six bodies in humans are in the same space and time, but are in different vibrational frequency levels.

1) The Astral Body is the energy source that drives human feelings and emotions. In dreams we usually travel in our astral body. The astral body can also be invaded by thoughts from others.

2) The Holographic Body extends out of the physical body usually 9 -10 feet in an average person; however, the holographic body of spiritual teachers, monks and saints usually goes beyond 10 feet in length.

3) The Auric Body extends outward from the body from 2 - 4 to 12 inches. This differs for each person.

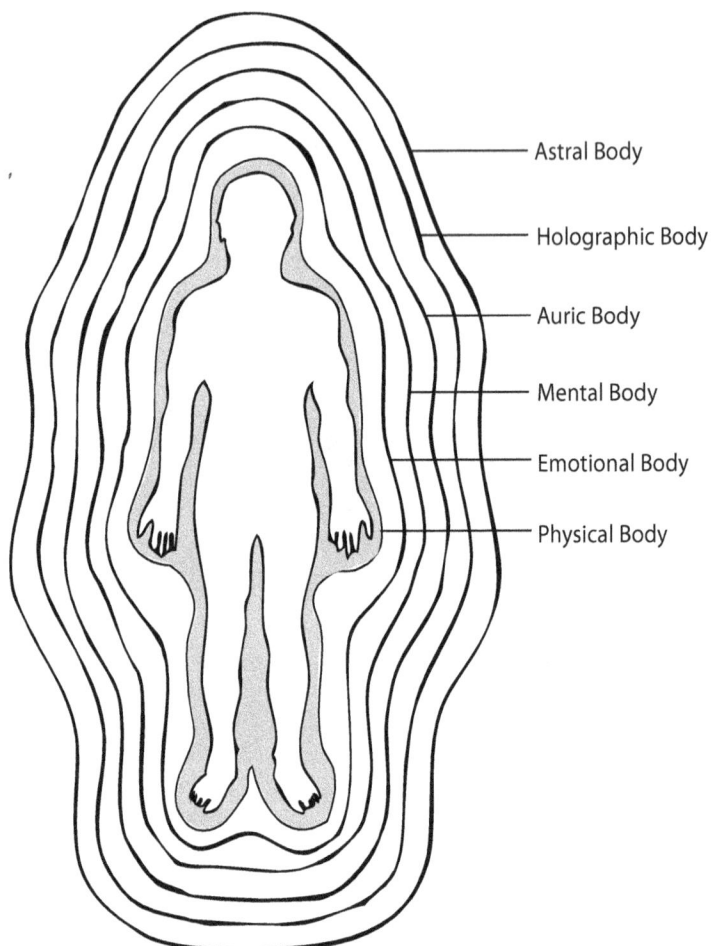

4) The Mental Body is the spiritual body. It is more subtle than the astral body. The mind is what moves the entire being, and is where thoughts originate.

5) The Emotional Body is located in an area of the mind where emotions are expressed as feelings.

6) The Physical Body is the densest frequency which allows our movement, in the material plane, going, coming back, playing and interacting with everything that has to do with the five senses.

In conclusion, the astral, holographic, auric, mental, emotional and physical bodies are constantly vibrating and producing sounds. It is imperative to note that in humans these bodies are in the same space and time, but at different vibratory frequencies.

The Healing Forces of Harmonic Sounds and Vibrations can have a powerful effect in balancing individuals' etheric, energetic, mental, emotional and physical bodies. It has been scientifically observed that the natural healing process is stimulated through specific harmonic sounds than can help a person obtain good mental, emotional and physical health.

Vibrational Medicine

Disease occurs when an individual's vibratory frequency has been altered by external or internal factors, or both. Vibrational medicine treats the cause of the imbalance by directing specific frequency tones that have resonance with the area of the body that is affected, so equilibrium can be restored.

Symptoms or diseases are not the cause of the problem, they are just effects. Vibrational medicine may be explained by the laws of quantum physics and the homeopathic principle of: "like cures like." (A similar vibrational frequency acts as a stimulus or medicine to the natural vital force response, giving it the encouragement it needs to complete its healing work.)

Today we are going through a revolution in medical systems. We are moving from a bygone era where most diseases were defined as "chemical imbalances," to an era of vibrational medicine, where natural forces are used to help reestablish the healing process of body, mind and spirit in a natural way.

Therapy through harmonic sounds and frequencies is one of the methods utilized. Homeopathy, music therapy and the use of modern technological equipment also provide specific frequencies to help stimulate natural healing responses in patients.

Many young doctors are aware of the benefits of vibrational medicine. They are becoming more receptive to exploring and implementing these forms of medicine, because they directly confront the origin of the disease and can correct imbalances in energy, frequency and vibration. Very similar to what Nikola Tesla said: "We live in an ocean of energy, frequency and vibration and we have to think in those terms."

12

The Law of Attraction

Thoughts generate vibrational frequencies and The Law of Attraction, thus the power of the mind can manifest its desires.

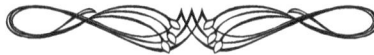

The Law of Attraction

We attract circumstances into our lives according to the vibrational energy generated by our minds. When we vibrate at a higher mental level we can attract positive health, happiness and great experiences. When we vibrate at a low, pessimistic and negative level the opposite can happen, and we can attract unpleasant experiences and disease.

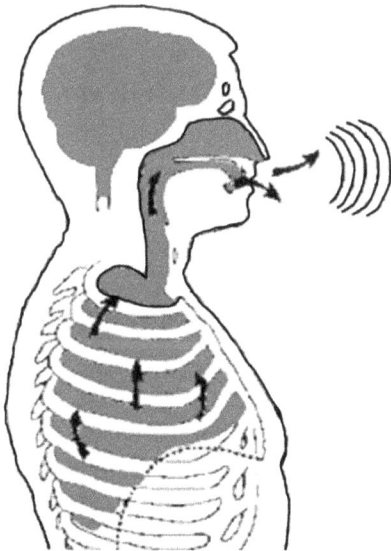

Illustration of the bio-mechanical process for the creation and expression of sound and the verb.

Thoughts Give Rise to Vibrational Frequencies and Sounds

When we generate a thought in our subconscious and conscious mind, we generate a vibrational frequency. When we talk about what we think, sound is produced. Speech is sound. Thoughts also generate sounds. Spoken sound emerges from unmanifested levels. Nothing can exist without sound.

In conclusion: everything that exists in the third dimension makes sounds.

The Origin of the Word at the Physical Level

At the moment we create a thought in the subconscious and conscious mind we bring forth a vibrational frequency that has not yet been physically manifested. The brain generates an electromagnetic energy pattern that moves through neural connections, traveling faster than the speed of light, from the subconscious to the conscious mind.

This process stimulates the left brain (objective, analytical, rational, logical, masculine,) the right brain (intuitive, feminine, holistic, subjective, transcendental,) and the cerebellum, at the same time that the vibrational frequency is traveling biochemically via the central nervous system. It activates the acetylcholine nicotinic receptors in neurons and stimulates the autonomic nervous system (sympathetic nervous system and the parasympathetic nervous system). Thus, the lungs inhale, the diaphragm expands and contracts, the air is expelled through the tubular conduit of the trachea all the way to the throat, the vocal cords vibrate, stimulate movements of the tongue and sound is expressed in words.

The sound that gives rise to the word is recorded at the DNA level in the individual's cellular memory and it is also recorded in the cellular memory of beings that hear that sound and word. Sound generates the word, and the word has the power to alter the atomic structure of matter.

That fascinating process takes place faster than the speed of light. It could be compared to the **Tachyon energy** that is generated by the pyramid, which also moves faster than the speed of light and in turn, is the energy that directly interacts with the universe.

In philosophical terms we could say that the mind is an integral part of the universe, and gives rise to thoughts and words which can create or destroy and also has the power to manifest.

The Power of Mind, Thoughts and Words

Thoughts and words generate a vibrational force. Loud sounds can affect the body's functioning at the cellular level, and in daily life.

Thoughts are vibrational frequencies that can manifest sickness or disease and can create or destroy. Only a positive thought can erase a negative thought. The power of the mind has no limits.

The subconscious and conscious mind generate vibrational frequencies that affect each sub-atom, atom, molecule, cell and DNA of one's body, and can also affect the person's energy field.

Modern science has acknowledged what ancient sages had been trying to teach us through spiritual teachings and sacred books. Words are the manifestation of our inner world. Words are the manifestation of our level of consciousness. By taking care of our language we can purify our inner world.

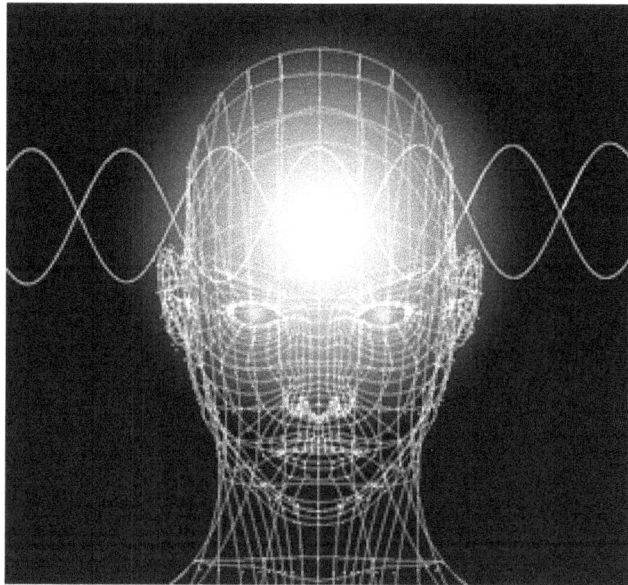

Illustration of the mind, the concept of the subconscious and the generation of vibrational frequencies which are produced by means of thoughts.

Watch your thoughts, for they become words. Watch your words, for they mark your destiny.

Words are alive, they bless or curse, encourage or discourage, create or destroy. One kind word can smooth things over. A joyous word may light up the day. A loving word may heal and give happiness.

Words can be powerful. Words can destroy what we have been building for a long time, or can manifest what we want to achieve. If our words are positive, constructive and creative, the echoes we hear will also be the same.

The Philosophy of the Buddha

The Buddha recognized the power and vibrational frequency generated by the mind thousands of years ago. Through his powerful philosophical messages and quotes, the Buddha taught that we become what we think and with our thoughts we can change the world.

All that we are is the result of our thoughts. Everything originates first in our mind. If a man speaks and acts with a pure thought, happiness will follow him like a shadow that never leaves. Since everything is a reflection of our thoughts, everything can be changed by our minds. Do not dwell in the past. Do not dream of the future. Concentrate the mind on the present moment.

Life is short. Time passes hastily. Discover your true nature. Purify your mind and heart to achieve happiness. Be kind, be merciful, be generous, do good. Concentrate, open yourself to the power of understanding, and wake up, be aware.

The Philosophy and Wisdom of the Buddha teaches us that man is a victim of his thoughts. Our minds create a powerful vibrational energy that gives rise to the creation of all things we desire to manifest in our life.

Messages written in the Bible and the teachings of Jesus of Nazareth, the Christ, concerning the Power of the Word

The Master of Teachers and central figure of Christianity, Jesus of Nazareth, the Christ, said the words we say are actually the overflow of our hearts "…for the mouth speaks from the fullness of our heart," see Matthew 12: 34-35. He never wrote about his teachings but his disciples wrote detailed accounts about his legacy in the New Testament of the Bible.

Words are more than sounds caused by air passing through our larynx. Words have real power. God spoke and thus activated the existence and creation of the world by the power of the Word. (Hebrews 11:03).

The power of our words can actually destroy one's spirit, arouse hatred and violence, and incite wounds. Humans are the only beings on this planet that have the ability to communicate through spoken words. The power of using words is a unique and powerful gift of our Universal Creator.

"Our words, despite being a gift, have the power to destroy, the power to build and create" (Proverbs 12:06). The writer of Proverbs tells us, "The tongue has the power of life and death, and those who love it will eat its fruit." (Proverbs 18:21) We use words to build or to destroy the people. Words can be full of hate or love, bitterness or blessing, complaints or compliments, lust or love, victory or defeat. In the same way that tools can be used to help us achieve our goals, words can cause us to spiral into a deep depression.

The apostle Paul wrote in Ephesians 4:29: "Let no evil word proceed from your mouth, but words that are good and useful for edification will impart blessing to those who hear them." In this passage, Paul is emphasizing the power of positive thinking, which can generate creative words. This is the opposite of negative thoughts which can generate destructive words.

"For in many things we all stumble. Anyone who does not offend in word, this one is a perfect man and able also to subdue his whole body" "Behold, we put bits into the mouths of horses that they may obey us and we turn around their whole body." (James 3: 2-3).

Romans 3:13, "Our words are filled with blessings when the heart is full of blessings." So if we fill our hearts with the love imparted by the Master Jesus Christ of Nazareth during his mission on Earth, only truth and purity can come out of our mouths.

Matthew 15: 11-20: "It is not what enters into the mouth which defiles a man; but what comes out of the heart and mouth; that is what defiles a man."

Jesus of Nazareth, who is considered the son of God by Christians, and Buddha, an enlightened being, were aware of **the ability of words to generate powerful sounds that can activate vibrational frequencies, wich alter the atomic structure of matter.** The Christ's mission was to raise humans' consciousness and awareness of the regenerative and creative power of love, which can stimulate our mind to originate the thoughts and words that create the harmonious sounds that impart grace, unity, balance and collective healing to all beings that listen to it.

Degenerative mental energy can affect the body and create emotional, physical and mental stress. Degenerative mental energy activates vibrational frequencies that disharmonize all systems of the body and disease originate.

Energy is Vibration – the Universe and our Minds have an Unlimited Supply of Vibrational Energy

One of the fundamental laws of physics is the conservation of energy. Energy is neither created nor destroyed. Energy generates vibrational frequencies that enable our minds and biophysical systems to perform many vital functions.

Energy fluctuations create vibrational frequencies that change all the time. We can consciously observe changes in the digestive system, respiratory system, and cardiovascular system when we exercise. However, we are often unaware that many of the changes that occur inside of us are caused by the complex process of the power of our mind, our thoughts, beliefs and words.

The energy generated by our thoughts can activate vibrational frequencies that ondulate and travel through the universe in all directions, similar to the waves that occur when a stone is cast into a lake.

The magnetism of our beliefs is based on the unlimited reserve of energy from the universe, which supplies us with the means to create many things in our life. Each one of us is here to learn the lesson of responsible co-creation.

Our thoughts and beliefs create and attract specific vibrational frequencies.

Some frequencies can be beneficial to our bodies and minds, while others may be harmful. Harmful frequencies limit, restrict and delay our evolutionary process. Thoughts are a tremendous vibratory energy force that can modulate and also affect all our affairs.

Our bodies are an extension of our thoughts, and maintain a vibrational frequency that is relative to the energy we generate through our minds. Both mind and body are in constant interaction with the energies and vibrational frequencies coming from the universe. Like an instrument in an orchestra, our thoughts and actions are but a small movements within a much larger body of vibrations.

In a state of optimal health a body's frequency, the vibrational energy of a person is clearer and it is in tune and in harmony with the energy of the universe. Such harmony and resonance operates as an electromagnetic field and the frequency remains clear and strong unless something disrupts the electromagnetic field. In this state one can live in good health, with vitality, energy, happiness and be open to new experiences.

Conversely a chaotic or sick mind is one that is not in harmony with the universe; the body of such a person will suffer from dissonance. It can be compared to a mistuned note that stands out above all other notes in a chorus that would otherwise be in perfect harmony. The mind that is not in tune with the universe or its surrounding environment, can suffer a state of vibrational shock. These vibrations form an energy field around the body that resonate through the cells, and cause them to vibrate.

When cells are vibrating from negative beliefs, the vibrational energy created by the negative beliefs outweighs the higher positive harmonic frequencies. Over time this can cause physical diseases, mental disorders, mood swings and personality changes.

The only way humans project and direct their energy is through their thoughts, beliefs and the thought structures they create. The thoughts that occur in our minds are not images that appear from nowhere and disappear into ether. Thoughts actually have real existence, they are an option as real as a rock, are chosen and accepted as true or false by our minds, and get recorded in the cellular memory of our DNA.

The thoughts that we accept lead to larger structures of thought called beliefs. These large structures are a more rigid form of the original idea, and in turn often lead into future thoughts that validate the initial theory.

Thus, our thoughts reveal much about the mental structures we have created in our lives. Every thought that we do not challenge will become an accepted belief. Accepted beliefs can conflict with other thoughts, or can complement and perhaps enhance our thinking process.

Thought directs emotions, and emotions generate vibrational frequencies in the same manner as thought. Each emotion emits its own unique, corresponding frequency. Now, we shall consider the frequency of love versus the frequency of fear.

Imagine thoughts of love as a vibrant sounds with clear, loud tones. These are sounds of creation and being. Our thoughts of love, acceptance, openness, empathy, unity and forgiveness are clear harmonic variations of the loud and clear sounds of life, that keep our bodies and minds in harmonic resonance with the universe.

On the contrary, emotions of fear are low, clumsy and confused sounds that collide with each other and produce dissonance. These vibrations do not fuse with life's vibrancy. These dissonances cause disruptions at many levels in the body and then cause the mind to suffer. A mind in such a state may think that this dissonance is desirable or inevitable and creates belief structures based on these thoughts. Thus, the mind becomes conditioned to vibrate with dissonance and reinforces chaos and fear.

Expectations are formed from thoughts and beliefs that are reinforced. Our thoughts have a **magnetic vibrational propensity** to attract events, people and situations that fit those thoughts. Thoughts of fear and death can attract terrible experiences that validate this type of thinking. That is the nature of creation, and is a fundamental precept that most of us have been taught to ignore and fear. The vibration of fear is instinctive for the preservation of life, but it can become a source of limitation. It has been used against us to enslave the mind. This is because fear is born of uncertainty and discord.

Our Thoughts Create Perception and Experience

Our thoughts create our own perceptions and experiences. We have been taught to distrust the mind and the power of intuition that expresses through our thoughts. This design has been perpetuated through the social elite that understands the nature of the power of thought and mind of human beings. Most of us have gone through mental programming from the fetal stage, during the nine months of gestation in the womb, through birth and throughout our lives.

Dr. Alfred Tomatis in his scientific studies showed that all sounds, vibrational frequencies and experiences that the mother is exposed to and experiences during pregnancy is amplified by the amniotic fluid that surrounds the fetus. These sounds are recorded in the cell memory of the baby's DNA because sound in water travels four to five times faster than in air.

We must also take into consideration that as we grow and evolve in the journey of life, communication systems such as television, radio, the press and other media, have been used to send vibrational frequencies that limit the development of the creative power of the mind and have manipulated the truth distorting the consciousness of unity.

Many systems have been used to activate frequencies of fear in people. Much of the fear in the world comes from lies, ignorance and guilt. This can stimulate the left side of the brain, causing individuals to become more analytical and only accept reality as what is perceived physically. Thus, the power of the right brain, which controls intuition, creativity and perception, is suppressed. The right brain can perceive what is beyond the physical.

Some educational and political systems, media commentators, television programs, press articles, and movies, frequently supply subliminal frequencies with violence, hostility, war and other topics that can induce fear. Because of this the frequency of fear is increasing worldwide. This can lead to a massive reaction of fear which can block people's creativity, induce negative thoughts, distrust, doubts, and promote separation among humans.

Advertising campaigns use techniques that incorporate rapidly changing colors, specific sounds, and accelerated and exaggerated movements in television commercials. These methods send subliminal messages which encourage viewers to consume the advertised products. Radio programs use the same methods in the commercials and news they broadcast, which fosters consumerism.

An effective way to counteract the frequency of fear, is to make changes in our lives. Affirmations, creative visualization, mantras, prayer, and meditation are beneficial. Harmonic vocal sounds in the diatonic harmony and the ancient solfeggio tones can also activate our natural healing power. Other ways to enrich our intellect include listening to harmonic sounds, classical music, Gregorian chants, harmonic music with constructive messages, listening or doing meditations with **The Healing Forces of Harmonic Sounds and Vibrations CD;** watching constructive documentaries, reading literature with positive content, and avoiding media programming and commercial tactics that influence people to become slaves of their programming systems.

The negative energy of fear generates vibrational frequencies that can cause depression, anxiety, stress, and imbalance of the body's organs and biological systems. In addition, environmental factors and unhealthy foods can also contribute to diseases.

Avoid giving your power to the negative frequencies of fear generated through the programming and communications systems that are promoted through television, radio and the press.

13

The Benefits of Harmonic Sounds

**Benefits of the healing forces of harmonic sounds and vibrations.
The intrinsic relationship between mind and heart**

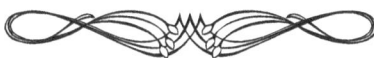

***

Benefits of The Healing Forces of Harmonic Sounds and Vibrations

The sound waves produced by **The Healing Forces of Harmonic Sounds and Vibrations,** pure quartz crystals bowls, silver bowls, Tibetan bowls, the human voice, the power of intention and creative visualization have beneficial effects for many conditions including organ imbalances, toxins in the body, anxiety, fear, depression, and insecurity. Using sound wave methods can help one establish a better sense of direction and gain mental clarity.

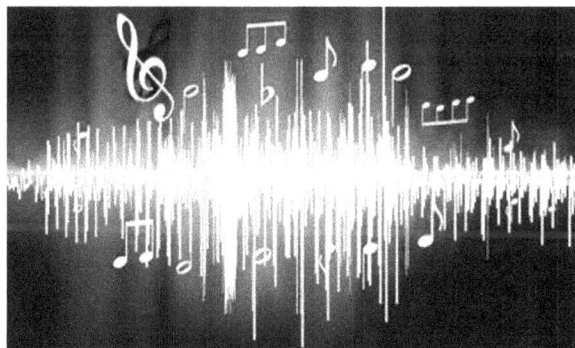

Ilustration of harmonic sounds and their vibrational frequency waves.

The Healing Forces of Harmonic Sounds and Vibrations stimulate individuals to advance in life by creating positive changes that increase the vibrational frequency of the mind and encourage the person to have a creative life.

Using affirmations, mantras and **The Healing Forces of Harmonic Sounds and Vibrations,** one can transform and restore a positive resonance of health and creativity in mind, body and spirit.

85

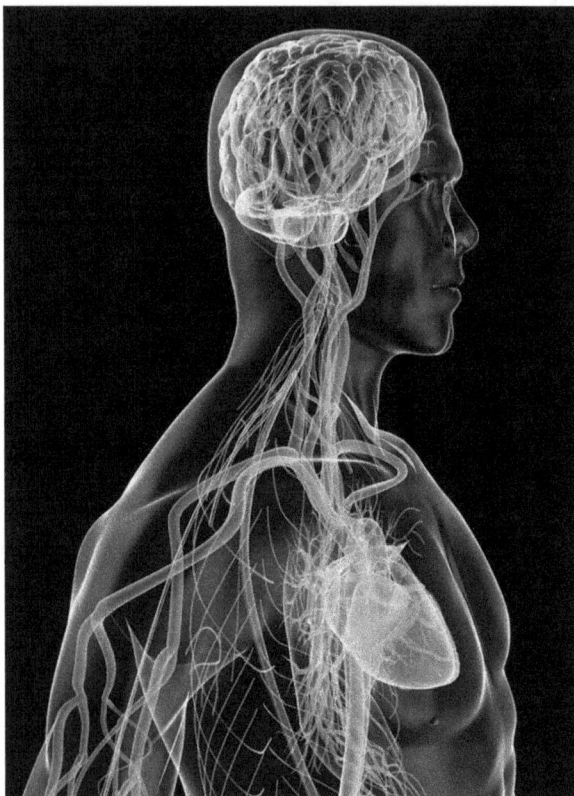

Illustration of the intrinsic connection of brain and heart in the human being.

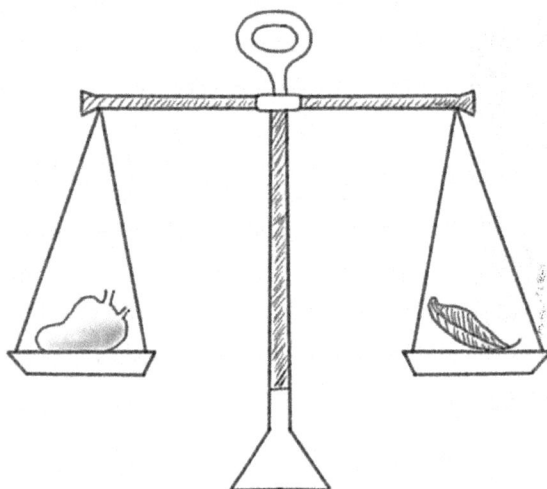

Illustration of the weighing of the heart in the scale, against a feather, as portrayed in Egyptian mythology.

The Intrinsic Relationship Between the Mind and the Heart

There is an intrinsic relationship between the mind and the heart. The heart is the first organ to form during fetal development. Every thought in a human's mind emits electromagnetic vibrational waves which are also generated from the base of the heart. The process of generating thoughts involves the bio-physical functioning of the mind and the heart. The heart is the generator of the strongest vibrational electromagnetic fields in the human body.

It is important to know this information because we believe that the brain is where the action is. It is true that the brain also generates vibrational electromagnetic fields, but they are weaker than those generated by the heart. The process of creating thoughts involves the mind and the heart and through these, a powerful electromagnetic vibrational frequency is generated. This produces powerful sounds which stimulate the heartbeats and can alter the atomic structure of matter when the thought is expressed by speaking.

The Heart is the Pivotal Point for the Soul and the Personality

It is through the heart that we learn the truth. The heart has its own intelligence and it is as obvious as the intelligence of the brain. The Egyptians believed that the heart and not the brain was the source of human wisdom. The heart was considered the center of the soul and personality. It was through the heart that divinity was expressed. The ancient Egyptians imparted their knowledge and called it **The True Way of Being.**

The Egyptians had a passion for life after death. For them the existence of the spirit or Ka energy, is infinite and not limited to the time we live on Earth. Measuring the weight of the Heart was represented in the hieroglyphics and was also found in several papyri discovered in Egyptian temples. At the time of the final judgment after death, the heart was weighed against a feather on a scale and if the weight of the heart was equal to, or less than the feather, it meant that the owner of that heart had lived a noble and generous life.

In other words, that pharaoh, priest, or person had gone to the other side of life, after death, with a light heart. That meant he/she had a good life. He/she was a person who had contributed good to the existence of life on Earth. This represents a universal or archetypal stage experienced by people in the process of awakening to the inner chamber of their heart.

The Egyptian concept of the intuitive intelligence of the heart reminds me about a dear lady who was like my own family, who many times brought to my attention; we perceive the minds of people through their words, but not through their hearts. Make sure to sharpen the intuitive senses of your heart to perceive the true nature and intentions of people. Learn to develop the natural wisdom of intuition and discernment of the heart which is more precise and accurate than the mind.

When we feel the power of love, when we connect our outer world with our inner world, then everything becomes one. That is the way which opens our hearts to perceive the music of the spheres.

The creative force of the universe, the universal intelligence or God is within each one of us. It is a true and natural state. The "I am that I am" means that God is in Heaven, in the Universe, throughout, and is also here, inside of me. I am here on Earth what I am in the universe. God dwells inside each one of us.

When we focus inward to the essence of our being, the heart energy activates and opens a direct path that leads to self-knowledge and self-realization through the power of love.

Rumi and his unforgettable poem dedicated to the heart

Rumi was a 13th century Persian poet. His work is associated with Sufism and the Mevlevi Order, recognized internationally as the Dervish Dancers. He taught "God should be celebrated through poetry, song and dance." His poetry transcended its Persian roots and is recognized as beautiful illuminated spiritual writing by many people of all different religions, all over the world.

Rumi, in one of his unforgettable poems, wrote "Only through the heart we can touch heaven."

Ancient sages knew that the heart is our very nucleus, the Seat of the Soul, the fount of love and the source of our creativity.

Ancient Scriptures Speak of the Importance of the Heart

"As he thinketh in his heart, so is he." (Proverbs: 23: 7) (The Bible).

But the LORD said to Samuel, "Do not look at his appearance or on the height of his stature, because I have rejected him; for I do not see as man sees; for man looks on the outward appearance, but the Lord sees what is on the heart." (ISamuel 16: 7) (The Bible).

In the hieroglyphics and ancient Egyptian writings, they believed that when a person dies, the person is put through a ceremony where "his heart is weighed in the scale." In this Egyptian ceremony of Judgment, the feather of Maat Goddess of Truth appears on the opposite side of the scale. The meaning is clear and simple: "To enter heaven you need a completely clear heart as light as the weight of a feather!"

The ancients had good reasons for their beliefs. Today we are beginning to discover that ancient people had a lot of knowledge about the heart's importance.

The heart is fragile. The subconscious mind is responsible for keeping the heart strong. Body organs generate vibrational frequencies that are perceived as emotions, and there is a direct connection between the brain and the heart.

We often create a **wall or shield in our hearts** which can block our ability to give and receive love. When a shield or wall is created in the heart, emotions of depression, isolation, and insensitivity can block the chances for achieving success.

Science is beginning to discover that the wall or shield of the heart is involved in heart disease, heart attacks, blood pressure problems, chest pain, neck pain, shoulder pain, and upper back pain. It can also lower the defenses of the immune system, which can cause vulnerability to infection and diseases.

The wall or shield we create in the heart can affect the thymus gland resulting in imbalances in the production of T cells. The thymus is located in the center of the chest above the heart.

The wall or shield we create in the heart can also make the natural healing process difficult and we are more prone to illnesses. The ability to succeed in our projects and enterprises are blocked by such heart wall or shield.

Many people have had success after removing the heart wall or shield. The heart wall or shield consists of trapped emotions that do not allow us to forgive ourselves or our neighbors. We may never have peace until we learn to do so.

If we do not eliminate anger, hate, resentment, jealousy and envy, a vibrational frequency of destructive energy can cause disharmony, invade the body, mind and spirit, and attract diseases and negative situations.

It is imperative to forgive ourselves and others in order to eliminate the heart wall or shield. Doing so can restore vibrational frequencies of peace and inner harmony, good health, productive energy, creativity and happiness. The act of forgiveness is a virtue that leads to a creative and fulfilling life.

The heart is the primordial center for the expression of unconditional love. When the vibrational frequency of love is activated, it regenerates atoms, molecules, cells, organs and systems. Love is the most powerful force in the universe, and it can activate healing and create miracles.

*By changing and elevating the frequency of our heart, we will ignite the spark of love that will illuminate and change the world. - **J.E.M.***

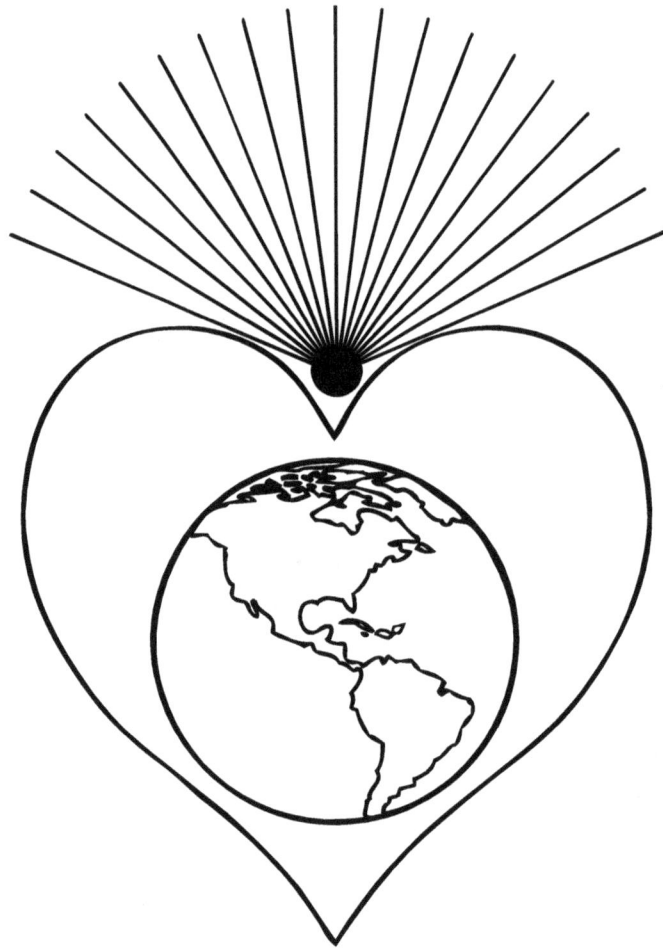

*To heal the planet and all that exists, we must vibrate in the frequency of love. - **J.E.M***

14

The Origin of the Art of Healing by Harmonic Sounds

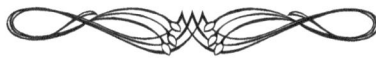

Where did the art of healing through harmonic sounds and vibrations originate?

The art of healing by sound is known as the oldest form of healing and goes back to the time of the continents of Atlantis and Lemuria.

The civilization of Atlantis was the first to incorporate the use of sounds, harmonic vibrations, crystals and minerals to cure diseases, physical and mental imbalances.

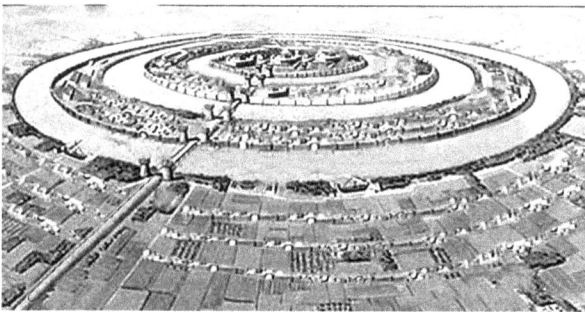

Illustration of the great continent of Atlantis.

A Brief Description of the Continent of Atlantis

It is estimated that the continent of Atlantis in 48,000 to 28,000 BC was located above the equatorial line of Earth, in the center of the Atlantic Ocean. Atlantis islands covered a long stretch of land, located parallel to the left side of North and Central America and parts of South America. To its right was Europe and a large part of Africa. It is said that Atlantis underwent sinking during three different time periods. The first sinking took place in approximately 28,000 years BC, the second, in approximately 18,000 BC, and the third one, which was its final and total destruction, in approximately 13,000 to 10,000 BC.

The tectonic plates of Atlantis in 18,000 AD were located in an unstable region for a long time. Two tectonic plates moved apart which caused disturbances in the delicate crust of the landmasses, and activated earthquakes and volcano eruptions. After the second flooding, Atlantis separated into five islands. The three major islands were known as Poseida, Aryan, and Og. The two smaller islands were known as Ataly and Eyre.

During its Golden Age Atlantis displayed pyramids of three and four faces. The Pyramids were made of marble, granite and complex crystals. The three-sided pyramids were used as antennas to amplify and send energy to a grid of poles, used to power homes, factories and create other energy fields, for diverse uses. The four sided Pyramids were temples of great complexity.

Some of the temples had domes and spheres that generated vibrational frequencies of sound and light. They resonated with the chakras of the human body, and amplified the ability to learn.

Poseida was the principal and largest island in Atlantis. It had temples and pyramids that activated the most complex vortices of the energy of that era. Its many temples included The Temple of Sound and Vibration, The Temple of Healing, The Temple of Regeneration, and The Temple of Knowledge.

Poseida housed most of the major institutions of higher learning in Atlantis. These educational centers were in Poseida because of its strategic location near geodetic networks and beneficial electromagnetic energy surges, that spiraled upward from the Earth's core.

The Atlanteans used sounds, crystals and minerals to heal their patients' physical, emotional, and mental conditions. For rejuvenation they applied frequencies generated by crystals. They also used crystals to make musical instruments that produced exquisite harmonic sounds and primarily to stimulate healing.

Crystals were used for meditation, to amplify mental capacities, and for storage and retrieval of information. Their technology was similar to, but more sophisticated than, the computer hard drive technology we have today.

Antlantean teachers and priests attained a high consciousness. They knew a big Earth change was coming and started survival preparations 200 years before the cataclysms that caused Atlantis to sink.

Three groups from Atlantis were believed to have migrated to different points on Earth

One group of Atlanteans migrated north, to England and Scotland, and founded the Druids. Another group migrated to North Africa and founded the Egyptian Civilization in the Giza Plateau. Another group emigrated to Central America, the territories now known as Guatemala and Mexico, and founded the Mayan civilization.

When Atlantean teachers and priests emigrated to new lands, they brought along the teachings of Thoth (Father of Wisdom.) Besides the teachings, they also brought icons, artifacts and powerful technological instruments from Atlantis.

The Atlanteans also brought the concepts of harmonic sounds and vibrations, and the natural healing power of crystals and minerals to the new places where they emigrated.

Teachers of Atlantean origin may have influenced the development of ancient civilizations. The Mayans speak of Pakal, a god who had the appearance of a white man, was tall, and similar in appearance to depictions of Quetzalcoatl.

Quetzalcoatl is the Sun God, or Feathered Serpent, worshipped in Mexico by the Mayans, Aztecs and other tribes. Bartolomé de las Casas (born 1474) writes that Quetzalcoatl, the feathered serpent, was white and tall, had a rounded beard, came from the East by sea, and said he would return. (see Anthology of The Indians of Mexico and New Spain, Editorial Porrúa, Mexico, SA, 1982, pp. 54, 218, 223).

Pyramids were also constructed in Peru, and there is talk of an Atlantean Master known as Manco Capac, also white in appearance, and with great knowledge of astronomy. The physical appearance of these characters was very similar. Some of them were white, tall, bearded, and with knowledge of astronomy. They taught great wisdom to the people, in the many places they visited.

Oral tradition of indigenous American tribes say that these teachers came from Atlantis, migrated to new lands, and brought the teachings of Thoth. They taught concepts of healing through harmonic frequencies of sounds, they used crystals and minerals, and used concepts of astronomy and sacred geometry when building temples and pyramids. They brought powerful icons and tools from their Atlantean civilization.

They built pyramids to create a network of electromagnetic energy that would preserve the ancient wisdom of Atlantis and benefit future generations with their teachings.

Pyramids were originally built and used in Atlantis more than 13,000 years ago and were built anew in Egypt, Guatemala and Mexico by the migrants of this continent. The construction of pyramids spread to other areas with additional concepts from Atlantis, such as astronomy, healing through harmonic sounds and vibrations, and also healing through the power of crystals.

The Possible Discovery of Atlantis According to Scientists Paul Weinzweig and Dr. Pauline Zalitzki

Scientists Pauline Zalitzki and Paul Weinzweig were searching for oil reserves in the ocean area adjacent to Cuba in July 2000. The project was undertaken by the governments of Cuba, India and China. During their search, they discovered a submerged ancient city in the depth of the ocean at about 600 feet deep. According to Dr. Zalitzki, the engineer Paul Weinzweig, and their team of researchers, the discovery coincides with the legend of Atlantis.

They estimated that the city sank over 10,000 years ago and faces the north eastern coast of Cuba and the limits of the Bermuda Triangle. Several unexplained events occurred in the Bermuda Triangle, and is a place of mystery to this day.

Using an underwater robot, the scientists were able to observe and confirm a gigantic city of antiquity on the ocean floor. The images captured by the robotic device show various sphinxes, several sculptures, engraved monoliths, and monumental buildings, including four pyramids, one of which appears to be made of glass.

It has been confirmed that the Pyramids and the stones found in the submerged city in the Atlantic Ocean were cut, carved and polished to make them fit and form larger structures. They are similar to Egyptian hieroglyphic inscriptions which are abundant and found in almost all parts of the field but little understood.

The submerged city covers an area of 20 square kilometers, or approximately 7.8 square miles and was found in an area of white sand. The city was built using a pattern of straight lines where faults exist, near a river bed and an extinct volcano.

According to scientists, the complex existed during the pre-classical period of Caribbean and Central American history and was inhabited by an advanced civilization, similar to that of Teotihuacan, Mexico.

The scientists Pauline Zalitzki and Paul Weinzweig returned in July 2001 to the same place where they found the city submerged in waters adjacent to Cuba, but this time they were accompanied by the geologist Manuel Iturralde, researcher of the Museum of Natural History of Cuba. On this occasion, they were equipped with a Remote Operation Vehicle to film and examine the structures. They obtained images of large stone blocks resembling carved granite, which measure approximately 8 to 10 feet. Many of the blocks appeared to have been cut and placed one above the other and others appeared isolated from the rest. Pauline Zalitzki commented that the images seemed to reflect the ruins of a submerged city, but that it is necessary to do more research before arriving at a conclusion.

Information about these underwater findings and the possible relationship with the Atlantis Lost Continent were quickly published in the media worldwide. However, Weinzweig and Zelitsky made no comment or statement confirming that their findings have anything to do with the Atlantis Continent. They said, it appeared to be the remainings of a local civilization that was about 100 kilometers away from Cuba towards the Yucatan peninsula in Mexico. The Cuban geologist Manuel Iturralde mentioned that the Yucatecan natives and the Mayans spoke of an inhabited island that sank underwater and they believe that they are descendants from this civilization.

Atlantis was first described by the Greek philosopher Plato. He wrote of legends that tell of the disappearance of Atlantis, due to to great flood, earthquakes and a volcanic eruption that occurred more than 10,000 years ago. However, besides Plato's dialogues, The Sanskrit writings of ancient India contain several descriptions of Atlantis, originally described in the Mahabharata as an island in the far West, and even assert that Atlantis was destroyed as the result of a war between the gods. Herodotus, the "father of history," mentions Atlantis by name in referring to the body of water into which it sank. In the Greek text, a portion of Clio (History, Bk I, 202) appears that the waters beyond the straits of Gibraltar is said to be known as the Atlantis Sea.

The discovery of the engineer Paul Weinzweig and Dr. Pauline Zalitzki about the city submerged in the ocean floor near Cuba might be related to the possible existence of the advanced civilization of Atlantis. However, future investigations will confirm whether it is a legend or a true civilization that existed thousands of years ago.

15

Ancient Cultures and the Healing Power of Sound

Ancient cultures knew the healing power of music and harmonic sounds.

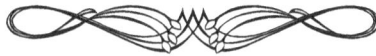

The history of the use of harmonics as a method of healing by ancient cultures

Most ancient cultures used the seemingly magical power of sound to heal. Healing through sound had almost disappeared in western medicine before 1930. After 1930, investigators discovered the medicinal properties of sound, and incorporated its medical uses with acoustic ultrasound.

With this discovery, research in healing through sounds has flourished and is fast becoming a new science. There is a lot of research on the healing benefits through sounds and infrasound, including using sound to break up kidney stones and to shrink tumors. Besides infrasound, audible sound is recognized as a potential healing method.

Which cultures have recognized the importance of the healing power of music and sounds?

Many past cultures recognized the importance, therapeutic value, and healing power of **harmonic sounds and music**. Most ancient cultures used sound and harmonic vibrations in their rituals and ceremonies. They used sounds and harmonic vibrations to encourage balance and harmony in the physical body, mind and spirit.

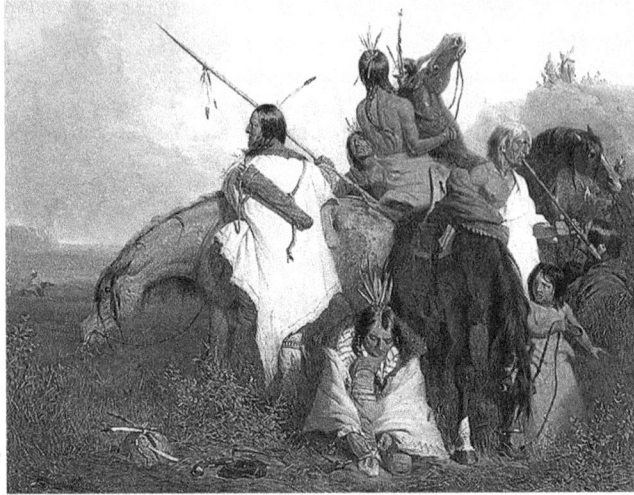

Native americans.

Australian Aborigines and Native North and South American Indigenous Cultures

The Australian Aborigines and Native North and South Americans led by their shamans, use repetitive vocal sounds in combination with instruments created by Mother Nature in their rituals and ceremonies.

Aboriginal Australians are considered one of the earliest known cultures which incorporated the use of sound to heal. For about 40,000 years, the Australian Aborigines have

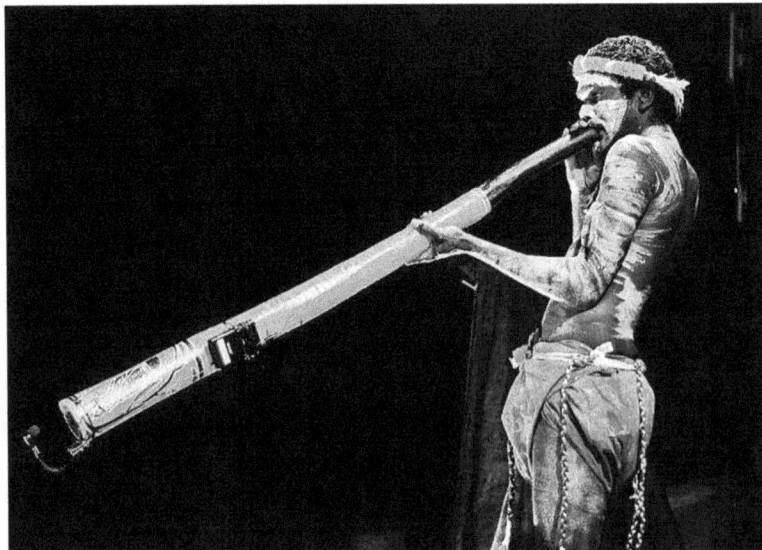

The oldest of all healing tools: The Yidaki (didgeridoo)

used an instrument now called a didgeridoo, as a healing tool.

Australian Aborigines have healed fractures, tears and muscular diseases of different types with this enigmatic musical instrument. Interestingly, sounds created by the didgeridoo (Yidaki is its' ancient name) are in alignment with the modern technology of healing with sound. It is becoming evident that our ancestors' wisdom was based on sound principles.

Tibetan Lamas and Monks

The power of sound and vibration is widely used by Tibetan monks, who incorporate meditation, music, vibration, prayer and mantras in their rituals and medicinal healing.

The main focus of Tibetan monks is the use of sounds, mantras and meditation. Meditation regulates the sympathetic nervous system which allows us to feel safe, calm and happy. In that space the body can achieve balance, increase energy and regenerate.

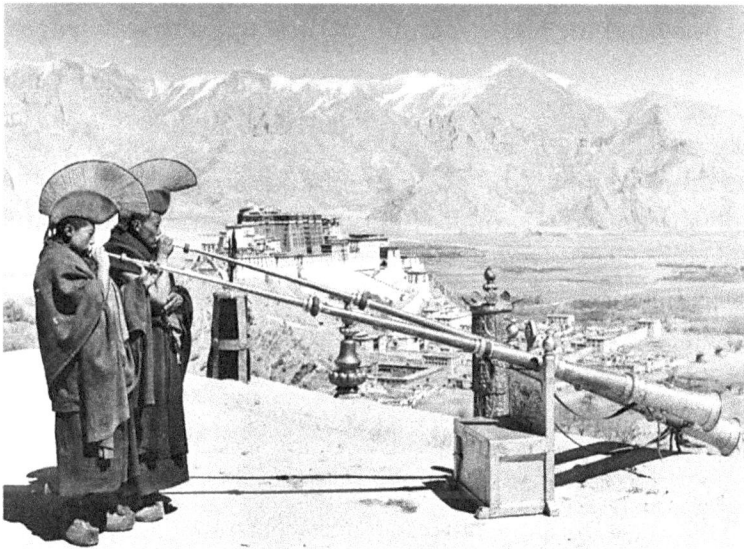

Tibetan lamas and monks with the instruments used in ceremonies and rituals.

Tibetan monks understand that our whole being is in a constant state of vibration and produces sounds. Our bodies' molecules, cells, bones, organs, tissues and fluids produce specific sounds and vibrations. Negative thoughts, beliefs and emotions can create harmful vibrational energies that alter the subtle energy field that surrounds the body which can cause disease and deterioration of the physical body.

Tibetan monks still use singing bowls in ceremonies to facilitate meditative states. They use bowls, chimes and bells made of seven metals, and they also use wind instruments. The alchemical composition of the bowls, bells and chimes is usually of seven metals: gold, silver, mercury, copper, iron, tin and lead. The vibrational resonance of the bowls sends specific tones to the body and brain, which help release tension, inflammation, and energy blockages in the meridians.

Monks recite mantras and sing low vocal tones to generate harmonic frequencies in order to activate collective healing on Earth. One of their powerful mantras is **"Om-Ma-Ni-Pat-Mi-Houm."**

Tibetan monks believe that the sound and tones produced by the human voice is the most powerful way to generate vibrational frequencies for healing. By using song, sound intonations, prayers and mantras in their rituals and ceremonies, negative and disharmonizing energies can be eliminated before they can physically manifest. By consciously executing different tones, they can stimulate electromagnetic fields of individuals exposed to these sounds. The deeper and low vocal tones stimulate healing of the physical body and the higher harmonic vocal tones have an effect on the subtle body's energy.

Tibetan monks recommend that we explore their techniques by making buzzing or humming and other sounds through the mouth, voice and throat. Buzzing sounds create powerful vibrations that produce internal movements through the mouth, throat and skull. They stimulate the pineal and pituitary glands, which begin to regulate the body's hormonal functions. This process also influences the brainwaves of Gamma, Beta, Alpha, Theta and Delta, and stimulates the natural healing process of body, mind and spirit.

The Priests of Ancient Egypt

Ancient Egyptians understood the power of sacred harmonic sounds and mantras. They knew that harmonic sounds and mantras activate powerful vibrational frequencies that stimulate higher levels of consciousness. They called those levels of consciousness Sheta Ren. They incorporated breathing techniques in combination with specific sounds to strengthen the energy centers we know as the chakras. This practice emphasized the importance of the reproductive chakra and sexual energy, which gives rise to our divine and creative power center.

Priests of ancient Egypt knew that using certain vowels in combination with specific harmonic hues would stimulate electromagnetic energy. This would transmit healing vibrational frequencies through the human nervous system, and meridians to harmonize the chakras.

When Egyptian priests sang hymns to the gods they used seven vowels in succession. This information was recorded by a Greek traveler, Demetrius. In around 200 B.C., he wrote that the Egyptians used powerful vocal sounds in their healing rituals and ceremonies.

The Egyptians, like the Babylonians , used drums and rattles, two musical instruments well known in ancient times. The drums and rattles generate a low frequency that can accelerate the healing process and that has been recognized scientifically.

The Corpus Hermeticum is a book that contains references to the use of sounds and words by Egyptians. This book was probably written in the first century of the Christian era, but it is believed that its origins date back to 1400 B.C.

Egyptians believed that vowel sounds were sacred, so much so that their language in its hieroglyphic writing has no vowels. We therefore assume that the powerful vocal sounds and songs used in religious and healing rituals had profound meaning to their priests.

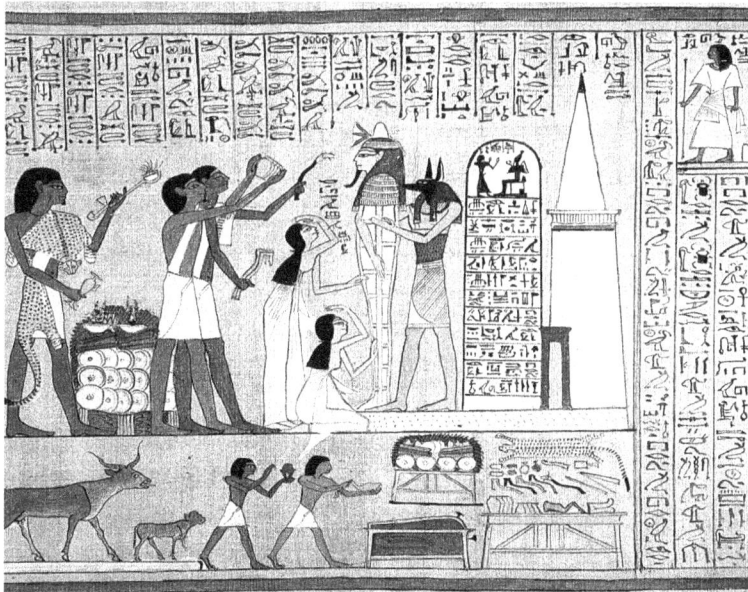

Egyptian priests performing rituals in the pyramid.

Egyptian priestesses used a musical instrument called the sistra. The sistra had rattling metal discs which created a pleasant tinkling sound and also generated an ultrasound frequency.

Ultrasound is a diagnostic and healing method that is currently used in the medical field. It is quite possible that Egyptian priestesses used sistras in their ceremonies not only with the purpose of producing powerful sound effects, but also as a healing means to improve people's health conditions.

Ancient Egyptians incorporated musical scales and sacred geometry in the construction of their buildings, pyramids, tombs and temples. The most common ratios used in the proportions of Egyptian temple building, correspond to harmonic musical intervals.

There are reports that certain chambers of the pyramids and particular rooms in Egyptian tombs enhance the resonance of tones, sounds, or music in these chambers, temples, galleries and rooms.

The chapel of healing in Deir el-Bahari in Thebes was dedicated to Amenhotep, son of Hapu, a saint who cured and was deified and closely associated with "Imhotep." Imhotep was recognized largely under the title of "Doctor." The reputation of Imhotep was well known, and 1,500 years after his death the Greeks identified him with the God of healing, Asclepius. The two deified names "Amenhotep, son of Hapu and Imhotep" were usually worshipped together in the same Egyptian healing temples.

Egyptians designed chapels and burial chambers with perfect resonance, in order to amplify the acoustic sounds of the chants and mantras used in their rituals. It is believed that the Egyptians knew the properties of sound healing long before the Greeks.

In the Egyptian Temple of Dendera, there are hieroglyphics on the walls that portray musicians. There is a specific glyph that reads **"The sky and its stars are singing with us."** Scholars of ancient Egypt concluded that music was intrinsic to the structure of the heavens and planets. The song of the cosmos, better defined as **The Music of the Spheres**, reveals the deeper unity of creation and confirms that eberything is in a constant state of vibration and producing sounds.

Chinese Buddhist Priests and Monks

Chinese Buddhist priests and monks use gongs, drums, string instruments and flutes in their ceremonies with the intention of sending mystical and spiritual messages to uplift and illumine the spirit. In the practice of Chi Kung (Qi Gong) in China, six healing sounds that resonate with vital body organs are used to attune the body.

Priests and Buddhist monks use Chinese chants and mantras in their spiritual ceremonies to establish a state of spiritual elevation during meditation. The chants and mantras are also used to help heal the sick. Chanting mantras can uplift the spirit, express feelings of love and unity, and connect man and the universe.

The Sufis of Islam

Sufism originated in Islam. The core of Sufism is to live a normal life and become one with God, truth and knowledge. This is manifested in their ceremonies through the use of music, song and dance. They incorporate a spiral rotating dance into their celebrations, as if to create a whirlwind. Through this trance-like movement, they enter a state of meditation in motion, that they claim connects them with the Divine.

The music, singing and spiral dancing can open the heart to live freely. The concept of separation ceases to exist. This practice creates a sense of union with the cosmos and the dancer feels that he or she becomes an intrinsic part of a living universe.

The symbol of the union with all existence is exposed in the well known ceremony called Mevlavi, where the Sufis perform a spiral dance as if in a whirlwind. This practice was inspired by the Persian poet Rumi, and partly by Turkish culture.

The music, singing and dancing allows the dervishes to release their egos and mind-conditioning. The experience is mystical and psychedelic, without the use of drugs or intoxicants. Love, music, song and dance are the only techniques used.

Sufis say that the existence of the creation of the universe is forever in motion, constantly vibrating and rotating. Electrons, protons, neutrons, atoms, stars, planets and their satellites revolve in a cosmic dance. In living beings the movement of blood circulates through all the arteries and veins of the body activating the flow of life. Life is a revolution that originates from within Earth and returns therein, with music, chants and whirlpool as natural as life itself.

Sounds and vibrations are the fundamental building blocks of the universe. Sound

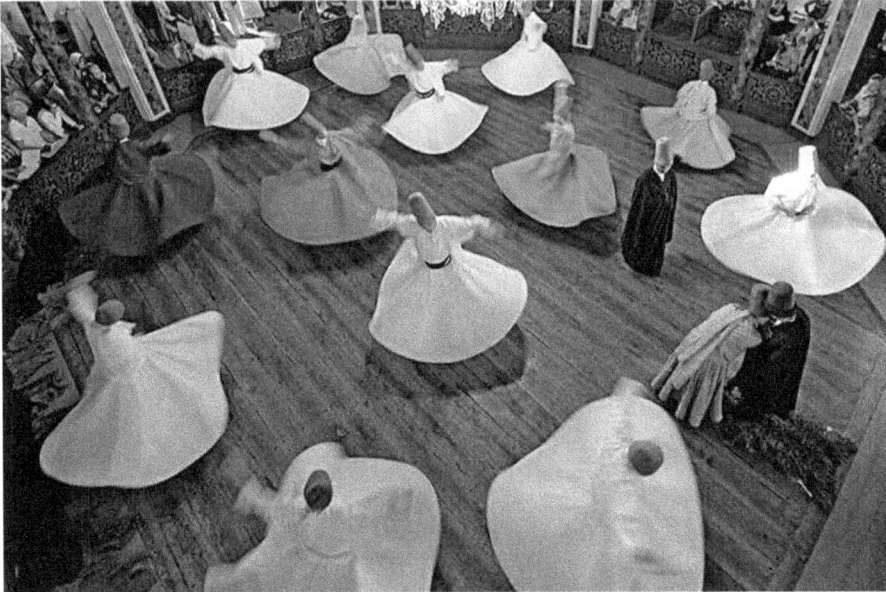

Image of Sufi dervishes dancing with Sufi music.

builds the mind, the body is shaped through sound, and sound gives form to everything that we see and perceive.

The Mayans

The Mayans used a trumpet known as a **Hompak** for therapeutic healing and to stimulate special states of consciousness. The sounds produced by the **Hompak** were used in Mayan ceremonies, rituals, dances, battles and hunts. The **Hompak** is a wind instrument or trumpet made from elongated hollow tree bark with a pumpkin at one end to amplify the sound. The **Hompak** is similar in look and sound to the Australian Aboriginal musical instrument Yidaki (Didgeridoo.) Both instruments have been used for relaxation, to activate spiritual connections, and to make healing music that harmonizes the chakras.

The **Hompak** and Digeridoo have been used by different cultures for over 40 thousand years. In 1568 the Spanish Friar Diego de Landa documented and described The Mayan Trumpet (La Trompeta Maya) or **Hompak** in his work "The Relationship of Things in Yucatan."

The **Hompak** was also called Incus Utop Chek (which means tree blossom trumpet) by the Mayan Lacandons. The **Hompak** can be made from dried kiote or maguey flowers, giving it lightness. In the murals of Bonampak, and in its walls, are images of Mayan natives using their **Hompak** trumpets during celebrations and battles.

The Mayans loved music. They used music in their dances, rituals and ceremonies as an inseparable element for their magical religious world. The **Hompak** was one of the main instruments of the Mayan culture of antiquity. However, they also had other musical instruments, such as whistles made of deer bones, large snails, Xul indigenous cane flutes made in tubular form and globular flutes. The drums called Tunjul and Teponaxtle were made from tortoiseshell turtles that were abundant in lakes and ponds. They also made drums from stone, metal and clay. The vigorous rhythm of the music and drums created a hypnotic effect that was important to the Mayans.

Therapeutic Benefits Produced by the Didgeridoo and the Hompak.

The circular breathing of the person who produces sounds with the Didgeridoo or the **Hompak** is the "magic" that allows the potential for self-healing, therapeutic benefits for the musician and the listeners.

The sounds are from a wide range of low frequency ultrasound waves (under 20 Hz) that relieve tension and muscle aches, improve recovery from injuries and illnesses, cleanse the chakras, promote emotional and physical release, and rejuvenate. The unique sounds of these instruments allow experimental deep meditation and stimulate the Delta, Theta and Alpha brainwaves.

Listening to the sounds can be compared to receiving a massage that promotes healing, provides relief for muscular and joint pain, and accelerates the healing of bone fractures and trauma from post-operative implants.

The sound frequencies generated by the Didgeridoo and the **Hompak** activate vibrations that produce a positive sensation of tingling throughout the body. This stimulates the cells and nervous system, relieves arthritis pain and bone injuries, and contributes to a state of peace and happiness.

In a recording made of the sound produced by Earth's rotating motion, NASA reported that the sound produced was similar to the sound of the Didgeridoo.

The Jews, Christians, Greeks & Romans

Since ancient times music occupied an important place in the life of the Hebrews Jews, Christians, Greeks and Romans, especially in their worship of God. Music was used in religious ceremonies, royal court, weddings, family gatherings and in the grape and grain harvest festivals. It was known to elevate the mind, the spirit and make prophets spiritually receptive. In "2 Kings 3:15" it was mentioned that Elisha was divinely inspired after he heard the sound of an instrument. ("But now bring me a musician." And when the musician played, the hand of the LORD came upon him.")

Revelation 5:9; 14:3; 15:2, 3 reveals that music was given to mankind by God to help express their thoughts, emotions and feelings ("And sang the song of God's servant Moses and of the Lamb"). Music is a heavenly gift to the world. (James 1:17, "Every good and perfect gift is from above, coming down from the Father of the heavenly lights, who does not change like shifting shadows.")

The Bible describes that music and singing originated in the Celestial Spheres

Angels, Cherubims and spirits sang and played instruments like harps and flutes when praising the Lord. The Universal Creator through the spoken word made the sound that originated the creation of the universe and gave birth to **"The music of the spheres"** and also implanted music in the unit of life, the DNA of all sentient beings that inhabit Earth. Humans, birds, dolphins, whales, Sumatran rhinoceros, frogs, the coquies, cats and many others produce musical sounds. God created us to be instruments with the ability to sing and make music.

Jews and Christians inherited the musical influence from King David. King David was a young shepherd who lived about 3,000 years ago. He was divinely inspired to write music Psalms which he used to sing with the harp when worshiping God. King David expressed his mystical experiences, feelings and compositions in words and music when singing psalms. He narrated his daily life, mystical experiences and the history of the Israelites of his time.

The Bible; **Psalm 150:1-5** describes the **different instruments utilized by the Israelites to worship God.** 1 Praise the LORD. Praise God in his sanctuary; praise him in his mighty heavens. 2 Praise him for his acts of power; praise him for his surpassing greatness. 3 Praise him with the **sounding of the trumpet,** praise him with **harp and lyre.** 4 Praise him with **timbrel** and **dancing,** praise him with the **strings** and **pipe,** 5 Praise him with the **clash of cymbals,** praise him with **resounding cymbals. Zephaniah**

3:17 "The LORD your God is in your midst, a mighty one who will save. He will rejoice over you with joy. He will calm you in his love. **He will rejoice over you with singing.**

Unaccompanied vocal music continued to be the norm in Christian worship for many centuries through Chorales, Gregorian Chants and priests singing Bible scriptures a capella in Latin during mass services. By the 15th century, organ music was widely accepted in the **Roman Catholic religion** from Occident or the West and eventually by the Orthodox of the East or Orient. The Coptic and Ethiopian churches, by contrast, had their own musical tradition, which made use of ancient percussion instruments.

In the 16 Century, the **Lutheran movement** loved music and in the reformation in Europe, they warmly welcomed music. Luther said **"God announces the Gospel through music also,"** the Gospel being the Word incarnated in Jesus Christ. Luther wanted the service to be centered on Christ, and thus had new hymns composed that preached the incarnation, the cross and resurrection. Their music compositions were named **"Lutheran Chorales."** The Reformed went further in reforming music and banned any reminder in stranglehold in sacred music used in Roman Catholic Ceremonies. Choir-stall organs were even done away with. The Lutheran worshippers sang a capella, in unison and without the help of instruments. The reformed repertoire also consisted of Psalms.

Unaccompanied music like the Gregorian Chants goes back to ancient times and they were an important part of the Churches Christian Chorales Ceremonies until about 1050 AD when they mysteriously disappeared. The Gregorian Chants were sung with the original Solfeggio frequencies in the music tuning of 432 of that time, and they had the capacity to transform peoples' lives. By the middle of 1970 a naturopathic physician Dr. Joseph Puleo examined the Bible Genesis "Chapter 7, Verses 12-83. He found a pattern of six repeating codes around a series of sacred numbers, 3, 6 and 9. When deciphered using the ancient Pythagorean method of reducing the verses' numbers to a single digit, the codes revealed a series of six electromagnetic sound frequencies that correspond to the six tones of the ancient Solfeggio scale. I dwell on this topic more broadly in other chapters. Music is holy and an important part of worship and praise to God. Harmonic music has the power to alter the atomic structure of all matter and can activate spiritual transformation and healing on a mental, spiritual and physical level.

The most influential book of Christianity, the Bible, contains many verses and quotes in the holy scriptures about music. Music has always been used by many religious people like Jews, Romans, Greeks and Christians in their ceremonies for worshiping and praising God. **Music is the universal language of mankind.**

I share the idea that the Master of Teachers "Jesus the Christ" left a legacy of powerful teachings to humanity and the purpose of his mission was to unify the human race in the frequency of love, peace, harmony, compassion, collective prosperity, good will and divine order. **"Union among man and not division."** If all people on Earth, regardless of religion, unite their hearts in prayers, affirmations and singing Jesus' teachings, we will raise the frequency and illuminate the collective consciousness of all beings on Earth. When this happens, Earth will be the new Shining Star in the Universe.

"Music, sounds and harmonic vibrations activate the energy of high spheres, activate frequencies that transform the mind, creatively alter the structure of all matter, manifest the music that elevates the spirit, and is the universal language that unifies all beings." - J.E.M.

"Music is the language that harmonizes the collective universal consciousness." - J.E.M.

16

Healing with Sound in Modern Times

The effects of sound and music, and the effects on humans in modern times.

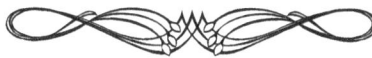

⸎

How healing with sound has re-emerged in modern times

Scientific studies of healing through sound first re-emerged in 1928 when the German scientist Erwin Schliephake discovered that sound could accelerate healing. Schliephake created an acoustic device known as the Novasonic which is still in use today.

In 1938 another German scientist, Raimar Pohlman, demonstrated therapeutic benefits through ultrasound in a physiotherapy clinic in Berlin. Until 1950, ultrasound was a healing modality used by many health institutions. However, the underlying healing mechanism of this therapy has not yet been completely understood.

A British osteopath, Peter Guy Manners, developed a healing modality with audible sound during the 1950s that is now called Cymatherapy. International Cymatherapy bought the rights to Mr. Manners' technology, and manufactures the Cymatherapy machine in the United States.

The new version uses advanced computers to create ultra-pure tones, especially in groups of five. Cymatherapy consists of 700 codes that address a wide range of injuries and disease. There are many new machine modalities, including a version of a computer program designed to be used with RIFE frequencies that stimulate healing through sound. Many ultrasonic machine technologies are manufactured in several countries including China, Korea, Japan, Germany, and Norway. They are becoming widely available in holistic centers throughout the world and are also purchased by individuals who want to use sound therapy in the privacy of their own homes.

What is sound and how does sound energy move?

Sound is defined as everything that moves and vibrates from the sub-atom and atom to the smallest molecule in the universe. Sound energy moves through the vibration of air and water molecules. A chain reaction activates the vibration of the air (or water) molecules and the vibrations are perceived by the human ear as sound. The same procedure occurs in water; however, the sound in water travels 3 to 4 times faster than in air.

The sound is not moving, rather it is the air or water molecules. When movement occurs, or a musical instrument is played, or we make vowel sounds, a vibration is created that moves air molecules and broadcasts sound.

The air and water molecules become agglutinated, or bonded tightly together, so when one molecule moves, it stimulates the movement of the surrounding molecules and causes the propagation of sound energy.

What is Music?

We define music as the science of organized harmonic sounds. It is the arrangement of sounds in time by which a continuous composition occurs, unified and evocative through the use of melody, harmony, rhythm and timbre.

Music affects the mind and body, and has been used to influence us in many ways. Music is used in ceremonies and celebrations, in the marches of soldiers who go to war, and to celebrate peace. Music soothes the soul, and can calm or lull a child to sleep.

In all cultures around the world, music has been used to heal. Music is as old as humankind. More than forty thousand years ago, Neanderthals played the flute and used rocks to produce percussion sounds. The voice used as music is an innate human characteristic. Our cells, organs, systems and bones respond to musical sounds; our biological systems resonate to specific notes in the diatonic musical scale, and also with the harmony of the Ancient Solfeggio musical tones.

The Effect of Music on the Emotions and Behavior of Individuals

Music is a powerful tool that can directly affect individuals' behavior and mental and emotional states. Young people are influenced and motivated by the lyrics, rhythms and melodies of current music. Music can directly affect a person's brain and emotional state. When a song makes you cry it is because the song stimulated a certain area of your brain and produced biochemical changes. Our relationship with music is deeper than we think. The rhythm and sound of music produces resonance in the brain and stimulates brain waves. When we hear a song, our breathing and heartbeats engage the rhythm of the song.

Humans, dolphins, whales and birds are the only beings that synchronize the beat of a song with their breathing and heartbeat. When we listen to soft music, serotonin is produced and encourages relaxation. Soft music has a therapeutic effect that can balance the body's chakras and organs.

When we listen to soft music our brain produces **serotonin** and has a strong effect in many of our body's biological functions. Serotonin is synthesized in the brain and the intestines. The majority of the body's serotonin, between 80-90%, can be found in the gastrointestinal tract. It can also be found in the blood platelets and the central nervous system. When the brain produces serotonin, tension is eased. Serotonin is the main brain chemical responsible for **making us feel happy, relaxed and self-confident.**

It's believed that **low serotonin levels** are responsible for our current epidemics of depression and anxiety. Beside mood, serotonin also plays an important role in our sleep, sex drive, and digestive health. In fact, depression is a consequence of the scarce production of this hormone.

Serotonin is released when the brain is **"positively shocked",** especially **when we listen to soothing music** like classical, new age, music, flute music and the music **"The Healing Forces of Harmonic Sounds and Vibrations"** can have a nourishing effect in all our biological systems.

For instance: **When we listen to soft music** the brain lets off a certain amount of serotonin which arouses and maximizes pleasant feelings. Music's rhythm can also stimulate other natural cadences of the body, resembling the heartbeat, or the Alpha-rhythm of the brain, and this effect is used to counter the development of clinical depression.

Soft music melody is the "Sparkle" that can also help to catalyze the creative process in our minds. **"Music therapy"** has been scientifically validated as a powerful natural method that can help people overcome depression, anxiety, insomnia problems, digestive problems, can influence the maturity and development of the mind and especially for good health maintenance.

The effect of singing on the brain and the nervous system

Recent scientific researchers are beginning to discover that **singing is like an infusion of the perfect tranquilizer.** It soothes the nervous system, elevates the spirit and treats

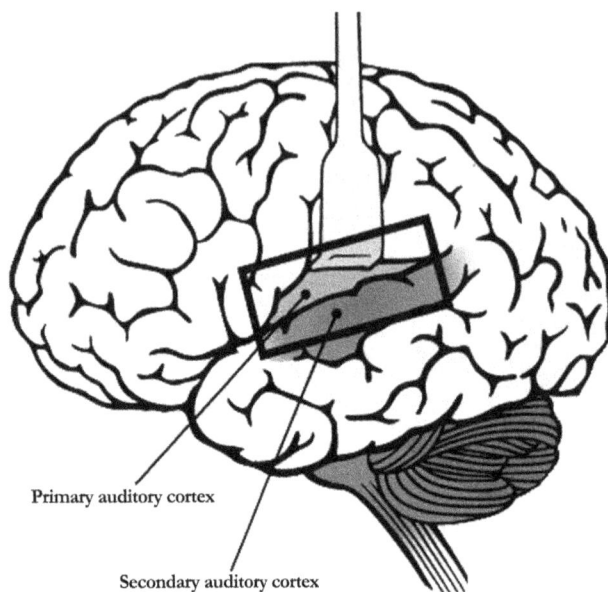

Primary auditory cortex

Secondary auditory cortex

Illustration of the auditory cortex of the brain.

depression. When we sing, we release **endorphin hormones** that biochemically make us feel good. This explains the emotional response that so many people have when they hear their favorite music or song.

Endorphins are among the brain chemicals known as neurotransmitters, which function to transmit electrical signals within the nervous system. At least 20 types of endorphins have been demonstrated in humans. Endorphins can be found in the **pituitary gland,** in other parts of the brain, or distributed throughout the nervous system.

These natural peptide chemicals produced in your body interact with receptors in your brain to help you feel focused, **less impacted by pain and put you in a better mood.** In fact, **endorphins** have a lot in common with **prescription anti-anxiety drugs** and opiate painkillers. While it might seem scary to know that endorphins work in a similar way to mood-controlling drugs like morphine, rest assured that they provide the benefits without all the risks. **Singing boosts the production of natural endorphins** helping us to reach a healthier mental state, without the risky side effects of drugs.

Another hormone released when we sing is **oxytocin.** This hormone is produced during childbirth and also when having an orgasm, which generates feelings of intimacy and connection.

The neuropeptide **oxytocin**, released by your pituitary gland, is a naturally occurring hormone in your body with incredibly powerful, health-giving properties. The more oxytocin your pituitary gland releases, the better able you are to **handle life's stressors.** Oxytocin decreases the level of stress hormones (primarily cortisol) your body manufactures and lowers your blood pressure response to anxiety-producing events. Oxytocin has also been found to reduce the cravings of drug and alcohol addiction, as well as for sweets. Oxytocin speeds the healing process in the body and helps people to heal more quickly from illness, addictions and chronic diseases. It could be why more studies have found that **singing** lessens feelings of depression, loneliness and helps to maintain a healthy mind, body and spirit.

Scientific studies demonstrated that people that sing frequently have **lower levels of cortisol** in their bloodstream, which is a stress related hormone and has inhibitory effects on the immune system.

A recent study showed that the synchronization of multiple heart rates during group singing has a calming effect similar to that which occurs during meditation.

Singing can produce satisfactory and therapeutic sensations even when the sound produced by the person's voice has mediocre vocal quality. If you are suffering from feelings of loneliness or depression, use the powerful tool of singing, and through the emission of harmonious vocal sounds you can stimulate the production of **endorphins and oxytocin** that will help you overcome the emotions that can cause serious illness.

The Effects of Music on the Brain: Stimulus and Response

Music is a regular activity that is processed by the two hemispheres of the brain. Each person has either a left or right dominant hemisphere of the brain. However, individuals that study, play, or arrange music in any form tend to use both hemispheres of the brain at the same time. Such individuals have clear and acute minds that enable them to solve problems clearly and with mental ease.

Music stimulates the brain the same way food, drugs and sex stimulate the brain. In the auditory area of the cerebral cortex, melodies, notes, and songs are assimilated. The auditory cortex of the brain is involved with the learning process, and long- and short-term memory. The auditory cortex has some capacity for short term musical memory but long-term memory is dependent on the variety of musical styles.

When an individual listens to music, the auditory function of memory and learning are integrated in the hippocampus which is located below the brain's auditory cortex. The hippocampus is involved in controlling our temporal orientation in space.
Listening to and interpreting music can generate complex patterns that activate hippocampal neuronal pathways. This can lead to more efficient functioning of our neurons and stimulate new synaptic connections.

The hippocampus is responsible for long-term past memories. When we hear old songs, forgotten memories may be activated. Listening to old music helps people suffering from Alzheimer's or dementia to recover the memory of their forgotten past life.

Many patients suffering from Alzheimer's have been able to recover lost memories by listening to certain types of music. The brain's processing of music can help recover lost memories. One can therefore speculate that there is a connection between the brain's memory centers and the centers of the brain that process music.

Another interesting phenomenon is the effect of music on patients with Parkinson's disease. Some Parkinson's patients who have been immobilized have risen and walked after hearing music. It is not yet known why this response happens, but certain types of music can enhance and stimulate complex motor centers in the brain.

Certain types of music can synchronize brain wave function and help the neural pathways involved in complex behaviors, such as walking or running. Thus, it is possible that emotional arousal produced by music can ultimately cause both recovery of memories and the desire for movement.

The involvement of emotion in the process of interpretation of music is very important. Certain melodic and harmonic elements are more pleasing to the brain. The brain is primarily an organizer. The information that is organized normally, produces some type of pattern or structure which is related to the melody's overall pattern.

The frontal lobe and limbic system are the areas of the brain that cause emotional responses in music recall, deciphering, and learning.

Festive music can produce well-pleasing emotions that animate and awaken individuals. The production of endorphins is the fundamental cause of pleasure and displeasure of music.

Anecdotal evidence suggests that music activates areas of the brain's limbic system that releases endorphins, and produces pleasant effects. Endorphins can alleviate certain forms of depression, such as the seasonal disorder which afflicts many people during the winter when there is reduced sunlight.

Physiological effects are also produced by positive emotional responses to music. The type of music a person hears can influence the person's emotional state. Music can raise or lower our emotional states.

The dysfunction or malfunction of some areas of the brain can affect the perception of music. If the affected area of the brain involves the processing of music, it could result in a huge loss of perception.

The integration of all areas of the brain is crucial to the emotional response involved in the brain's processing of music. This information is leading to interesting possibilities in the

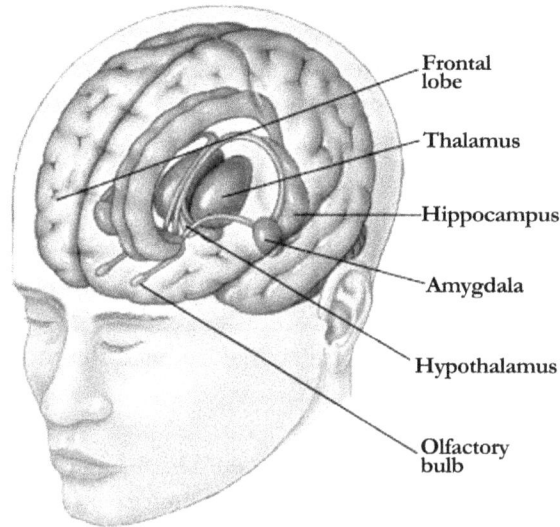

Illustration of the limbic system, the area of the frontal lobe and hippocampus of the brain.

field of music therapy.

Harmonic Music as medicine and Therapy

Researchers are exploring how music therapy can improve health outcomes among a variety of patient populations, including premature infants and people with depression and Parkinson's disease.

Daniel J. Levitin and his postgraduate research fellow, Mona Lisa Chanda, PhD, found that **harmonic music improves the body's immune system function and reduces stress.** Listening to soft music was also found to be more effective than prescription drugs in reducing anxiety before surgery (**Trends in Cognitive Sciences, April 2013**).

In the book **"Your Brain of Music"** (Plume/Penguin, 2007) Daniel J. Levitin (psychologist and neuroscientist), author of this book, points out how music influences health. Playing and listening to harmonic soft music promotes relaxation. Researchers also found that harmony music increases the body's production of the **antibody immunoglobulin A and natural killer cells (NK Cells)**, the cells that attack invading viruses and boost the immune system's effectiveness. Harmonic music also **reduces levels of the stress hormone cortisol.**

Scientific studies have also found out that harmonic soft music can help soothe pediatric emergency room patients (JAMA Pediatrics, July 2013). Researchers from Alberta University found that patients who listened to relaxing music while getting an IV inserted reported significantly less pain and less distress, compared with patients who did not listen to music. Two-thirds of the health care providers reported that the people that listened to music were very easy to administer the IV's in comparison with 38 percent of providers treating the group that did not listen to music. (IV's intravenous is a common procedure utilized in hospitals).

Lisa Hartling, PhD and professor of pediatrics at the University of Alberta says that there is scientific evidence that demonstrated that the brain responds to music. Children that listen to music during painful medical procedures react much better than the ones that do not listen to music. Listening to music can make a big difference in children and adults during painful medical procedures.

Lauren K. King of the Sun Life Financial Movement Disorders Research and Rehabilitation Centre at Wilfrid Laurier University, in Waterloo, Ontario, in 2009 found that short-term use of **vibroacoustic therapy with Parkinson's disease patients** led to improvements in symptoms, including less rigidity and better walking speed with bigger steps and reduced tremors (Neuro Rehabilitation, December 2009). In this study, the scientists exposed the Parkinson's disease patients to low-frequency 30-hertz to 40-hertz for one minute to 30 minutes three times a week for four weeks, followed by a one-minute break. The patients have reported excellent improvement in their conditions.

Rather that viewing music only as a cultural and art phenomenon, music therapy can be implemented as medicine protocol for vibratory stimulus that attend to deficits that may result from many neurological conditions. Harmonic and soft music generates vibratory frequencies that expand memory dimensions and serve as a therapy for specific neurologic functions.

Music can stimulate the immune system and can reduce the production of harmful hormones

Dr. Ronny Enk, an expert in neurocognition at the Max Planck Institute, and the leader of scientific investigation aid: **"We believe that music can induce a pleasant state that leads to favorable physiological changes, reduce stress and improve the immune system."** When 300 people listened to pleasant dance music for 50 minutes. **Their immune defense systems were stimulated, their antibody levels increased significantly and their stress hormone cortisol decreased.**

The researchers, from the University of Sussex and the Max Planck Institute in Leipzig, Germany, in an unpublished study, also found that playing **soft and pleasant music** while patients were under anesthesia helped **reduce the levels of harmful stress hormones.** This study scientifically proved that music helps accelerate the recovery process in hospital patients.

17

Using Musical Sounds for Manipulation

What defines vibration, musical harmony, diatonic harmony and old Solfeggio?

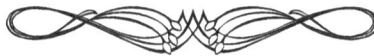

How can certain types of music be used for manipulation?

Listening to music above 95 dB (decibels,) reduces mental capacity, and physical reactions are reduced to 20%. It is imperative to take into consideration that music in clubs is usually played over 120 dB (decibels.) The loud music in clubs may influence people to consume more alcohol than normal. Loud music and dissonant frequencies have negative effects. The high volume de-harmonizes brain-waves and brain chemistry, and can also affect behavior and the body's physical functions.

Music can be used to manipulate people's minds. During the past several decades, the recording industry has acquired financial power and enrichment through CD sales and other media outlets. The quality of the music and its messages contain very little substance that can influence humanity positive and creatively.

Much of current music's themes, rhythms and structures often can impair human values. The music's subliminal messages can affect human behavior, especially in youngsters.

It is beneficial to listen to harmonious music that contains constructive messages, which can stimulate the natural healing process and help activate creative energy and positive thoughts. The mind and body are influenced by thoughts, sounds and vibrational frequencies daily.

What is vibration?

It is the effect produced by the pulsations and rapid changes of intonations and sounds. Rapid pulsating changes and sounds produce an emotional response.

What is musical harmony?

Musical harmony occurs when simultaneous combinations of musical tones are mixed in a chord that sounds pleasing. It is also occurs when we agree with our emotions and actions, which produces harmony between tones and melodies.

What is diatonic harmony?

The Greek prefix **dia** means through or across (as in the words diameter and diagonal.) In musical notation, the **tone** is the center of a key. Diatonic means through a tonal center or through the notes of a key.

Diatonic harmony is reflected in almost everything that exists. **Diatonic harmony** is composed of a musical scale of 5 full tones and 2 semitones, major tones, minor tones and other modalities resulting in a total of seven basic musical notes.

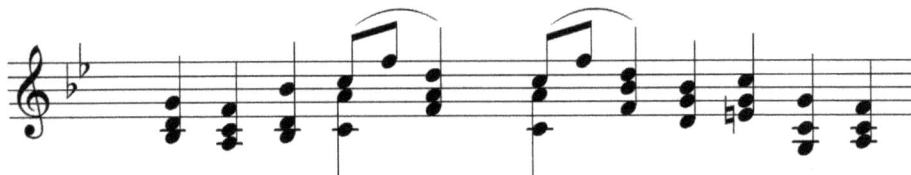

(Do, Re, Mi, Fa, Sol, La, Si)
(C, D, E, F, G, A, B)

7 musical notes in the diatonic harmony and their vibrational frequencies in Hertz in the old solfeggio:

C (UT) (Do) frequency = **396 hz = 9,** resonance with the root chakra.
D (Re) frequency = **417 hz = 3,** resonance with the reproductive chakra.
E (Mi) frequency = **528 hz = 6,** resonance with the solar plexus chakra.
F (Fa) frequency = **639 hz = 9,** resonance with the heart chakra.
G (Sol) frequency = **741 hz = 3,** resonance with the throat chakra.
A (La) frequency = **852 Hz = 6,** resonance with the third eye chakra.
B (Si) frequency = **963 Hz = 9,** resonance with the crown chakra.

The sum of the frequencies in Hertz of the notes in the diatonic harmony, originates chord values of 3, 6, and 9, which can alter the atomic structure of matter and contribute to the natural healing process of the body, mind and spirit. These chords are known as **Sacred Chords.**

The third of the six notes of the sacred and old solfeggio, the **E** note, which generates the 528 Hz frequency, is the frequency used by genetic engineers to repair DNA. Dr. Lee Lorenzen, a renowned American biochemist, declared that the frequency of **528 Hz** offers many benefits to maintaining good health, including the prevention of aging in DNA and cells. He did research on geometric hexagonal crystallizations of water with the purpose of stimulating the rejuvenation of DNA.

Seven has significance in terms of the time space continuum; There are seven musical notes in the musical scale, the human body has seven chakras or energy centers that resonate with chords of musical notes in the diatonic harmony, the rainbow has seven colors spectrum, planet Earth has seven continents and one week has seven days. The number 7 appears in many systems of creation, including in mystical books like the Bible and means a termination of some kind. "A divine command that has been fulfilled." It is the symbol of the whole universe created in 7 days (3 days heaven + 4 days Earth), it expresses the creation within which man evolves.

Dr. Joseph Puleo and harmonization of the chakras through old solfeggio frequencies

Dr. Joseph Puleo is an American naturopathic physician and herbalist. In his search of the musical scale of the **Lost Old Solfeggio**, he was inspired to study the Bible, where he discovered in Genesis, Chapter 7, Verses 12-83, a repeating pattern of six codes from a series of sacred numbers 3, 6 and 9.

When they were deciphered by the old method of Pythagoras and by reducing verse numbers to a single digit, the codes showed a series of six sound frequencies corresponding to the lost six missing tones of the **old solfeggio** scale.

The Old Solfeggio musical scale was used by monks in Gregorian chants in the original 432 Hz pitch and codes 3, 6 and 9. Eventually, the use of that frequency used in these songs, was archived in the vaults of the Vatican. The effectiveness of this sacred music activates a high state of awareness in people and ceased to be used in ceremonies in its original form.

In recent years a powerful healing tool, **The Ascension through the Ancient Solfeggio Frequencies,** has been reintroduced. Dr. Puleo and Dr. Leonard G. Horowitz, known for their work on AIDS research and vaccines, wrote about this topic in their book **Healing Codes for the Biological Apocalypse.** Dr. Joseph Puleo rediscovered that the **Old Sacred Solfeggio Tones** play an important role in stimulating the natural healing process of the body, mind and spirit. **Old Sacred Solfeggio Tones** can also help people reach an elevated state of consciousness.

Since its launch, Dr. Horowitz has continued his research on Old Solfeggio Tones. He believes that Old Solfeggio Frequencies can activate healing in all of mankind's ills. He has called this musical old solfeggio, the **Cycle of Perfect Sounds** because of its impeccable symmetry with mathematics and sacred geometry whereby three perfect triangles are produced.

Through geometry, mathematical practices, esoteric practices and Genesis, Chapter 7, Verses 12-83 in the Bible, it was found that the vibrational frequencies produced by the **Old Solfeggio** sounds may hold the keys that would give rise to the superconsciousness of man (superhumans,) to longevity, accelerated healing and dimensional travel. It has been said that the **Old Solfeggio** frequencies possess the power of creation, have effects on all matter and has the power to transform the conscience of human beings.

The solfeggio has 18 tones and 6 of them have been used for a long time in multiple environments with good results, even long before science made use of them.

Every human cell, organ, tissue, system, and thought generates a vibrational frequency, electro-magnetic energy, thermal energy (heat or cold) and sound. Our body systems need an adequate energy balance. Everything is about balance (**Yin & Yang.**) The balance of chakras depends on the way we think, speak, act, eat, care and behave in our daily lives. When the chakras are balanced and the vibrational frequencies are properly harmonized, they perform their functions normally and we attain good health.

Our minds and voices are powerful healing instruments. Each of the **Old Solfeggio** tones contains the exact frequency necessary to balance our chakras. Many secrets lie within the sound frequencies produced by the **Old Solfeggio**. It is said that the sound frequencies produced by the **Old Solfeggio** have the power to create and transform.

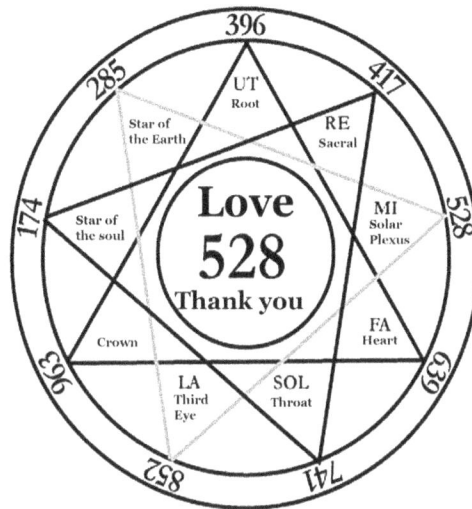

Illustration of the three triangles of the cycle of perfect sounds.

The frequencies of the Ancient Solfeggio are related to Sacred Geometry, and the numbers representing them are mathematically linked in a sequence very similar to the Fibonacci Sequence, or Fibonacci Numbers. They are basically 6 chords of ancient sacred sounds that were used in ancient Gregorian chants, and when sung imparted powerful uplifting frequencies and may influence in the process of ascension. These powerful frequencies corresponded to the syllables of the hymn to Saint John the Baptist and were rediscovered by Dr. Joseph Puleo in the mid-1970s. These frequencies have the power and the ability to alter the atomic structure of all matter, and the consciousness of living entities.

The 6 frequencies of the Old Solfeggio, the 7th frequency TI and its effects on emotions:

1. **UT (DO) (C)- 396 Hz - Releases fear and guilt.** This frequency is related to the **root chakra.** The conventional piano keyboard has 88 keys and does not offer the exact frequency of 396 Hz, but the closest note to that frequency in the piano is key 47, G4-g note, frequency 391.99 Hz.

2. **RE (D) - 417 Hz - Undoing of situations and facilitating changes.** This frequency is related to the **reproductive chakra.** The conventional piano keyboard of 88 keys does not provide the exact frequency of 417 Hz, but the closest note to that frequency in the piano is key 48, Note G #4/A b 4 - G#'/A b, frequency 415.30 Hz.

3. MI (E) - 528 Hz - Transformation and Miracles (DNA repair). This frequency is related to the **solar plexus chakra.** The conventional piano keyboard of 88 keys does not provide the exact frequency of 528 Hz, but the closest note to this frequency in the piano is key 52, Note C5 Tenor C - C" 2, eighth line, frequency 523.251 Hz.

4. FA (F) - 639 Hz - Connection and relationships. This frequency is related to the **heart chakra.** The conventional piano keyboard of 88 keys does not provide the exact frequency of 639 Hz, but the closest note to this frequency on the piano is key 55, Note D#5/Eb 5 - d#"/eb", frequency 622.254 Hz.

5. SOL (G) - 741 Hz - Activation of intuition, solve and clean. This frequency is related to the **throat chakra.** The conventional piano keyboard of 88 keys does not provide the exact frequency of 741 Hz, but the closest note to this frequency on the piano is key 58, Note F#5/Gb5 - f #"/gb, frequency 739.989 Hz.

6. LA (A) - 852 Hz - Returning to the spiritual order. This frequency is related to the **third eye chakra.** The conventional piano keyboard of 88 keys does not provide the exact frequency of 852 Hz, but the closest note to this frequency on the piano is key 60, Note G#5/Ab 5 - g#"/ab, frequency 830.609 Hz.

7. TI (SI) (B) - 963 Hz - The highest frequency of the solfeggio. This frequency is related with the **crown chakra. Waking to the most perfect state.** The conventional piano keyboard of 88 keys does not provide the exact frequency of 963 Hz, but the closest note to this frequency on the piano is key B5 987.77 – A#5 932.33 Hz.

Summary of the chords of an 88-key piano and their relationship with the musical resonance frequency of the chakras with the six frequencies of ancient solfeggio and the seventh frequency TI:

Musical note G4 = (391.99 Hz) = Root Chakra (C = 396 Hz)
Musical Note G#4/Ab = (415.30 Hz) = Reproductive Chakra (D = 417 Hz)
Musical Note C 5 = (523.251 Hz) = Solar Plexus Charka (E = 528 Hz)
Musical Note Re#5/Eb5 = (622.254 Hz) = Heart Chakra (F = 639 Hz)
* Musical Note F5 = (698.46 Hz) = Thymus Chakra (690 Hz)
Musical Note F#5/Gb5 = (739.989 Hz) = Throat Chakra (G = 741 Hz)
* Musical Note G5 = (783.99 Hz) = Cerebellum Chakra = (796.5 Hz)
Musical Note G#5/Lab5 = (830.609 Hz) = Third Eye Chakra (A = 852 Hz)
Musical Note B5 = (987.77 Hz), A #5 = (932.33 Hz) = Crown Chakra (B = 963 Hz)

* = Frequencies in Hz are included in the thymus and cerebellum chakra as references, but those two chakras are not included in the frequencies of ancient solfeggio.

When raising our vibrational frequencies we are able to activate healing at all levels. The **E Old Solfeggio note,** the frequency of **528 Hz,** is important because it allows transformation, miracles, and DNA repair. By raising our frequency and focusing on activating healing and concentrating our minds positively to achieve favorable changes, transformations and miracles manifest.

18

History of the Old Solfeggio

History of the Old Solfeggio, the Frequency of 432 Hz and the Fibonacci Spiral

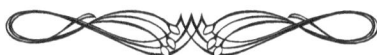

The origins of the ancient solfeggio

The origin of the ancient solfeggio begins with a very remarkable man who lived about 3,000 years BC, King David, he was given six tones that were created with the strings of an instrument that he used to make music, known as a lyre. The lyre was a harp made of wood. David was a man endowed with many talents, he was a musician, instrument maker, poet, composer, singer and is credited with writing more than half of the psalms. King David used the six tones of the ancient solfeggio in his musical compositions of the psalms and sang them in his praises to God. David passed the knowledge of the tones of the ancient solfeggio to Solomon.

The mathematics of the ancient solfeggio tunes coincides with the gematria and mathematics of the psalms. Solomon used those tones and gematria in the creation of the most sacred of the psalms "Song of Songs" or "Song of Solomon," but at some point, after Solomon, the tones were lost.

The ancient solfeggio has also been known as the sacred solfeggio and as the secret solfeggio. During the creation of the Gregorian chants, the tones of this solfeggio were rediscovered, which consisted of five notes and later a sixth note was added. These were based on the discoveries of Pythagoras and his harmony "The music of the spheres", but also they were lost.

In the 1990s, Dr. Josep Puleo received the secret of the gematria of the lost ancient solfeggio reading the Bible and discovered in Genesis Chapter 7, Verses 12-83 that there is a pattern of six repetition codes from a series of Sacred numbers 3, 6 and 9. Using the ancient method of Pythagoras and reducing the numbers of verses to a single digit, obtained the codes of six sound frequencies that correspond to the tones of the lost solfeggio, also known as the ancient solfeggio, the sacred solfeggio or the secret solfeggio.

History of Old Solfeggio versus the diatonic harmony

The origin of what is called **Old Solfeggio** emerged from a medieval hymn to John the Baptist, which has the peculiarity that the first six lines of the music begin, respectively, in the first six successive notes of the scale. The first syllable of each line was sung to a note and higher degree than the first syllable of the line that preceded it.

Gradually these syllables were associated and identified with their respective notes and as each syllable ended in a vowel, they were adapted for vocal use. Therefore **UT** was replaced by **C (Do).**

Italian Guido d'Arezzo, (995 AD - 1050 AD) was a Benedictine monk. In 1026, he introduced the staff, the original scale of the Old Solfeggio and invented the writing of the notes C(Do), D(Re), E(Mi), F(Fa), G(Sol), A(La). The Old Solfeggio was used by singers to learn songs more easily. He was a medieval music theorist whose principles served as a foundation for modern Western musical notation.

To create the musical scale, Guido d'Arezzo, used the first syllable of each verse of a hymn that was dedicated to St. John, which is attributed to Paulo the Deacon and says:

> **Ut** queant laxis,
> **Re**sonare libris,
> **Mi**ra gestorum,
> **Fa**muli tuorum,
> **Sol**ve polluti,
> **La**bii reatum, Sancte Joannes

The hymn dedicated to St. John was written in Latin.

Later, due to difficulties in singing **UT**, it was changed to **DO (C)**. It took until the sixteenth century (five centuries) for the musical scale to be completed as we know it today. The same hymn that Arezzo used in the XI century with the initials of Saint John was written **Sante Ioanes** and formed the seventh note **SI (B)**; the eighth note was the repetition of **DO (C)**.

Guido d'Arezzo was the first to embrace change in the old solfeggio in the XI century. To complete the series, Le Marie, a French musician from the XVII century added **Si (B)** as the seventh note of the musical scale.

Other research also indicates that after **Pope John I** (523-526 AC) was canonized as **St. John**, the musical scale of the old solfeggio was changed. The seventh note **SI (B)** was added in his name and later became **TI.** These changes significantly altered the frequencies in the songs used in masses and ceremonies in churches of that time. Today, the letters **A B, C, D, E. F,** and **G** are used to designate the musical notes.

The most common names of the sounds are:

English: C, D, E, F, G, A, B
German: C, D, E, F, G, A, H
Spanish, Italian, French: Do, Re, Mi, Fa, Sol, La, Si

Alterations of the old solfeggio notes weakened the spiritual impact of the church's hymns. The music was arranged with harmony and mathematical resonances, and the frequencies provided inspiration in getting closer to God. The changes influenced changes in conceptual thinking, affecting and distancing mankind from God.

The old solfeggio was destined to be music for the soul and the **Secret Ear.** The changing notes altered the matrix of thoughts that elevated and connected the spirit to higher spheres. To a large degree, there was a negative change that altered the original purpose of the harmony of the old solfeggio.

The original scale of the **Old Solfeggio** was **UT, RE, MI, FA, SOL, LA.** According to definitions found in Webster's Dictionary and the Greek Apocrypha, these original frequencies could turn pain into joy, repair DNA , help connect with spiritual family, resolve situations, increase intuitiveness and to help return to a spiritual order.

432 Hz Frequency

432 Hz frequency resonates with all harmonic principles of nature and is found everywhere in nature and history. Nada Brahma, as written in the ancient **Vedas** means **"The universe is sound."** Sound is the sacred element of the universe that permeates all living and non-living things to reach the structure of DNA. Before 1930, instruments' intonations fit in the sacred Harmony of **432 Hz.** After 1930 instruments' intonations were changed from **432 Hz** to **440** Hz.

The **432 Hz** frequency vibrates and oscillates with natural principles and the propagation of harmonic sound, and unifies the properties of light, time, space, matter, gravity and electromagnetism. The Sun, Saturn, Earth and Moon oscillate and vibrate with the same frequency of **432 Hz.**

The **432 Hz** frequency has a positive effect at the body's cellular level and at the level of consciousness. Atoms and DNA vibrate and oscillate in resonance with the **PHI** spiral.

Great musicians, such as Mozart and Verdi, used pitch and tone of LA=432 Hz (A=432 Hz) in their music, concerts, operas and compositions. Although 432 Hz is only 8 vibrations per second different from the standard tuning of 440 Hz, the slight difference seems to have a remarkable effect on our consciousness.

There is a growing movement in the field of music and metaphysics that is attempting to recover optimal integrity in the music industry through the use of the 432 Hz tune. In 2008, Dutch journalist Richard Huisken founded a committee called "Back to 432

Hz." They argue that this original pitch was used in ancient cultures and in high quality musical instruments as the Stradivarius violin.

According to Richard Huisken, music tuned at 432 Hz is smoother, brighter, clearer and easier to hear. Many people who listen to music tuned at 432 Hz can achieve a very good state of meditation and relaxation of body and mind. The natural musical tone of the universe at 432 Hz gives a more harmonious and pleasant sound than the pitch currently used at 440 Hz.

The pitch and tone at 432 Hz seems to work on the heart chakra (feelings), so it could have a positive influence on the spiritual development of the listener. Some people who are not able to distinguish the difference of 8 Hz say that music is more pleasant. This is due to its greater wavelength.

432 Hz provides greater clarity than 440 Hz so there is no need to play music at 440 Hz. This can reduce noise and hearing damage, as long as the volume is not too high. Researchers and musicians, such as Coreen Morsink (pianist and music teacher), report that they feel calmer, happier and more relaxed when they play music at 432 Hz.

Music based on the pitch of 440 Hz produces blockages and stagnant emotions. Lowering just 8 Hz in tone and pitch can help a person to feel more flexible and spontaneous. 432 Hz tuning produces energy and brings the person to a state of natural relaxation.

Where does the pitch and tone of 432 Hz come from?

According to Ananda Bosman, researcher and international musician, ancient Egyptian instruments unearthed from Egyptian tombs are largely tuned in pitch of A = 432 Hz. The ancient Greeks tuned their instruments and sang predominantly to 432 Hz. Within the Eleusnian Greek Ancient Mysteries, Orfeo, the God of Music, Death and Rebirth were the guardian of the ambrosia and music that activated transformation. Ananda Bosman's instruments were tuned and pitched at 432 Hz.

Italian composer Giuseppe Verdi placed the note LA (A) exactly at 432 Hz because this pitch is ideal for the voices of opera singers. Jamie Buturff, a sound researcher, noticed that some Tibetan monks tuned their handmade instruments in pitch and tone of 432 Hz. He played a CD with Tibetan bowls music, and with a Korg tuner discovered that they were tuned at 432 Hz.

This musical tuning can be found along various religions and cultures of the ancient

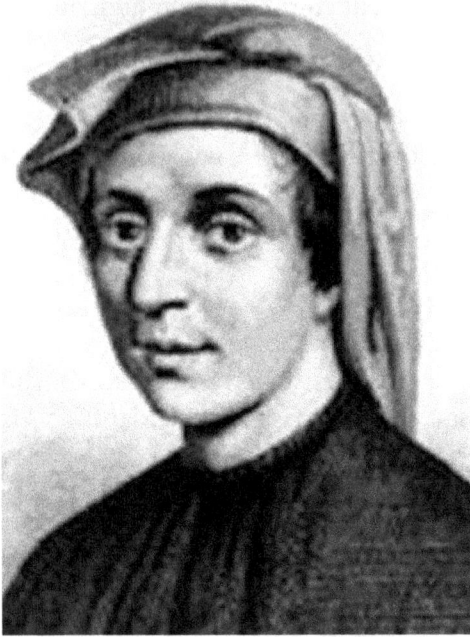

Leonardo Pisano Bigollo Fibonacci.

world. Even today, many musicians have reported positive effects when tuning and pitching their instruments at 432 Hz. They feel more relaxed during performances and claim there is a better response from the audience.

Why did the modern world forget the pitch and tone at 432 Hz?

In 1885, it was decided that the 440 Hz pitch was standard. A year earlier, Giuseppe Verdi wrote a letter to the Music Commission of the Italian government stating: "Since France has adopted a standard pitch, I advise that we also follow the example and formally request that the orchestras of several cities in Italy, including the Scala of Milan, to lower the tuning pitch to a pitch that fits the French rule. If the institute and the musical commission of our government believe that by mathematical requirements we must reduce the vibrations of the tuning fork from 435 Hz to the tuning fork of 432 Hz of the French tune, the difference is so small, almost imperceptible to the ear, I agree willingly with this." - *Giuseppe Verdi*

Unfortunately, Giuseppe Verdi was unsuccessful in his attempt. The American Federation of Musicians accepted the LA 440 (A440) as the standard pitch in 1917. Around 1940 the United States presented 440 Hz worldwide, and finally, in 1953, it became the standard ISO 16.

It is theorized that the change of 432 Hz to 440 Hz was dictated by the Nazi propaganda minister Joseph Goebbels. He used it to make people think and feel a certain way and to make them prisoners of a certain consciousness. The theory about Joseph Goebbels is certainly interesting, but the real reason for the change to 440 Hz has not been clearly explained.

It is said that the change of pitch from 440 Hz to 432 Hz will not be an easy task, and not due to the influence of any nefarious organization. The reason is trivial. Most musical instruments can be adjusted and tuned at 432 Hz, but this is not easy for all instruments. For example, most wind instruments cannot play at 432 Hz because it would change their internal harmonic structure. The change would require the construction of new instruments.

Many ancient instruments were built and tuned to 432 Hz because the tone is closely related to the universe. Each of us has to search, discover and feel the universal and natural sound of 432 Hz, which is directly related to the natural frequencies of our micro and macrocosmic universe.

Intonation and tuning of 432 Hz directly resonates with nature and can generate healthy effects to listeners. It brings natural harmony and balance of the third dimension and connects people with a higher consciousness. The pure and clean energy of 432 Hz eliminates mental blocks and can open wide paths towards a fuller life.

The musical tone of 432 Hz is consistent with the golden ratio PHI. It can unify the properties of light, time, space, matter, gravity and magnetism with biology and DNA. The natural pitch of 432 Hz can have deep effects at the cellular level and on consciousness.

The musical tone of 432 Hz connects to the numbers used in the construction of a variety of ancient works and sacred places. An example is in the sophisticated construction of the Great Pyramid of Cheops in Egypt, which method remains unknown to architects and engineers. The 432 Hz musical tone is softer, brighter, easier and more beautiful for human ears than the tone of 440 Hz.

If we transform musical instruments to the 432 Hz intonation and use the 432 Hz pitch at concerts instead of 440 Hz, our atoms and DNA would resonate with the spiral nature of Phi.

The spiral nature of Phi, the 432 Hz pitch and its relationship with Fibonacci's sequence.

To understand Fibonacci's spiral sequence we must understand how it was originated. The story began in Pisa, Italy, in 1202 (XII century) when Leonardo Pisano Bigollo Fibonacci was in his twenties. He discovered a simple numerical sequence that is the basis of an amazing mathematical relationship behind Phi.

From 0 and 1 each new sequence number is simply the sum of the two previous numbers: 0, 1, 1, 2, 3, 5, 8, 13, 21, 34, 55, 89, 144...

The ratio of each successive pair of numbers in the sequence approximates to Phi

(1.618), where 5 is divided by 3 = 1.666...and 8 divided by 5 is 1.60.

The following graph shows how the ratio of successive numbers in the Fibonacci sequence changes to Phi. After 40 numbers in the sequence, the ratio is accurate to 15 decimal places (1.618033988749895...)

The Fibonacci sequence produces spirals and similar curves and is known as the **golden ratio**. This fascinating phenomenon has been appreciated for its beauty, but no one can explain why it occurs so clearly in the world of the arts, nature and the universe.

The most famous and beautiful examples of the Fibonacci sequence in nature are spiral structures in a variety of trees and flowers. Many flowers have the mystical spiral shape of Fibonacci's sequence. A daisy has a central core consisting of small pins arranged in opposite spirals. There are usually 21 petals that spiral to the left and 34 to the right. A mountain aster can have 13 spirals to the left and 21 to the right. Sunflowers are the most spectacular example because they typically have 55 spirals inclined in one direction and 89 in the opposite direction and they express the Fibonacci number sequence 89 + 55 = 144.

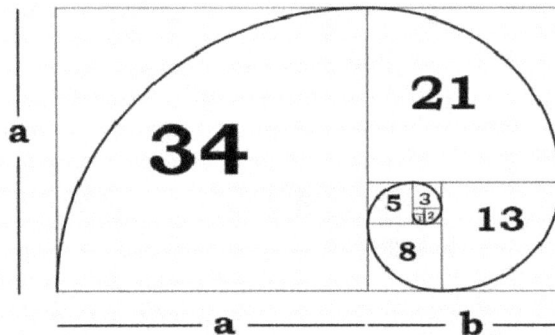

Why does the Fibonacci sequence have a spiral shape?

Mother Nature must have found an evolutionary advantage in the organization of plant structures in spiral shapes showing the Fibonacci sequence.

There is no exact answer. In 1875 a mathematician named Wiesner provided a mathematical demonstration of the spiral arrangement of leaves on a branch. The proportions of Fibonacci's spirals offer the most efficient way for plants and flowers to receive the maximum amount of sunlight.

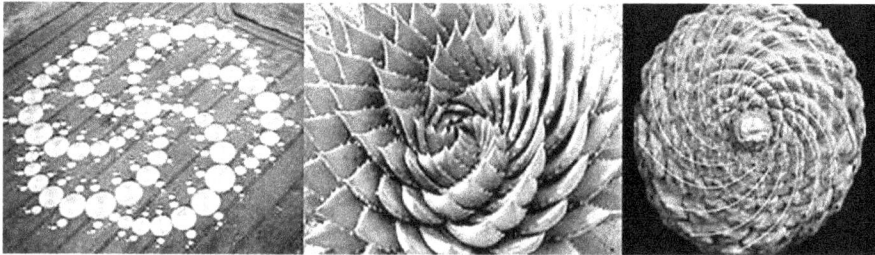

The golden ratio and the spiral recurring in nature and the universe.

Recently, a botanist at Cornell University, called Karl Niklas decided to test this hypothesis in his laboratory. He discovered that Fibonacci's spiral allows almost all reasonable arrangements of leaves and flowers to have the capacity to receive the same amount of sunlight.

The movement of electrons and protons around the atom, the movement of galaxies and planets, and our DNA all move in spiral form, produce sound frequencies and are in a constant state of vibration.

Storms, hurricanes, tornadoes, sound waves and water when we throw a stone into a lake all move in a spiral shape.

In conclusion, there is a close relationship between music in the intonation of 432 Hz, the spiral nature of Phi and the Fibonacci sequence. These three are directly related to the natural frequencies of our micro and macrocosmic universe.

Music and the Fibonacci Sequence and Phi

The Fibonacci series appears in the foundation of aspects of art, beauty and life. Even music has a foundation in the series, as: There are 13 notes in the span of any note through its octave. A scale is composed of 8 notes, of which the 5th and 3rd notes create the basic foundation of all chords, and are based on a tone which are a combination of 2 steps and 1 step from the root tone, that is the 1st note of the scale.

Musical frequencies are based on Fibonacci ratios. The scales of the actual western Chromatic and Diatonic music are based on natural harmonics that are created by ratios of frequencies. The ratios found in the first seven numbers of the Fibonacci series (0, 1, 1, 2, 3, 5, 8) are related to key frequencies of musical notes.

Musical instrument design is often based on phi and the golden ratio. Violins crafted by the master Luthier Antonio Stradivari are famously known for their exquisite tonal quality and aesthetic form. Genuine Stradivarius violins are highly sought after and are the most valuable instruments in the string-playing world because of their unmatched sound. However, what is most amazing about his violins is that they were designed and built around the Golden Ratio. The current design of high quality speaker wires are also designed and built using the Golden Ratio.

The Golden Ratio or Golden Section is a mathematical ratio that artists, architects, and musicians have also used to craft their art for centuries. The famous Leornardo Da Vinci futuered the Divine Proporcion in many of his paintings mainly because **"it is a natural way"** of dealing with balance, dimensions and divisions of time.

The Fibonacci sequence also known as the Golden Ratio has captivated scientists, mathematicians, designers and artists through history. Its fundamental characteristic demonstrates its functionality in nature.

The number of **petals in a flower** consistently follows the Fibonacci sequence of Phi 0.618034 allowing for the best possible exposure to sunlight and other factors. **The head seeds in sunflowers** are produced at the center and migrate towards the outside to fill the space in a spiral shape. The **seed pods on a pinecone** are arranged in a spiral pattern. Each cone consists of a pair of spirals, each one spiraling upwards in opposing directions. The shape of **some spider's webs, some horns of goats, snail shells** as well as the **human inner ear** follow the spiral logarithmic shape. The angular speed rotation of **galaxies and the Milky Way** follow the spiral logarithmic patterns of about 12 degrees. Hurricanes also have a spiral shape. The human face and also non-human face, mouth and nose are positioned at a golden ratio distance between the eyes and the lower part of the chin. The eyes and the ears also follow a spiral shape. Leonardo da Vinci's drawing of the old man and the Mona Lisa painting show the squared inside the Golden Rectangle in the face of the old man and in the Mona Lisa's body.

Famous Artists that Incorporated the Golden Ratio in their Art Compositions and Designs

Leornardo da Vinci, "The Last Supper," and "The Annunciation," **Michelangelo's** painting of "The Creation of Adam" on the ceiling of the Sistine Chapel in the Vatican, **Rafael** "The School of Athens," **Botticelli** "The Birth of Venus," **Pierre Seurat** the French impressionist "attacked every canvas by the golden ratio," **Edward Burne Jones**

"The Golden Stairs," **Salvador Dali** "The Sacrament of the Last Supper," and others.

The golden ratio offers opportunities to connect and to understand the conceptions of ratio and proportion to geometry expressed in the universe, in nature, in art and music.

The Infinite Healing Power is within each of us

How we live life,
And express our thoughts and words,
During each second and
Through our daily actions,
Influence immensely on our internal ability,
to achieve peace, harmony, prosperity, and happiness,
And activate the internal natural healing process in our atoms, molecules and cells.

The level of consciousness is expressed through our thoughts and actions,
and It is the life force that influences in everything that we attract to our life's.
It is the universal law in which for every action there is a reaction.
Releasing negative thoughts, fears, anger, selfishness, hatred, resentment, envy, lust and guilt,
The spark of light activates the heart,
With the immutable cosmic energy of love and light
Which raises consciousness and the mind,
Healing and miracles manifest. - J.E.M.

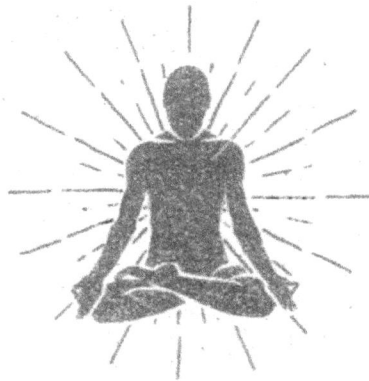

When we sing harmonic vocal sounds, do prayers, mantras, affirmations,
listen to soft music and meditate, we free the mind,
And it is the best medicine and natural therapy that helps in the
recovery for any condition and that leads us on the path to a creative, productive and
happy life. - JEM

If you dedicate to yourself just a few minutes of the twenty-four hours of the day to do this
practice, you will transform your life. - J.E.M.

19

432 Hz, 8Hz Frequencies and Schumann's Resonance

The secret of the 432 Hz pitch, its relationship to the frequency of 8 Hz and Schumann's resonance.

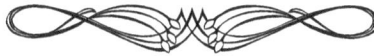

⁂

The secret behind the tuning and intonation at 432 Hz.

To understand the healing power of 432 Hz, we must first learn about the 8 Hz frequency. It is said that 8Hz is the fundamental rhythm of our planet Earth. Earth's heartbeat is best known as **Schumann's Resonance** and it is named in honor of physicist Winfried Otto Schumann who presented this mathematical discovery in 1952.

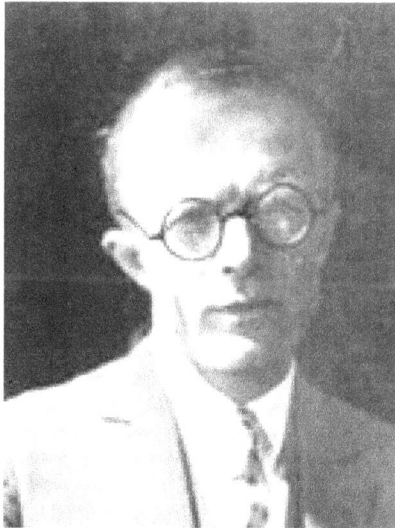

Dr. Winfried Otto Schumann

Schumann's Resonance is a global electromagnetic resonance that has its origin in electrical discharges of lightning produced within the cavity between Earth's surface and the ionosphere. This cavity resonates with electromagnetic waves at extremely low frequencies of about **7.86 Hz to 8 Hz.**

Thought waves originated by humans have a range of 14 Hz to 40 Hz. This waveband only includes certain types of dendrites on the brain cells of the nervous system, especially in the left hemisphere of the brain (the more rational side), which is also the center of activity.

If the cerebral hemispheres are synchronized at **8 Hz,** they work with more harmony and with a maximum flow of information. The **8Hz** frequency seems to be the key to the brain's maximum efficiency.

The **8Hz** frequency is also the frequency of the double helix in **DNA** replication. Melatonin and pinoline work in DNA, inducing an 8Hz signal to enable replication of DNA and meiosis. One form of the body's superconductive temperature is evident in this process.

What is the relationship between 8 Hz frequency and 432 Hz intonation and tuning frequency?

In the musical scale where A has a frequency of 440 Hz, the C note is approximately 261.656 Hz. On the other hand, if we take 8Hz as a starting point and we follow up by five eighths (the seven notes of the scale five times), we arrive at a frequency of 256 Hz in the note A whose scale has a frequency of 432 Hz.

According to the harmonic principle by which any sound produced automatically resonates with other multiples of the frequency, when we play C at 256 Hz, the C note of the other octaves vibrates synchronously and activates the 8Hz frequency. This is why the musical tone of 432 Hz is also known as the **Cientifica Tuning.**

The tuning setting and 432 Hz tone was approved unanimously in the Congress of Italian Musicians in 1881 and was recommended by physicists Joseph Sauveru and Felix Savart, and Italian scientist Bartolomeo Grassi Landi.

Conversely, the 440 Hz tuning frequency was chosen in London in 1953 as the reference frequency from which all music has been adapted. However, it has been defined as inharmonious because it has no scientific relationship with the physical laws governing the universe.

According to the above information, playing and listening to music that has been tuned at 432 Hz would have natural resonance with our bodies and environment. This would fill us with a sense of peace and well-being.

Listening to music that has been tuned to the **Scientific Frequency of 432 Hz** would benefit all beings and the planet. The opposite occurs when listening to music in tune with the **inharmonious frequency of 440 Hz** which generally produces stress, negative behavior, and unstable emotions.

Listening to music in pitch and tone of 432 Hz has direct resonance within the body, releases emotional obstacles and expands consciousness. Music in pitch and tone of 432 Hz, harmonizes the body and mind with the natural vibrational frequency of the universe and can expand consciousness and knowledge.

The vibrational frequency of the Earth or the heartbeat of our planet known as Schumann's Resonance is changing.

In 1952, German physicist Winifred Otto Schumann, found that Earth is surrounded by an electromagnetic field at the bottom of the ionosphere. This expands 65 miles above us and generates a global vibrational frequency electromagnetic resonance.

This electromagnetic field (**Schumann's Resonance**) has a resonance of about 7.83 Hz. The fundamental rhythm of Earth is about 8 Hz. This rate key is also defined as Earth's heartbeat.

Similar to a pacemaker, it is responsible for the balance of the biosphere, the environment and all forms of life on Earth. All vertebrates and the brain have the same frequency of 7.83 Hertz.

For thousands of years, Earth's vibrational frequency, also known as Earth's heartbeat, had the same pulse rate, and life unfolded in relative ecological balance. However, from the 1980s, and more sharply from the 1990s, the frequency increased from 7.83 Hz to 11 Hz, and from 11 Hz to 13 Hz respectively and has continued to rise.

Empirical evidence shows that human health declines outside the natural biological vibrational frequency of 7.83 Hertz or 8 Hertz. Whenever astronauts made space travel out of the vibrational frequency of **Schumann's Resonance,** they got sick. If they were subjected to the action of a Schumann's simulator, they would recover balance and health.

There is a recurring argument among cosmologists and biologists about whether Earth is a living superorganism; whether Earth and humanity form a single entity. Human beings are made from Earth's elements, and can feel, think, and love. Since humans have the same bioelectrical natural vibration they are surrounded and affected by **Schumann's Resonance Frequency.**

The increase of Schumann's electromagnetic vibrational frequency from 7.83 Hz to 13 Hz is activating changes on Earth. Earth's heartrate increased from 7.83 Hz to 13 Hz from 1980 to 2000 and continues to increase. This is causing ecological imbalances, climatic disturbances, volcanic activity, rising bodies of water and tsunamis.

Schumann's electromagnetic frequency also produces changes in the bioelectric environment and can affect humans' brain waves. This can also affect human behavior and create tension in the world.

Due to overall acceleration, a 24-hour day is actually about 16 hours, as if time were collapsing. The perception that everything is happening too fast is not illusory. This could be due to changes in the vibrational frequency of Schumann's electromagnetic resonance.

As the solar system and Earth move to new paths and dimensions, changes occur in the vibrational frequency of Schumann's electromagnetic resonance. Earth's heartbeat is constantly changing and can affect the planet's inhabitants. Gaia, that living superorganism that is Mother Earth, may be looking for ways to return to its natural balance...

20

528 Hz Frequency and its Effects on DNA

528 Hz is the frequency of miracles and love.

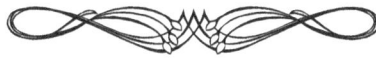

528 Hz frequency and how it affects DNA

Our DNA is not written in stone; it can be transformed. According to Dr. Leonard Horowitz, the 528 Hz frequency has the ability to heal damaged DNA. Dr. Horowitz learned about this from Dr. Lee Lorenzen. Dr. Lorenzen formulated his theories about repairs to DNA when he was using the frequency of 528 Hertz to create clustered water.

The clustered water is broken down into small stable rings or groups of small rings. Our DNA is found in the cell nucleus and has a membrane that allows water to flow through it clear and free from impurities. Because clustered water is grouped into smaller rings than regular water, it passes quickly through the cell membrane and takes less time to remove impurities. When there is a high agglomeration of water molecules within the cell, waste products remain within the cell and it is more difficult for them to exit through the cell membrane. The same applies if there is a high agglomeration of water molecules outside the cell – it is difficult for nutrition products to pass through the cell membrane and enter the cell.

The agglomeration of water molecules inside and outside the cells leads to disease because the detoxification process is affected.

Richard J. Saykally, from California University (UC Berkeley) explained that structured clustered water molecules confer special properties to DNA and are essential for the proper functioning of DNA. Properly hydrated DNA has more energy than when dehydrated.

Professor Saykally and other geneticists at the University of California, Berkeley have shown that a slight reduction in the energy of water affects the DNA matrix.

Dr. Lee Lorenzen and other researchers found that clusters of six-sided molecules of water, which form hexagonal crystals, support the matrix of healthy DNA.

Depletion of the DNA matrix is a fundamental process that adversely affects each physiological function of the body. Biochemist Steve Chemiski says that hexagonal groups of clustered water vibrate at a specific resonance frequency of 528 Hertz and benefit the double helix of DNA.

These revelations do not mean that the sound frequency of 528 Hz will repair its DNA in a direct way. However, the 528 Hertz sound frequency is effective in separating the molecule clusters of water. The frequency of 528 Hz can help eliminate impurities at the cellular level, balance the metabolism, and contribute to good health.

How can music and the 528 Hz frequency affect DNA?

Sounds and vibrations can activate DNA. In 1998, Dr. Glen Rein, from the Quantum Biology Laboratory Research Department in New York, conducted experiments with DNA in vitro. He put DNA into testing tubes and exposed them to rock and classical music. He included Sanskrit music and Gregorian chants, which have a frequency of 528 Hz. The sound of Sanskrit music and Gregorian chants were broadcasted through scalar audio waves.

The effects of the music were determined by measuring the absorption of ultraviolet light from the DNA samples after one hour of exposure to the music.

The results of the experiments showed that classical music caused an increase of 1.1% in absorption, and rock music caused 1.8% decrease in absorption, which indicated that there was no effect. However, Gregorian chants caused an increase in absorption of 5.0% and 9.1% in two separate experiments. Sanskrit chanting caused an increase in absorption of 5.8% and 8.2% in two separate experiments. This indicates that both types of sacred music, Gregorian chants and songs in Sanskrit, can affect the functions, balance and development of DNA. Glen Rein's experiment indicate that music can resonate with DNA in the body.

Classical music showed only an increase in absorption of 1.1% in this experiment. However, it has been shown in other scientific studies that have very favorable effects on brain states Alpha, Delta, Theta and Beta.

Music resonates with human DNA. Dr. Glen Rein's experiment indicates that sacred music and Sanskrit music can resonate with human DNA. Although these experiments were performed with purified DNA isolated in test tubes, there is a high probability that the frequencies associated with these forms of music can affect DNA in the body.

Another study entitled "Effect of sound waves in the synthesis of nucleic acids and proteins in chrysanthemum" concludes that some genes induced by stress can be activated under sound stimulation and the level of transcription increases.

If genes can be activated or deactivated by "sound simulations," then it is reasonable to conclude that DNA can be affected by sound frequencies.

Harmonic sound can have a positive impact on the body. The effect of sound frequency 528 Hz on DNA and cells of the body may have some scientific validity. However, it is necessary to do more research to demonstrate DNA repair.

528 Hz - Frequency of love

According to Dr. Leonard Horowitz, 528 Hertz is the fundamental frequency for the "musical-mathematical matrix of creation." More than any previously discovered sound; the "frequency of LOVE" resonates in the hearts of all beings. It connects our hearts and the essence of our spirit with the reality of spiral motion in heaven and earth.

The frequency of love is known as **the miracle note** of the original musical notation of the Solfeggio. It has been confirmed by independent researchers that these primary creative frequencies were used by ancient priests and healers of advanced civilizations to manifest miracles.

Mathematician Victor Showell described 528 Hz as the fundamental frequency of the mathematical constants Pi, Phi, and the golden ratio, which is evident in all designs of nature.

Victor Showell and John Stuart Reid (pioneers in acoustic research and cymatic measurements) have demonstrated that 528 Hz frequency is essential in the formation of circles and spirals in sacred geometry and it is also consistent with the structure and restructuring of Hydrosonic DNA.

528 Hz frequency is equal to 5 + 2 + 8 = 15, and 15 is equal to 1 + 5 = 6 (using the mathematical method of Pythagoras.) The number "6" is the spiral symbol traveling from heaven down to Earth and also forms the sacred hexagonal geometry shape of the structure of water molecules, which consists of two major triangles that give rise to "6" smaller triangles.

In fact, the frequency of love can be critical to the dissemination of all energy and matter in accordance with the laws of physics.

Dr. Joseph Puleo, naturopath and scholar of "The Bible Code", and Dr. Horowitz, speak in their book that the 528 Hz frequency is the note "E" in the original musical scale notation of the ancient solfeggio and means "Miracles." Physicists and mathematicians have published evidence that the 528 Hz frequency is defined as the frequency of love and is essential for the universal construction of Pi, Phi, the Fibonacci series, sacred geometry, the circle, the square, the hexagonal ring of organic chemistry and the world of biology. Plants grow due to the presence of chlorophyll, which has the 528 Hz frequency. The real Da Vinci code also has to do with these findings according to Dr. Horowitz.

Tone of miracles - 528 Hz

528 Hz frequency is known as the tone of **miracles,** which brings remarkable and extraordinary changes. Dr. Joseph Puleo analyzed the meaning of tone using Latin dictionaries and occult publications from the Webster Dictionary and found that the E tone is characterized by (according to the definition):

1. An extraordinary event that surpasses all known human powers or natural forces and is attributed to a divine or supernatural cause.

2. An excellent example of overcoming something, a wonder [1125-1175]; ME<L Miraculum = Mira (Ri) to marvel at. Fr. (French): sighting, with the aim of maintaining backlit. (Gestorum: gesture, movements to express the thought, excitement, any action, communication, etc. intended for effect.)

The 528 Hz frequency cleans contaminated water from the Gulf of Mexico

The tone of 528 Hz, which is associated with DNA repair, was used to clean the contaminated water in the Gulf of Mexico. In 2010 John Hutchinson, an expert in electromagnetic energy from Vancouver, BC, Canada, helped to purify contaminated water in the Gulf of Mexico after the BP oil spill. He and his research partner Nancy Hutchinson (formerly known as Nancy Lazaryan) used the frequency of 528 Hz and other G-F (Sol-fa) tones to lessen oil from the contaminated water.

The contaminated area was treated with the frequencies for four hours the first day, and the next morning the water had cleaned and looked clear. The test was completed with four additional hours of RF frequency. The machine generating the frequencies was about 25 meters from the waters of the beach.

The restoration of water vitality was confirmed by the return of fish, dolphins and barnacle crustaceans (crustaceans that grow on ocean rocks). Nancy said, "Water that was murky and brown had turned to light-green color. Two dolphins came to five feet of water and many fish stocks and crabs were active in those waters."

Oil and grease before the frequency treatment had 7 ppm (parts per million or milligrams per liter), while samples that had undergone frequency exposure had less than 1 ppm.

John Hutchinson's method of using sound and radio frequencies almost removes oil and toxins completely, and has no dangerous side effects. John and Nancy can clean contaminated waters within a mile radius in just one 24-hour session.

The Analytical Chemistry Testing Laboratory, Inc. (ACT) stated: "While the technology is not fully known by the undersigned, it is evident that the process can have an extreme value, and should be given the opportunity to be presented and tested at a greater scale."

The favorable effects of 528 Hz frequency

528 Hz frequency is the **bio-energy of health** and longevity. It is the divine voice and the harmonic vibration that elevates the heart in harmony with heaven. The world would be a place of harmony and peace if the love vibration of 528 Hz frequency coming from the sunlight rays that regenerate the air is active in the hearts of all beings on Earth.

Every day more people are awakening spiritually, mentally and emotionally and they choose to be in tune with the frequency of love 528 Hz. This is the healing frequency that helps the flowing of rhythm in perfect harmony.

The rays of the sun produce the sound, light, the rainbow and the green color of chlorophyll in 528 Hz (528nm) frequency and energizes air with oxygen restoring balance, health, and harmony.

The music on 528 frequency can help heal diseases, bring peace, harmony and can also help strengthen people's immune systems.

Researcher and music therapist "Lunartunar" in his recent research stated that John Lennon's song "Imagine" which sold and continue selling millions of copies was recorded on the musical tone of 528 Hz. Apparently, John Lennon, writer, singer, musician, peace activist and one of the main members of "The Beatles" group from the 1960's decade had knowledge of the power of 528 Hz frequency. The song and deep message of the song "Imagine" still continues impacting thousands of people in many countries in the world, producing the same feeling and strong vibration of peace, harmony, serenity and hope. The musical theme "imagine" promotes a powerful message for the activation of collective consciousness of love, peace and harmony in humanity. The 528 Hz musical tone generates exactly the frequency that imparts the powerful creative, regenerative and healing energy of love.

Chlorophyll is the most powerful biological healing pigment and vibrates in the 528 Hz frequency that is encoded in green grass and must vegetation on Earth. The animal kingdom survives consuming green grass and vegetation, and people that eat greens and organic vegetables regain good health. When consuming greens the 528 Hz frequency encoded in chlorophyll activates blood, cells and DNA with the healing frequency of love. The air we breathe, the 'prana' of life," or the "chi" as defined by Qigong Masters and in oriental medicine, is also filled with the vibrational frequency of love - 528 Hz.

Recent scientific findings have observed that "faithful prayer energizes the heart in C=528 Hz frequency," and people can manifest the objective desired and even produce miracles when comes with the power of intention and visualization from the heart and with faith. It is even more powerful especially when it is done musically through the recitation of prayers, affirmations, chanting mantras and singing songs in groups.

Almost all of our global economy is built on a foundation where conditions, illnesses and death have a great influence on people. The powerful sound of 528 Hz frequency can solve the world's problems. If we take initiative and use the frequency of 528 Hz, we could restore human consciousness in all is powers and potential.

Elevating Our Vibrational Frequency

We live in an ocean of Energy, Frequency and Vibrations. This concept was very well explained by the physicist and scientist Nikola Tesla. Everything in the macro-cosmic universe and in our microcosmic universe, inside and outside our bodies is in a constant state of vibration. Energy is being absorbed from many sources including the celestial bodies, space, sunlight, the moon's magnetic energy, water, air, Earth's magnetic energy and vegetation. Everything around and inside us is energy and is constantly generating vibrations and sounds. Earth's vegetation absolves the frequency from the cosmic sunlight's rays, and through photosynthesis oxygen is released to help restore balance, health and vitality in all life forms on Earth.

The Sun's light frequency is the main source of energy that sustains life in our planet, and has a strong effect on all life forms on Earth. According to Dr. Leonard Horowitz, the 528 frequency is the bio-energy of health, love and harmony and can assist with restoring equilibrium. It is the Universal Healer and is associated with DNA repair. This frequency is also present in the Sun's rays of light and encoded in vegetation.

When our spirit, mind and body is in tune with mother Earth, nature and its natural elements, our vibrational frequency is high and we enjoy regenerative energy, good health and vitality. But when we are not in tune with mother nature, our vibrational frequency is low and can result in diseases and a lower state of consciousness.

We can elevate our vibrational frequency by reciting or singing harmonic vowel sounds, mantras, Sanskrit songs, affirmations, prayers and positive lyric songs. We can utilize the Ancient Solfeggio Tones: C (Do-396 Hz), D (Re-417 Hz), E (Mi-528 Hz), F (Fa-639 Hz), G (Sol-741 Hz), A (La=852Hz) and B (Si-963 Hz) or we can use the Pythagorean or Johannes Kepler major scale Solfeggio Tones. However, the most important aspect is the positive power of intention and the power of love coming from your heart. I use the small master key chromatic pitch instrument in 440 Hz to do my vocal sounds and mantras in the 7 natural tones and 5 semitones every morning after I wake up to prepare myself for the work that I have to accomplish during the day.

It usually takes me about 35 to 40 minutes to vocalize the vowel sounds and mantras, while incorporating the dynamic and coordinated movements of my hands around my body. I do these exercises in a similar way to Qigong exercises but in my own style. I dwell on this topic more broadly in other chapters of this book and also in a new book that I am writing and CD Video entitled **"Harmonic Healing Sounds Qigong."**

This daily practice helps me to activate the Qi or Chi energy of life in combination with the power of harmonic sounds in my energy and physical body. After I do this practice, I do a meditation in lotus position for about 15 to 20 minutes. After I finish the meditation, I feel revitalized, full of energy, rejuvenated, alert and very focused. The whole process takes me about 50 minutes to 1 hour in the early morning every day. However, it can also be done at a different time during the day and by using the musical tones in 432 or 440 Hz, or using the Pythagorean or Johannes Kepler major scale Solfeggio Tones. You will have to select which is the best time for you and the best solfeggio tonality that works for you. This practice is the most powerful therapy and healing section that one can give to himself or herself every day. **We are all healers and "The Power is Inside Every One of Us." We need to learn to cultivate this inner power.** Only 50 minutes to 1 hour of the 24 hours of the day doing this practice can have amazing revitalizing and transformational healing effects. Dr. Glen Rein is from the Quantum Biology Laboratory Research Department in New York His experiments indicated that Sanskrit Songs, Gregorian Chants and music can resonate with DNA and can also have a positive impact on the body. Recent scientific researchers also discovered that singing is like an infusion of the perfect tranquilizer. It can calm the nervous system. It elevates the spirit and treats depression. When we sing and make harmonious vowel sounds, we release **endorphin hormones** and these hormones interact with receptors in the brain to help us feel concentrated, less affected by pain, and help us achieve better mood.

These daily practices can increase your vibrational frequency and consciousness and keep you in good health. When it is done with the power of intention of love, peace and harmony, and to heal yourself and the planet, you will energize your body, mind and spirit with a powerful electromagnetic vibration similar to a dynamo. This can also elevate the energy and frequency of people around you, and that frequency will be broadcasted to the atmosphere of the planet in general. **The Healing Forces of Harmonic Sounds and Vibrations,** the power of love, peace and the power of intention and meditation can move mountains and manifest miracles.

In order to elevate our vibrational frequency, it is important that we do not give in to negative thoughts or be influenced by pessimistic and negative people. Avoid alcohol, drugs, smoking, chemicals, pesticides and watching horror and violent movies. It is important to find a way to protect your body from the harmful electromagnetic energy frequencies from cell-phones, microwaves, Wi-Fi, radar, and radio signal antennas.

It is also imperative to consume natural organic greens, fruits, seeds, and legumes and avoid genetically processed food (GMO) and if possible eliminate food that contains gluten. Food is energy and when it is naturally organic and fresh, it contains high frequencies that will nourish the mind and body. In chapter 29 of this book you will find scientific evidence about the vibrational nature of thoughts, body and food.

Listen to classical music, **The Healing Forces of Harmonic Sounds and Vibrations music,** flute, instrumental soft music, Gregorian Chants, Vedic Chants and Sanskrit

Songs. Practice Qigong, yoga, Tai Chi and dance and sing every day. Laugh, smile, walk in the forest, meditate, express gratitude every moment of your life and do good to every being, animal and insect. Try to protect the natural resources of the planet, do not contribute to wasted contamination, reduce your energy consumption and if possible use natural solar and wind energy. When we do our best to do these things, we will elevate our vibrational frequency and gradually elevate the frequency on Earth.

21

Science and the Power of Sound

Great minds and scientists have had a great impact on the healing power of sound and harmonic vibrations.

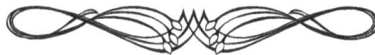

Who are the great minds and scientists who had great impact in the history about the healing power of sound and harmonic vibrations?

Edgar Cayce, Rudolf Steiner and Nostradamus predicted that by the end of the 20th century and the beginning of the 21st century, sounds and vibrations would be used to heal the body, mind and spirit (now known as Vibrational Medicine.)

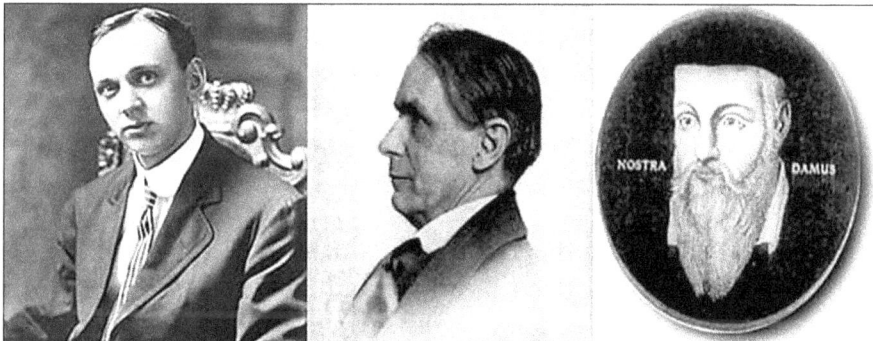

Edgar Cayce, Rudolf Steiner and Nostradamus.

Nikola Tesla (1856-1943) was born in Yugoslavia (Esmilian - Croatia) and immigrated to the United States at age 28 in 1884 and stayed until his death. He was an inventor and research scientist. He worked as a telephone engineer in Prague and Paris, where he conceived a type of electric motor operated by direct current (DC). He began to work with the rotating magnetic field and developed his early concepts of **alternating current.**

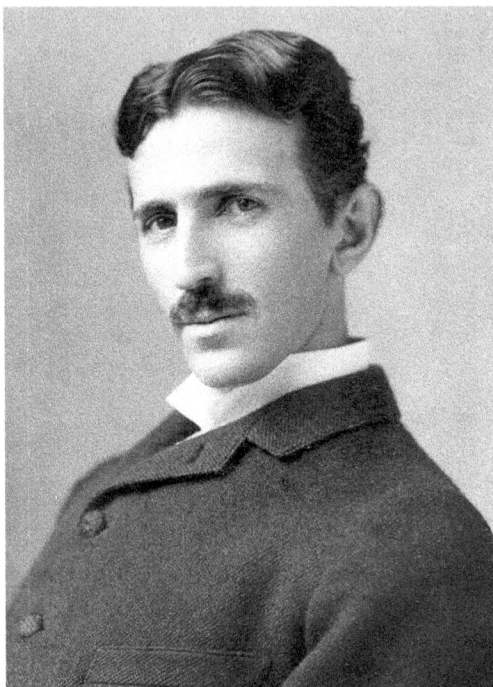

Nikola Tesla

He discovered that rotating magnets can produce a powerful magnetic field, which led to his invention of alternating current. It is currently used in almost all industrial machines. He worked for a short period with Thomas Edison under unpleasant circumstances. Nikola Tesla established his own laboratory and developed great inventions. He obtained patents for the polyphasic motor, dynamo and transformer which were used in his **alternating current** systems (AC).

Nikola Tesla said "if we want to find the secrets of the universe, we need to think in terms of energy, frequency and vibration." **We live in an ocean of energy, frequency and vibration.** Nikola Tesla also knew about the power of frequencies in codes of 3, 6 and 9, which are directly related to the Fibonacci sequence. He said, **"If you knew the magnificence of the codes 3, 6, 9, then you would have the key to the universe."**

Tesla understood the therapeutic value of high frequency sounds. He never patented in that area, but spoke of this invention with people in the medical community. Many inventions were patented and used by other scientists, based on concepts of **Tesla's high frequency sounds.**

His most known invention was the **Tesla Coil,** which is an oscillator that uses spiral wound cables through which electrical current frequencies pass. The Tesla Coil influenced scientists like Royal Rife and George Lakhovsky in their work and concepts of high vibrational frequencies that have therapeutic effects and activate the body's natural healing process at the cellular level.

The invention of the **Tesla Coil** influenced future scientific thought and led to the development of instruments that generate vibrational frequencies, sounds and radio waves used in **Vibrational Medicine and Electromagnetic Medicine.**

In early 1891, Nikola Tesla described the universe as a **kinetic system** full of vibrational energy that could be accessed and used naturally from many places. He was influenced by Vedic philosophy and used Sanskrit terms to describe the phenomenon of natural pranic energy coming from the universe.

For many years, his concepts were influenced by the teachings of Swami Vivekananda, one of the first yogis of India that brought Vedic philosophy to Europe and the United States. After meeting the Swami and after continuous studies on the oriental vision of the mechanisms driving the material world, Tesla began using Sanskrit words such as Akasha and Prana, and the concept of a luminous ether to describe the origin, existence and formation of matter.

This paper suggests the Tesla's understanding and development of **Vedic science,** his correspondence with Lord Kelvin on these issues and the relationship between Tesla and Walter Russel and other scientists of the 20th century who had knowledge of advanced physics.

Tesla also had a great influence on music, and not just because he created the technology that made possible the wireless transmission of radio waves, sound waves and electricity.

Tesla recognized that the human body performs biochemical functions through energy and frequencies that create sounds. He said that if we could remove certain external frequencies that interfere with our bodies, we would have greater resistance to disease.

After a long period of inactivity, Nikola Tesla introduced the concept that **we have to think in terms of energy, frequency, and vibrations. We live in an ocean of energy, frequency and vibration.** This inspired him to patent free energy systems through natural forces – the magnetic force from the Sun and Earth and natural elements such as water, air, ether and other elements, which are in a constant state of vibration thus producing sounds.

Nikola Tesla Concept about Music, Sound Frequencies and its relation with the Universe

Nikola Tesla was interviewed by **John Smith in 1899** and he revealed his extraordinary personality. **Nikola Tesla expressed in this interview his sensibility, admiration and knowledge about the amazing power of music, the forces of harmonic sound frequencies and its relationship with the Universe.** He told the interviewer John Smith that he wanted to illuminate the whole Earth. There is enough electricity to become a second sun. Light appears around the equator, as a ring around Saturn, but man is not ready for the great and good. In Colorado Springs I soaked earth with electricity. Water can give energy such as positive mental energy, **as in the music of Bach or Mozart, or in the verses of great poets.** When John Smith asked Tesla about the theory of relativity of Albert Einstein he said: "Remember, it is not curved space, but the human mind which cannot comprehend infinity and eternity! If relativity has been clearly understood by its Creator, he would gain immortality, even yet physically, if he is pleased. **I am part of a light, and it is the music.** The Light fills my six senses: **I see it, hear, feel, smell, touch and think.** Thinking of it means my sixth sense. **Particles of Light are written notes. A bolt of lightning can be an entire sonata. A thousand balls of lightening are a concert. For this concert, I have created a Lightning Ball, which can be heard on the icy peaks of the Himalayas.** About **Pythagoras and mathematics** a scientist may not and must not infringe on these two. **Numbers and equations are signs that mark the music of the spheres. If Einstein had heard these sounds, he would not create theories of relativity. These sounds are the messages to the mind that life has meaning, that the Universe exists in perfect harmony, and its beauty is the cause and effect of Creation. "This music is the eternal cycle of stellar heavens." The smallest star has completed composition and also, part of the celestial symphony. The man's heartbeats are part of the symphony on Earth.** Newton learned that the secret is in geometric arrangement and motion of celestial bodies. He recognized that the supreme law of harmony exists in the Universe."

Albert Einstein (1879 - 1955) was a scientist of Jewish-German origin who moved to the United States in the 1940s . Einstein said that imagination is more powerful and important than knowledge and intellect. "Imagination is a form of mental energy in a state of vibration."

Albert Einstein imagined riding in a beam at the speed of light which inspired him to create the formula of relativity of matter $E = MC^2$. This was the precursor to the **age of nuclear energy power and the atomic bomb.**

In 1905, Albert Einstein showed that matter can be broken into smaller components and move beyond the material realm to one of energy and vibration. This is the law of vibration, a natural law that says that **nothing rests, everything moves, everything is vibrating.** The lower the vibration, the slower the vibration, the higher the vibration, the faster the vibration. The vibration has a range from zero to vibrations of cosmic rays, which are extremely high (science is still unable to measure them.)

The philosophical and scientific basis of the law of vibration can be found in quantum physics and Einstein's theory of relativity. Energy is related to matter and the speed of

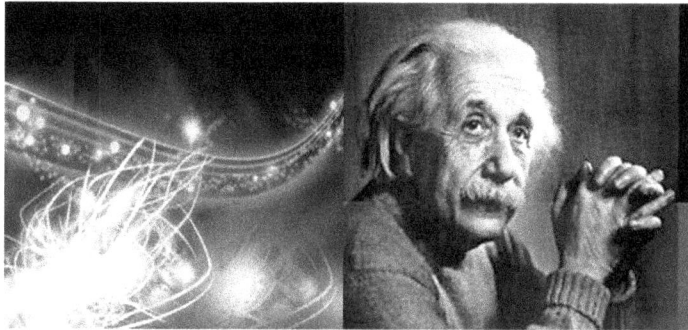

Vibrational frequency of light and Albert Einstein.

light. Einstein's famous equation is $E = MC^2$ (Scientists have failed to demonstrate the existence of mass because of the failure to demonstrate the existence of gravity.)

Albert Einstein was not only the leading scientist of the 20th century, but also a gifted enthusiastic musician. He said "If I were not a physicist, I would probably be a musician. Life without music is unconceivable. I often think in music. I see my daydreams in music. I see my life in terms of music and I get most joy in life out of music."

When Einstein moved to Aarau in Switzerland in 1895 to complete his studies, he dedicated a large part of his time to music. While there, Einstein worked intensively on Brahms' sonata in G-major for violin and performed it for the great violinist Joseph Joachim . Just before his 17th birthday, he fiddled for a review of the Cantonal Music School. The school's inspector reported that "a student named Einstein performed brilliantly, demonstrating a profound feeling and played an adage of one of Beethoven's sonatas very lucidly."

In addition to his prowess on the violin, Einstein also played the piano and loved to improvise. Music was not just a relaxation for Einstein, but also helped him in his research and scientific work.

His second wife, Elsa, gives an account of their life in Berlin. "When I was little, I fell in love with Albert because he played beautifully Mozart's music with violin." She also wrote: "Music helped Einstein in his scientific theories and research. He used to go to his studio to work, he came back and played some chords on the piano and then returned once again to his studio to continue what he was doing or writing."

Albert Einstein enthusiastically accepted invitations to perform in concerts that were scheduled to benefit philanthropic organizations. However, on one occasion an insensitive critic commented that Albert Einstein was an excellent musician, but there are many violinists as good as him. The critic concluded that his fame was undeserved because his recognition did not come from his music, but from his research and work in physics.

Albert Einstein had famous personal friends and chamber music partners in the world of classical music. Among them, Arthur Rubinstein, cellist Gregor Piatigorski and Bronislaw Huberman, one of the most outstanding violin virtuosos of the 20th century.

In 1936, Einstein was visited by Bronislaw Huberman at Princeton to discuss his plans to found the Israel Philharmonic Orchestra, with Einstein as one of its main and prominent sponsors.

Violinist Janos Plesch, a friend of Einstein wrote: "There are many musicians with better techniques than Einstein's, but none, according to my opinion, fiddles so sincerely and with deep feeling than Albert Einstein."

Towards the end of his life, Einstein began to lose the agility of his left hand and stopped playing the violin. However, he never lost his love for the violin and said, "The merriest and happiest moments of my existence have come from music and the violin."

Albert Einstein in the depths of his being, recognized harmonic music as one of the main factors that helped and inspired him in his great scientific discoveries. He recognized that harmonic music has the power to inspire, transform and stimulate creativity.

Georges Lakhovsky (1869 - 1942) was born in 1869 in the Russian Empire and died in New York in 1942. He was an engineer, scientist, writer and inventor.

Georges Lakhovsky was in France in 1929, where he wrote a book titled, **The Secret of Life.** In this book he tried to prove that good or bad health can be determined by the oscillations generated by the cells. If cell oscillations are corrupted by interference from oscillations produced by microorganisms such as bacteria and other pathogens, then disease and cancer occur.

In January 1924, with the help of D'Arsonval, he began building a machine he called the **Cellular Radio Oscillator**, also known as the **Multiple Wave Radio Oscillator.** This device was used in therapeutic applications.

His theory is based on living cells emitting and receiving electromagnetic radiation and vibrational frequencies of long and short wavelengths. These waves generate frequencies of sounds that are very similar to the measurable waves in Hertz. Sick cells produce weak vibrations. If they are exposed and stimulated by a field of multiple radio frequencies, they find their own frequency and start to oscillate normally through resonance.

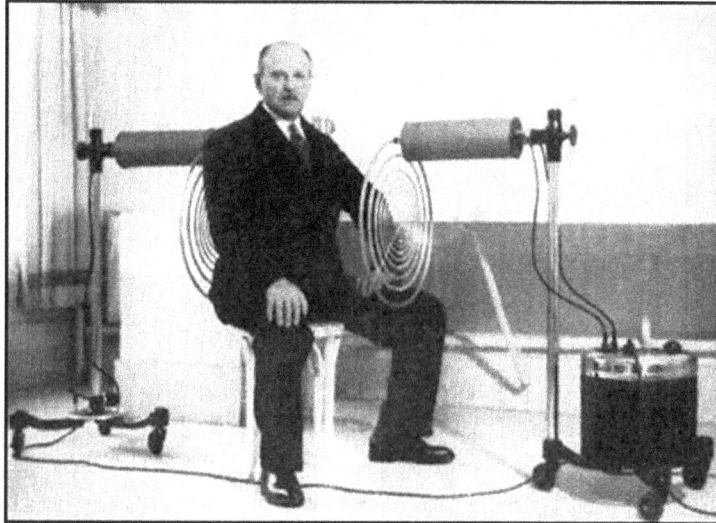

George Lakhovsky

The **multiple wave radio oscillator** generates electromagnetic waves of high vibrational frequency. It produces waves of two meters in length, which correspond to 150 million cycles per second.

Lakhovsky's theory is based on the following: Suppose a cell vibrates at a determined frequency and a microbe vibrates at a different frequency; the microbe attacks the cell through its radiation or vibration. Disease begins if the cell cannot repel the stronger vibrations coming from the microbe.

If the vibrational frequency of the cell is forced to diminish, the microbe gets strength, has control over the cell, and can cause disease and death. If the living cell vibrates with suitable frequency amplitudes inside and outside, the oscillatory attack from the microbe is repelled and the cell survives.

The invention of George Lakhovsky, the multiple wave radio oscillator, has been used in cancer research in plants. Plants have been subjected to treatments with ultra high vibrational radio frequencies, with wavelengths of two meters and also with shorter waves producing harmonic waves with favorable results in healing plants.

Today, similar experiments are performed with animals and people. The results have been favorable, activating the subject's natural healing process.

Georges Lakhovsky's invention, the multiple wave radio oscillator, is another important scientific achievement of vibrational medicine. This shows that the sub-atoms, atoms, molecules, cells, tissues, organs and systems of living organisms are in a constant state of vibration; generating sound frequencies and their electromagnetic energies can be balanced by radio waves, which generate vibrational frequencies and sounds.

Dr. Royal Raymond Rife (1888 - 1971) was an American scientist and researcher. He is considered one of the great scientific minds of the 20th century. He was known for two major scientific inventions:

1st. In 1930, Rife designed the **high visual magnification microscope,** where he

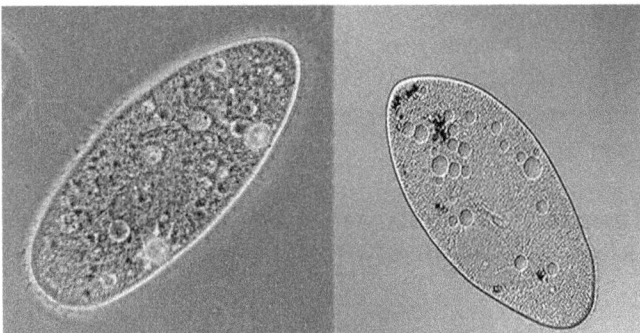

could observe extremely small microorganisms that could not be seen through existing technology of the time. This discovery was recognized by the Smithsonian Institute board of regents, in its annual report of 1944.

Images of bacteria.

2nd. In 1930 Rife invented a machine that could disable, destroy and disintegrate microorganisms or pathogens such as parasites, bacteria, virus and fungi. This machine uses electromagnetic radio vibrations with specific frequencies that generate sound waves. Rife discovered that microorganisms (bacteria, virus, fungi and parasites) and their chemical constituents have a specific resonance frequency, which can be neutralized, deactivated and destroyed with specific frequencies produced by sound waves.

The machine invented by Rife uses a unique combination of electromagnetic pulse radio waves, generating high and low frequency sounds that effectively deactivate and destroy microorganisms that cause disease. This discovery was demonstrated by Royal Rife in the 1930s.

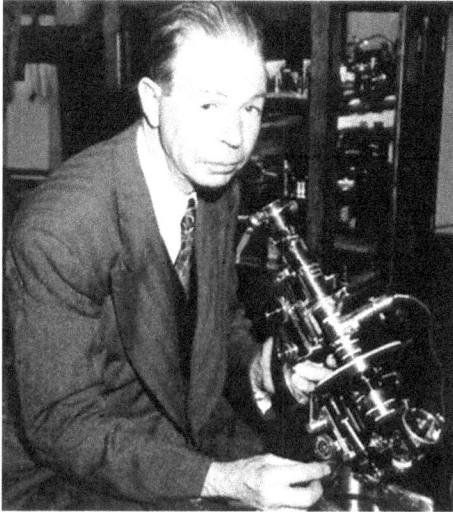

Dr. Royal Raymond Rife.

Royal Raymond Rife was sponsored by a wealthy gentleman from California. He provided the funds to build a Laboratory in San Diego, California. In this laboratory Rife worked intensively to build the most sophisticated light microscope of that time and today many scientists consider this invention one of the best instruments of this nature. Rife dedicated many years observing and studying microscope microorganisms, their nature, and their biological behavior. His research led him to find the frequencies that resonated with each of the microorganisms or pathogens.

His studies inspired him to create a machine that generates electromagnetic radio waves and frequencies that are caplable of weakening and destroying microorganisms or pathogens that cause disease. Today this machine is known as the **Rife Machine.**

Rife's discoveries and research started conflicts with theories and medical standards during the 1930s. Royal Raymond Rife discovered and facilitated the concept of electromagnetic radio frequency waves as an effective method to activate the body's natural healing process, but his discovery was not accepted by the medical sector of his time.

He is regarded as the man who discovered methods to treat diseases by simply using **vibrational energy.**

Through his scientific research, Rife found that all viruses, bacteria, parasites and other pathogens are sensitive to specific sound frequencies. These microorganisms can be destroyed by the intensification of sound frequencies until they explode, similar to an intense musical note that can shatter a wine glass.

The scientific method used by the Rife machine.

The Rife Vibrational Frequency Generator has the power to disintegrate microorganisms through frequencies and vibrations produced by radio waves. It generates specific sounds that deactivate and disintegrate pathogens. The generator quickly stimulates the natural process of cell detoxification and the regeneration of tissues, organs and body systems.

In Germany, Austria, France, Norway, Canada, Mexico, Japan, Russia and other countries, homeopaths, chiropractors and medical institutions use the Rife machine as a Vibrational Medicine method in their holistic practices for treatments for countless conditions and therapies with favorable results.

Treatments have no side effects and are not invasive.

The frequencies generated by the Rife machine are programmed in specific frequency ranges that disable and disintegrate parasites, bacteria, virus and fungi but they are not harmful to cells, tissues, organs and body systems. However, conventional medicine cannot be discarded because medication and surgical methods are often effective and necessary.

Treatment through vibrational frequencies does not damage the body's cells or normal tissue . It does not have any ionizing radiation, so it cannot damage tissue, the immune system, or DNA. No side effects have been reported from using the Rife frequency generator, and it has been used as an alternative method of treatment.

Rife incorporated the principle of resonance in the **Rife machine.** All objects have a natural resonance frequency. When the natural frequency of an object is output from another external source, such as a speaker, an instrument, or a voice, the object will vibrate at that frequency. If the sound intensity is strong enough, then it is possible that the vibrations become more intense than the structural properties of the object, to the point that the object can be manipulated or disintegrated.

That's exactly what happens when a singer produces a musical note in the same resonance frequency of a wine glass, thus breaking the glass. This same principle applies when a specific vibrational radio frequency produces a sound corresponding to that of a parasite, bacterium, virus or fungus, causing disintegration and destroying the microorganism or pathogen.

All types of microorganisms, cells and living entities generate specific electromagnetic frequencies. They are in a constant state of vibration, produce sounds and have an oscillating pattern according to each individual genetic map. The electromagnetic frequencies, vibrations and sounds that living entities produce are different for each one of them.

Royal Raymond Rife based his studies and research on specific electromagnetic vibrational frequencies producing direct resonance with parasites, bacteria, viruses and fungi, and also with frequencies that activate cancer and other conditions. He experimented with special frequencies to destroy these microorganisms and to eliminate many medical conditions including cancer and with good results.

Doctors, holistic centers and institutions that currently use the **Rife machine,** use it as an additional or complementary method of therapy in their practices and research purposes, to observe the effects of bioactive frequencies. They test the frequencies at the cellular and body system levels. They stimulate the natural process of healing in the body through vibrational frequencies to treat health conditions. **The users of the Rife machine do not claim that it can cure a disease. Its use is merely experimental.** The results may vary, but it is true that thousands of people have achieved excellent therapeutic benefits in the treatment of many conditions using bioactive frequencies generated by Rife's vibrational therapy.

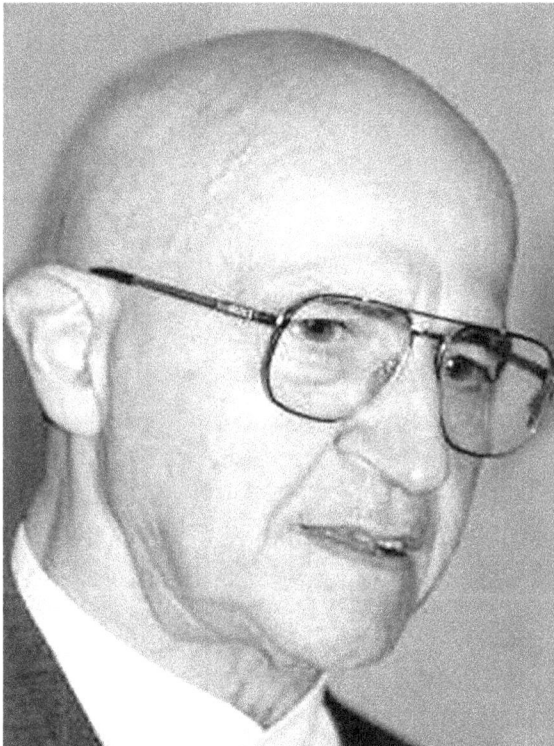

Dr. Alfred A. Tomatis

Dr. Alfred A. Tomatis (1920 - 2001)

Alfred Tomatis grew up in a family of musicians in Nice, France. His father was an opera singer, and he spent much of his childhood traveling with him and watching his presentations and theatrical performances. At an early age he and his parents decided that theater would not be his vocation and he proceeded to study medicine. He eventually became an ear, nose and throat specialist (otolaryngologist.)

Shortly after Dr. Tomatis started his practice, his father referred his colleagues with vocal problems to him. Dr. Tomatis soon discovered that traditional treatments were not adequate, and that there was little research in the area on voice. Based on this, he formulated the theory that many vocal problems occur due to hearing problems.

161

placenta

umbilical cord

uterus

cervix

fetus

uterine wall

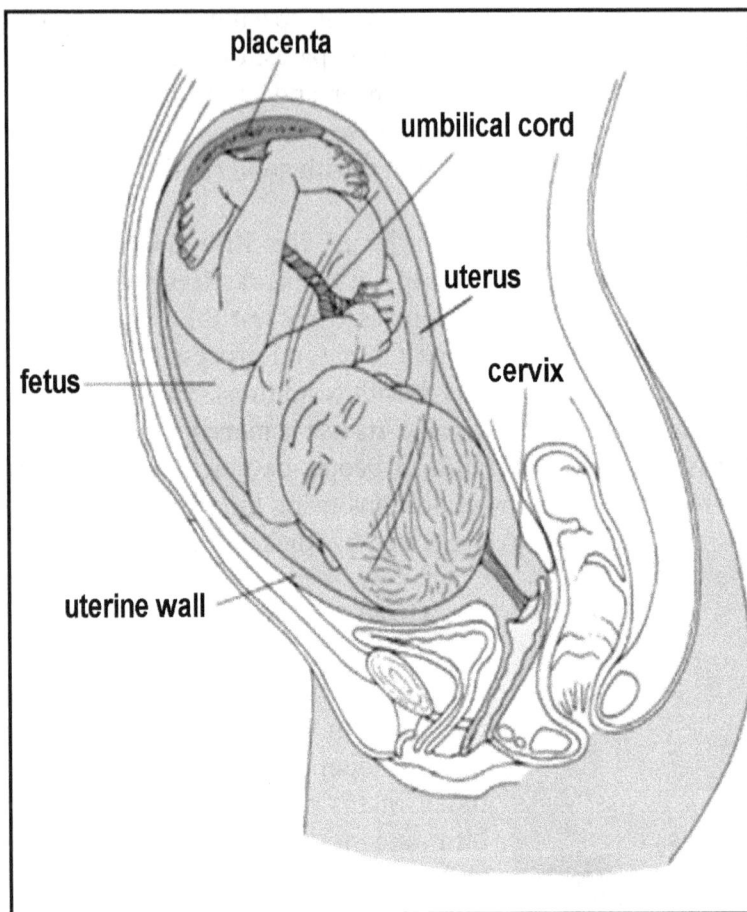

Dr. Tomatis became an internationally known otolaryngologist and inventor. He received his PhD in Medicine in Paris. He developed the Tomatis Method or Audio-Psycho-Phonology method based on his alternative medicine theories on hearing and listening. His work was the result of his curiosity about the vital influence of the human ear in the functioning of a healthy mind, body and spirit.

Dr. Tomatis noticed that the ear is one of the first organs that develop in the uterus and this enables the fetus to hear sounds and learn language from the mother's voice.

Tomatis concluded that much of human health has a direct relationship to the ear's health. He researched, developed and tested his theory that the voice only produces what the ear hears. His theory was confirmed independently at the Sorbonne University, in Paris, in 1957 and became known as the Tomatis Effect.

Tomatis summarized his theories based on three laws:
1) The voice contains and produces only what the ear can hear.
2) If the hearing process is modified, the voice is modified immediately and unconsciously.
3) It is possible to transform phonation when the auditory stimulation is maintained for a certain time (the law of duration and resonance.)

Tomatis imagined that through ear re-training one could recover hearing and hear sounds that are weak or not perceived by the ear, and he found a way to do this. Not being able to hear some sounds could be the result of a difficult pregnancy or birth, colds, childhood illnesses, accidents, living in an environment where there are loud sounds, emotional trauma and experiences that have altered how a person perceives sounds.

His curiosity led him to experiment with classical music and different sound ranges. He discovered that hearing problems are the cause of many learning problems. Based on his scientific research he developed an effective technique to solve learning problems, which he called **Tomatis Method.**

Dr. Alfred Tomatis demonstrated that we can hear sounds and vibrations not only through our ears but also through our body. Our bones are good conductors of sound.

Dr. Alfred Tomatis' studies conclude that we begin to hear sounds and vibrations from the early stage of fetal development.

Dr. Alfred Tomatis demonstrated through his scientific research that babies begin to hear sounds and vibrations inside the womb during fetal formation. He concluded that the sound of the mother's voice during gestation prepares the child to develop language skills.

Dr. Alfred Tomatis' scientific studies demonstrate that when we hear sounds within the uterus they get recorded in our cellular memory or DNA (cells' blue print.)

He also found that certain types of music can stimulate areas of the ear that control body movements of some areas of the body. Some sounds can also regulate and improve our motor skills area (e.g.: bicycling, standing straight, catching a ball.) He also found out that there are music and specific sounds that stimulate learning and adapting capabilities.

The mother's womb is a symbiotic environment filled with water. Water is the primary element that sustains life on Earth and is the most abundant element in our bodies. Sounds and vibrations travel 4 to 5 times faster in a watery environment. Because of this, sounds and vibrations have a direct effect on cellular memory and DNA. When a baby is in the womb, it is floating in water. We can be compared to amphibians at that stage because we are floating in water and the conduction of sound is accelerated and amplified.

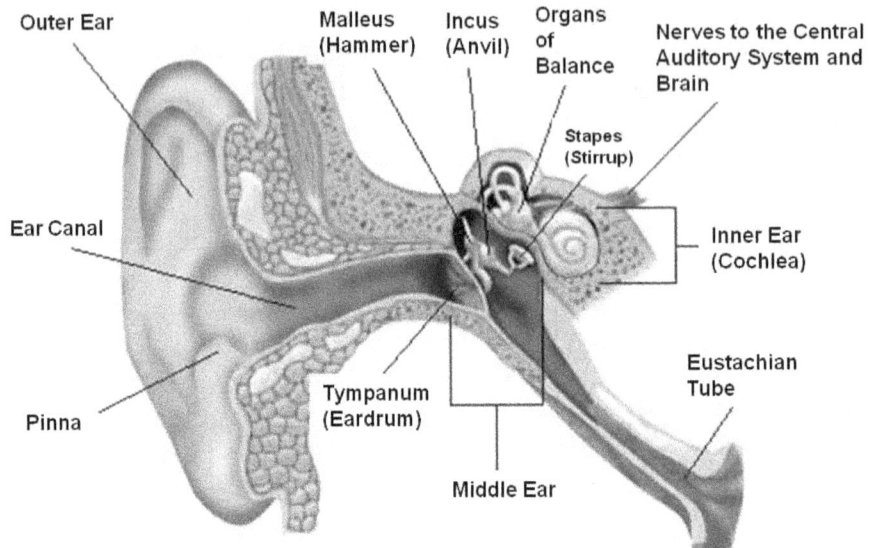

Illustration of human hearing.

The power that sound and vibration have on us is beyond our imagination. Our mental, emotional and physical development is affected by the sounds and frequencies generated in our environment, from the time we are conceived and throughout our lives.

22

Sound and Electromagnetism

The intrinsic relationship between the physical power of sound, music, resonance, magnetic energy and vibration.

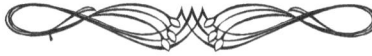

Effects of vibrational frequencies produced by magnetic fluctuations and how they affect all beings on Earth.

Fluctuations in the Earth's magnetic field are caused by solar flares and lunar cycles. These magnetic fluctuations produce sound wave frequencies that affect the Earth's magnetic field and also affect many biological functions of humans and all living beings on the planet.

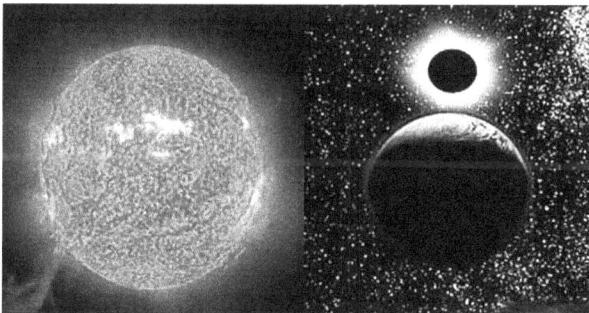

Images of solar explosions and effects of electromagnetic vibrational frequencies produced by the sun and moon.

The natural law of magnetic energy.

Our bodies and each physical body in this dimension have an electromagnetic field that produces vibrational frequencies. All the planets, our solar system and all celestial bodies in the galaxy, also have an electromagnetic field and produce vibrational frequencies and sounds.

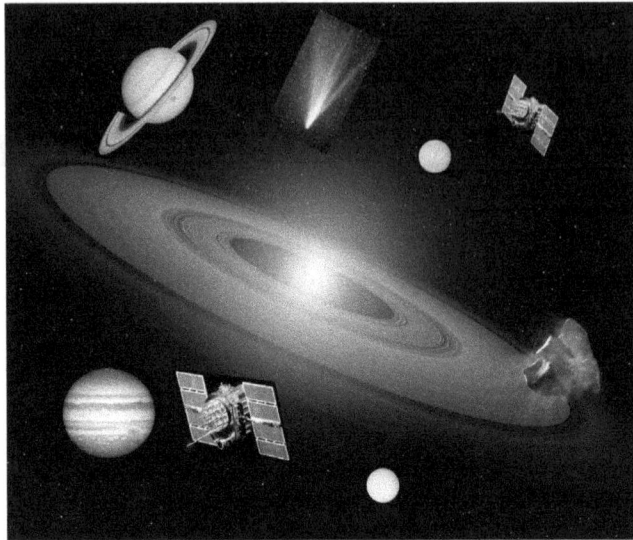

Illustration of celestial bodies, the sun, planets, satellites and the effects their vibrational energies have on all living beings on Earth.

Frequencies and sounds generated by cosmic vibrations and energies have a direct effect on our bodies' functions and all life on Earth.

What is electromagnetism?

Electromagnetism is a vibrational frequency that generates attraction or repulsion forces on metals, especially iron, which is abundant on Earth and is also the most abundant metal in the plasma of living beings. Earth's poles generate a negative and positive electromagnetic field.

Electromagnetism is essentially a mixture of sound and light that produces a vibrational frequency. Some examples are the frequencies of sound, light and video produced by your TV and its speakers. Sound from speakers can produce vibrations that stimulate physical changes and movement of objects through the law of resonance.

What is the relationship between sound, vibrations and magnetic energy?

The physical world is composed of protons, electrons, neutrons, subatomic particles, quarks and neutrinos. These particles are the basis of the material world we perceive. They generate electro-magnetic fields, sound frequencies and vibrations. The electromagnetic spectrum consists of a scale of 3 Hz to 100,000 billion Hz.

Neutrinos are neutrally charged subatomic particles of fermionic type that are constantly oscillating and vibrating. Scientific studies have confirmed that neutrinos have mass. A neutrino's value is not exactly known because it is so small, about 200,000 times smaller than an electron. Its interaction with other particles is minimal because it passes through matter without disturbing it. In fact, neutrinos travel through matter, regardless of how dense. They carry no electrical charge and are attracted neither to protons nor electrons, so they don't interact with electromagnetic fields.

There are three types of neutrinos: electron neutrino, muon neutrino, and tau neutrino. They are NOT affected by electromagnetic or nuclear forces, but they are affected by subtle, nuclear and gravitational forces. **These super-tiny subatomic particles are in a constant state of vibration and generate extremely tiny sound frequencies.**

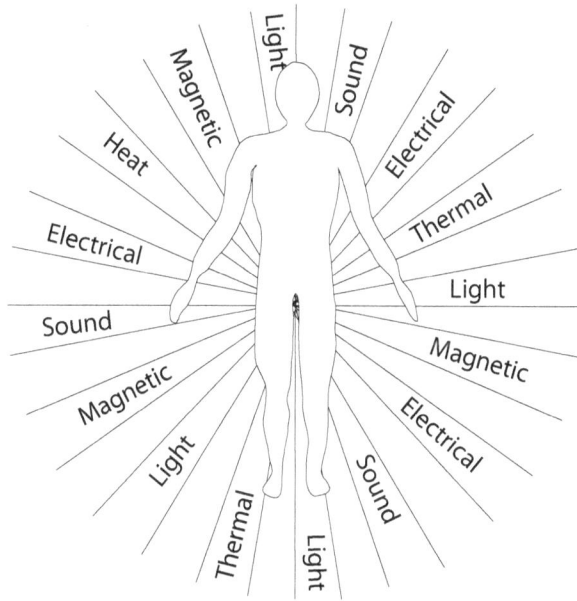

The human body emits a variety of energies.

The human body is a microcosmic universe emanating various forms of energy.

The human body is a microcosmisc universe affected by the universal laws of sound, vibration and magnetic energy (as above, so below.)

Sound, vibrations, magnetic energy, electricity and thermic energy (heat or cold)

Sound, vibration, light, and video signals can be recorded through magnetic energy on tape, cassette or CD.

Our emotions and thoughts are recorded in our DNA's memory and cells much like the way sound, light and video are recorded in a tape.

My goal is to show the intrinsic relationship between sound, music, resonance, magnetic energy and vibration. All these factors affect our energy bodies (auric body, holographic body, mental body, emotional body, astral body), and our biological systems (physical body.) These factors also govern the planet's physical laws .

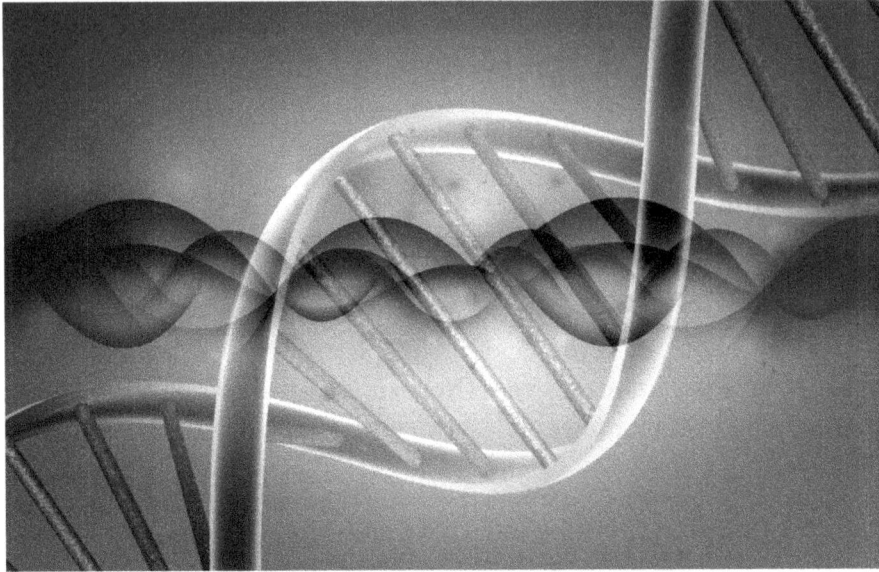

Illustration of the effect of the vibrational frequencies on DNA

The human body is a micro-cosmic universe composed of sub-atoms, atoms, molecules, cells, tissues and organs. It is a **magnificent quantum physical machine** that is in a constant state of vibration producing frequencies of sounds and vibrations. Each cell, tissue and organ of the body generates its own field of electromagnetic energy and emits electrical energy, thermal energy (hot or cold), sounds and light, and is affected by the fluctuations of the magnetic energy that is generated by the Earth, Sun, Moon and celestial bodies.

Each atom is just a probability wave, and most of the things we call physical matter are actually composed of empty space. **We are more empty space than physical matter; more vibration than mass.** Therefore, we can be strongly impacted - either positively or negatively - by magnetic energy, electrical energy, thermal energy and by non-harmonic or disharmonic vibrational sound frequencies. Quantum physics describes the macro-cosmic and micro-cosmic universe as vibratory energy waves. **It is the Creative Universal Intelligence force that manifests in every function of mind, body and spirit in all beings on Earth.**

Everything that moves and vibrates, from neutrinos, sub-atoms, and atoms to the smallest molecule in the universe produces sounds and is affected by the physical laws mentioned above. **The sound generates vibrations and frequencies that have the power to alter the atomic structure of matter.**

23

Magnetic Harmonic Vibrational Therapy

The power of intention and history of the bowls used to produce harmonic sounds.

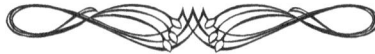

Magnetic Harmonic Vibrational Therapy.

Magnetic Harmonic Vibrational Therapy is what I call my technique to heal the body, mind and spirit through specific sound frequencies, musical tones, and creative visualization. The body's energy centers (chakras, organs, tissues and bones) vibrate in unique musical tones. The aim is to restore the harmony of tones and create suitable vibrational frequencies within the chakras.

Magnetic Harmonic Vibrational Therapy includes harmonic vocal sounds in the codes 3, 6, 9 of the diatonic harmony, and some shades of the chromatic harmony. This therapeutic method can stimulate and accelerate the body's natural healing process at the cellular level.

All our energy centers, chakras, organs and meridians respond to resonance. All our biochemical compositions, sub-atoms, atoms, molecules, cells, tissues and organs are in a constant state of vibration, produce sounds and vibrate in specific musical tone. **Magnetic Harmonic Vibrational Therapy** can assist in harmonizing the vital energy of the etheric body, aura and physical body.

What instruments are used in Harmonic Vibrational Magnetic Therapy?

Alchemist pure quartz crystal bowls, Tibetan bowls, and tuning forks are used in

Harmonic Vibrational Magnetic Therapy. The most powerful of all instruments that is also used: **the human voice in combination with the mental power of intention (the power of sound and speech).**

The Power of Intention

The power of intention is the most powerful vibrational force generated by the mind. The formula is as follows:

intention = visualization + (affirmations, mantras and sounds) + (have faith and believe) = manifestation

To be able to manifest something we want in our lives, we need to activate the power of intention. We need to make a clear mental image of what we want to manifest. Once visualized, the object or desired goal is activated. The power of sound produced by vocal cords, tongue movement, speech, affirmations and mantras expresses what we want to manifest.

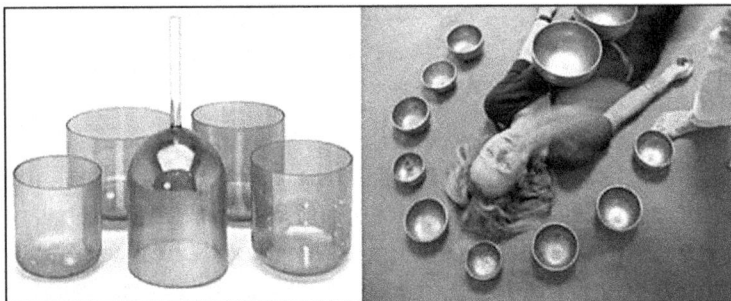

Alchemic pure quartz crystal bowls and Tibetan bowls.

We must believe from the depths of our hearts and have faith in what we want to manifest before expressing it verbally.

It is imperative that we have a firm belief in what we want to manifest. When the sound originates and releases from the mouth feelings activate and the desired object or goal materializes.

The sound that originates in our mind and comes out of our mouth produces a powerful vibrational frequency that has a direct effect on all matter. It is recorded on the body's memory cell, DNA, and on any object present. When we send a verbal message through harmonic sounds, we alter the atomic structure of matter and eventually manifest the desired objective.

What we want to manifest must be in harmony with the laws of the universe. This formula should not be used to manipulate or affect others, or alter cosmo-ethical laws.

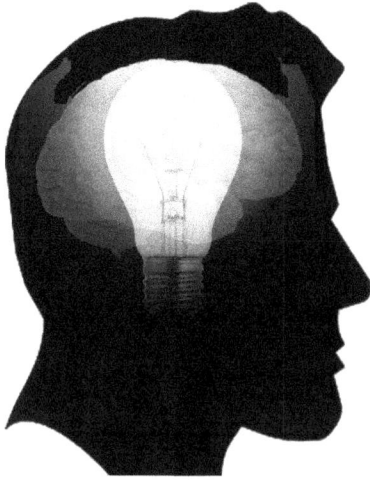

What the mind can conceive, man can achieve or manifest.

Laws of cause and effect govern the universe. To every action, there is a reaction. **Using knowledge and wisdom for self-benefit activates karma.** We must measure our actions to avoid counterproductive or negative effects.

Therapeutic effects of bowls that produce harmonic sounds and their history

The history of the bowls that produce harmonic sounds goes back before the Sakyamuni Buddha (560-480 BC). Their history is a mystery, but it seems that they emerged from the Bon philosophy, which preceded Buddhism in Tibet and India. There is a possibility that the Atlantis and Lemuria civilization existed approximately 38,000 to 11,000 years ago. It is believed that they were the first civilizations that incorporated the use of sounds and harmonic vibrations, in combination with the natural power of crystals and minerals, to cure people from their physical and mental imbalances.

The bowls were built from an unknown alloy of metals; later they were made from brass, glass, and pure quartz crystals. Archeologists have found bowls made of semiprecious stones such as amethyst, quartz ruby, citrine, and white quartz and other stones and minerals. Tibetans manufacture singing bowls that are made of seven metals: gold, silver, mercury, copper, iron, tin, and lead.

Alchemist crystal bowls made of precious, semiprecious stones and pure quartz

The company **Crystal Tones,** Crystal Singing Bowls, located in Salt Lake City, Utah, produces alchemist pure quartz crystal bowls alloyed with precious and semiprecious stones and metals, including diamonds, rubies, emeralds, gold, silver and copper. They also have a great variety of alchemist bowls made with other semiprecious stones.

The frequencies of sounds produced by the alchemist bowls generate pure and powerful sounds of great amplification that can activate balance and stimulate the natural healing process of body, mind and spirit. Alchemist bowls of pure quartz crystals, precious and semiprecious stones emit sound frequencies that produce vibrations corresponding to sound octaves within the etheric body.

Materials used to make alchemical pure quartz crystal bowls

Crystal bowls are made of 99.992% pure pulvertized quartz, also known as silicon quartz. It is similar to crystalline sand, found only in a few places in the world. It contains a high concentration of silica, which is pure crystal by nature. The crystal quartz bowls produce defined musical tones that have direct resonance with many structures of the body, including DNA, blood, bones and the colloidal liquid crystal in the brain.

The spiral structure of our DNA's double helix is similar to that of crystal quartz. The four molecules of silica (quartz) in each of our molecules enable pure crystal quartz bowls to resonate with our biological systems. When crystal bowls are played, resonance with crystalline substances, like silicates and the oxygen floating in the bloodstream, bones, muscles and tissues, is activated. When these elements are stimulated, the vibrational frequency is transported by conduction to different areas of the body. As a result, energy blockages in the meridians, central nervous system, organs and chakras are released.

Pure crystal quartz bowls generate sound frequencies which affect the brain. The resonance stimulates the neurotransmitters and contributes to the production of neurochemicals, endorphins and other hormones that help reduce pain, inflammation and balance the brain hemispheres.

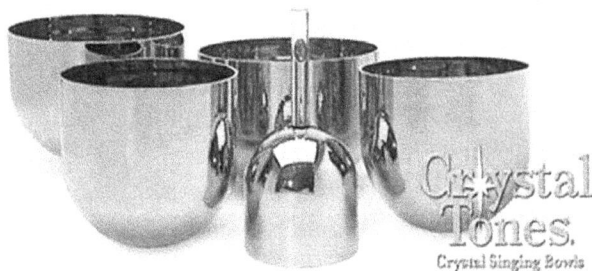

The sound of the bowls can produce a state of altered consciousness which allows one to reach the mental state of relaxation **alpha (9-14 Hz) and Theta (3.5 -7.5 Hz.)** In this state, the natural healing process of the mind, body and spirit accelerates. A state of deep meditation can also be achieved through the music and the harmonic sounds of the pure crystal quartz bowls sound frequencies and it is even more powerful when singing vowel sounds and mantras.

This can be likened to hypnosis, where an individual is brought to an alfa relaxation state between asleep and awake. In this state an individual feels relaxed, can overcome limitations and negative emotions, and can develop creativity.

Pure crystal quartz bowls construction

Refined, pure powdered silicon quartz is required to create a crystal quartz glass bowl.

The quartz powder is deposited into a mold, and mounted on a centrifuge in motion that has more than 4,000 0C. It can be compared with volcanic lava.

When the refined quartz is deposited into the highly accelerated mold with spiral movement, it begins to melt and expand throughout the mold surface and forms a bowl.

The molds are calibrated in a diatonic harmony, which consists of five complete tones and two semitones. Major keys, minor keys and other modalities result in seven basic musical notes **C, D, E, F, G, A, B.**

The molds are also manufactured with minor chromatic tones such as **C#/Db, D#/Eb, F#/Gb, G#/Ab, and, A#/Bb.** The pure quartz crystal bowls vary in size and are 6 to 24 inches in diameter. They have direct resonance with the chakras, organs, meridians and body sytems

The manufacturers of the pure quartz crystal bowls cannot accurately predict the musical resonance note the bowl will produce during the manufacrturing process. A digital instrument will identify the tone of the sound when the bowl is played.

Less-frequently manufactured bowls are those of whole tone, especially F (heart chakra) and E (solar plexus chakra). The C, D, G, A, and B tones are produced more frequently. Larger bowls usually produce an octave lower and deeper tones. Size does not determine the sound of the musical note produced by the crystal bowl.

Sounds produced by pure quartz crystals bowls directly resonate with the body's chakras, meridians, and tissues. The sound frequencies stimulate the brain and can achieve an Alfa state from 9 to 14 Hz. Then neurotransmitters stimulate the production of endorphins and other hormones that release in the bloodstream and contribute to pain relief, inflammation reduction and deep relaxation.

Pure quartz crystal bowls generate sounds that have powerful resonances that correspond to an octave of the sound and vibrations ngenerated by the etheric body or energy body of the human being (the auric body and the holographic body.) These sounds help us to align with the mathematical vibrations coming from the universe.

The quartz bowls' sounds are pure and harmonious. When the quartz bowls are filled with water and played, shapes form in the water. When the bowls are placed on a person's body, a similar effect should be activated within the person's body. Many people who have had vibrational therapy with the crystal quartz bowls have observed favorable changes toward higher and balanced health level.

The high vibration sounds produced by pure quartz alchemical bowls in combination with the human voice, the use of vocal sounds and sacred mantras can help to eliminate tension, negative emotions, stress, depression, and anxiety, and can accelerate the natural healing process of mind, body and spirit.

Tibetan singing bowls

Tibetan singing bowls first appeared in the Himalayas. The bowls are considered a symbol of "the unknown" and their vibrations have been described as "the manifestation of the universe's sound."

Tibetan singing bowls go back to the time of Buddha Shakyamuni (560- 480 B.C.) but the exact origins are a mystery. Some say they were a gift from the "Bon" religion, which preceded Tibetan Buddhism for centuries. Monks, nuns and lay Buddhists traditionally used the bowls in their rituals, prayers and meditations.

The bowls' sounds were supposed to transfer spiritual energy and teachings to help monks and lamas contact the Void. Lamas and Tibetan monks can perceive things that are beyond the tangible and melodic sounds produced by these wonderful instruments.

Tibetan singing bowls were located in sandlots and played during secret rituals by advanced meditation students to deepen their meditative abilities. The students experienced liberation from their physical bodies (astral travel), mental projections, visited other planets in the solar system and contacted spirits.

A common belief was that Tibetan singing bowls helped lamas, monks and advanced teachers in esoteric practices, and enabled them to get in touch with the sacred spiritual center of our planet, Shambhala.

It is speculated that as sound travels from the center of the bowl to the outside world, the experienced meditators hear the sounds of the bowls and through the chanting of mantras and the powerful sound frequencies and mantras, they were able to travel in the astral world without physically leaving their location.

The rituals were secretive and infrequent. The correct way of playing the Tibetan singing bowls was secret and has never been revealed to the public. Inexperienced monks would not participate in the rituals.

Those familiar with esoteric spiritual traditions know that sound generates vibrational frequencies and has the power to alter the atomic structure of matter.

There are over 50 types of Tibetan singing bowls. The technique to produce these bowls has been lost. Various sources claim that up to 15 different metals are used in the metal alloy. There is speculation that one of the metals used in the manufacture of the bowls is the iron found in meteorites.

According to local legends, meteorites found in Tibet traveled through a low-oxygen environment due to the altitude of the mountains. It is said that its composition differs from meteorites found in other parts of the world. Perhaps this could be one of the attributes of the healing powers of Tibetan singing bowls.

How to use Tibetan singing bowls for meditation

The sounds produced by Tibetan singing bowls are effective in establishing the Alfa mental state of meditation. The harmonic sounds encourage an inner peace that opens the mind to new ideas and concepts, promotes physical relaxation and relieves stress. The harmonic sounds can transport an individual to other dimensions and higher states of consciousness.

The best way to produce sounds with a Tibetan singing bowl is to move a wooden stick (mallet) clockwise around the outer edge of the bowl. Apply even pressure as you play the bowl and move the wooden stick. Increase the volume gradually. The sound coming out of the Tibetan singing bowl can serve as a point of concentration to focus your attention.

The sounds produced by Tibetan singing bowls offer benefits that are physically observable. They increase energy, balance blood circulation, help to rejuvenate the skin and relieve pain. Some people have obtained healing, transformation and release of psychic blockages and also have been freed from negative energies of the past.

The sounds of the Tibetan singing bowls can be used as a medical modality to treat stress disorders, pain, depression, emotional problems and many other conditions.

A very important rule: never play a Tibetan singing bowl counterclockwise. The proper spiritual direction and selfless attitude is movement to the right. When our chakras are balanced and healthy, they rotate clockwise, in the beneficial, right direction.

In conclusion, the sounds of pure quartz crystals bowls, the alchemist bowls made with precious and semi-precious stones generate patterns of specific frequencies that harmonize with the vibrational frequency produced by the sound of "AUM" or "OM."

The sounds generate frequencies that resonate with the sympathetic nervous system, and the brain waves synchronize with the vibrational frequency produced by the sounds of the bowls. The harmonic vibrations activate and stimulate the reflexes of the nervous system so that relaxation occurs. This slows the breathing and rhythm of the brain and heart. This dissipates pain, creating a deep sense of well-being.

Pure quartz crystals bowls, such as alchemy and Tibetan singing bowls are an essential part of sound therapy. These are all valuable tools that complement the holistic vibrational medicine of today and they are very effective especially when combined with vocal sounds. Through these techniques, we can produce powerful sounds generating vibrational frequencies that relieve stress, pain and stimulate the natural healing process in all systems of the body, mind and spirit.

"OM, Aum or Oum"

The Sound **"OM, Aum or Oum"** represents the light and sound of all matter. Singing the sacred universal sound of **"Om, Aum or Oum"** helps the seven centers of energy **"the Chakras,"** to expand and harmonize consciousness into Divine Oneness. The vowel or mantric sound of **"Om, Aum or Oum"** is universal and can be used as a powerful frequency to stimulate the natural healing process of the body, mind and spirit. This vowel sound or mantra is considered to have a high spiritual and creative power, but despite this, it is a vocal sound or mantra that can be recited by anyone regardless of religion and beliefs. When singing the powerful vocal sound **"OM, Aum or Oum"** in different harmonic diatonic or chromatic tonalities, it will activate a powerful vibrational frequency that can be felt in the diaphragm, chest cavity, throat and face. The frequency stimulates the pineal and pituitary glands in the brain, the segregation of endorphins, and oxytocin hormones, and reduces the levels of cortisol in the blood stream. The frequencies travel through the spine and the nerve system to every cell in the body. This simple **"Om, Aum or Oum"** vowel sound frequency, when recited for 5 to 10 minutes, has been scientifically demonstrated to have many beneficial effects harmonizing all biological systems in the body.

24

The Power of Resonance of the Human Body

Dr. Daniel David Palmer and chiropractic science.

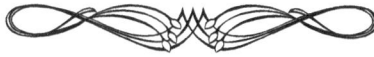

The human body has the potential to resonate.

The human body contains millions of minerals and crystals.

Our bones are made of calcium, magnesium, silica, folic acid and collagen, which is a protein in the form of a double helix intertwined around itself. These minerals form a structure of calcium phosphate crystals, called "apatite crystals."

Human bones have a natural biochemical composition of minerals and crystals which is very similar to the molecular structure of pure quartz crystal bowls.

Crystalline minerals travel through the blood inside the arteries, veins capillaries and all internal systems of the body. Our internal physiognomy is crystalline in nature; thus, sound vibrations and frequencies affect us, especially sounds produced by pure quartz alchemy bowls and bowls

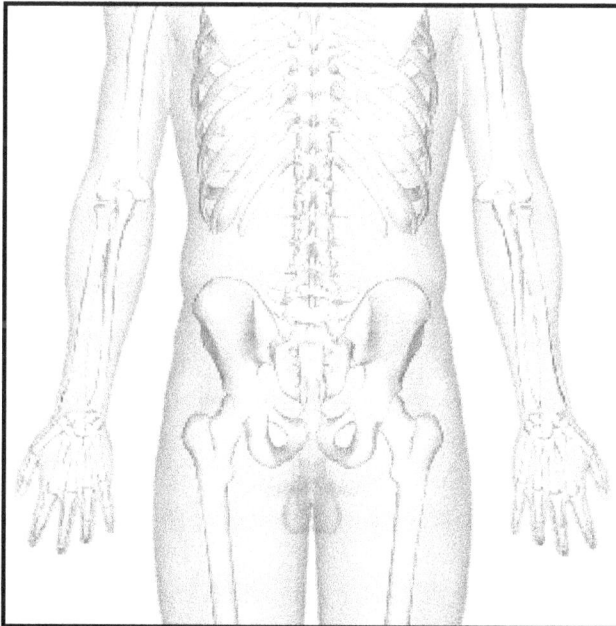
Illustration of bone mass of the human body.

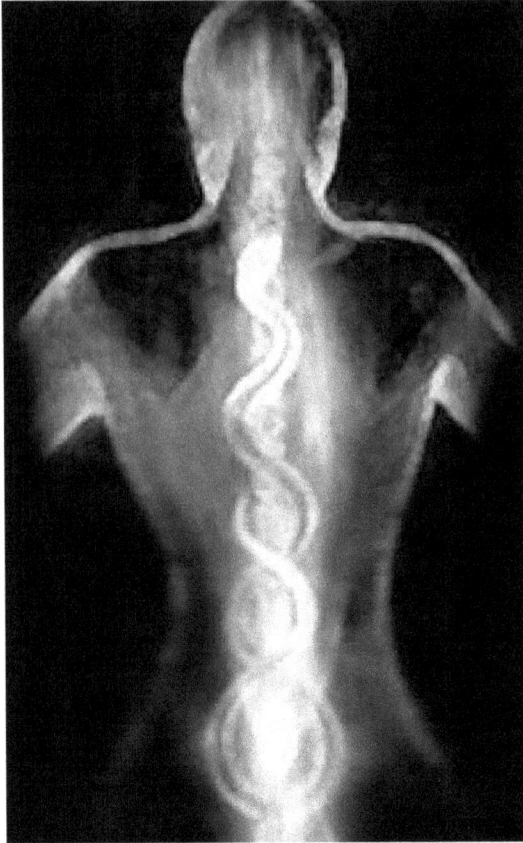

Illustration of the diffusion of vibrational energy through the central nervous system.

made with precious and semiprecious stones.

Frequencies and vibrations created by pure quartz crystal bowls, in combination with human vocal sounds can produce a powerful resonance in a bone's crystal structure.

The vibrations have a great effect on the spine, diffusing along the central nervous system to pathways, tissues, organs and body systems.

The vibrations also balance and activate the chakras, and have a direct effect on the blood, circulatory system, and endocrine system at the cellular level.

The human spine can be visualized as a musical instrument

Dr. Daniel David Palmer (March 7, 1845 - October 20, 1913) was born in Pickering, Ontario, Canada, where he studied and then moved to the United States in 1865.

Dr. Palmer is considered the father of Chiropractic Science; in the 1880's he said **"Chiropractic Science is based on tones and when the spine loses its original tone it results in a dislocation or subluxation of the vertebrae."** Palmer read the medical journals of his time, and followed developments throughout the world regarding anatomy and physiology. While working as a magnetic healer, he decided to find the cause of all disease, and his work led to the foundation of chiropractic. **His theories revolved around the concept that altered nerve flow was the cause of all disease, and that misaligned spinal vertebrae had an effect on the nerve flow.** He postulated that restoring the vertebrae to their proper alignment would restore health. Dr. Palmer said that in a white seance spiritism session, Dr. Jim Atkinso's spirit sent a message to him about the principles to found chiropractic science.

The Asian acupuncture science is also based on the principle that when there are blockages in the meridians, nerves, tissues and the central nerve system the Chi, Ki or Prana energy cannot travel efficiently from the neurovascular system (the brain) to the organs and can lead to serious body imbalances and diseases. Chiropractic science also shares a similar principle. However, it is primarily based on the misalignment of spinal vertebrae; When the vertebrae are properly restored to proper tone and aligned, the person regains good health.

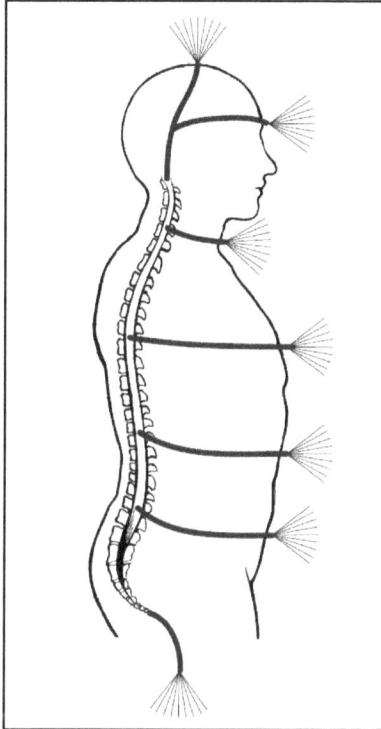

Illustration of the chakras and connection with the spine.

I have been studying and attending Applied Kinesiology workshops since 1999, with Dr. Paul T. Sprieser, D.C, DIBAK in New Jersey. Dr. Sprieser has taught the basic A.K. course since 1983 and has co-lectured with Dr. George Goodheart, the father of Kinesiology. I attended several seminars with Dr. George Goodheart and also met him personally on several occasions through my A.K. teacher Dr. Paul Sprieser and his wife Priscilla Sprieser, who also coordinated many of Dr. Goodheart's seminars.

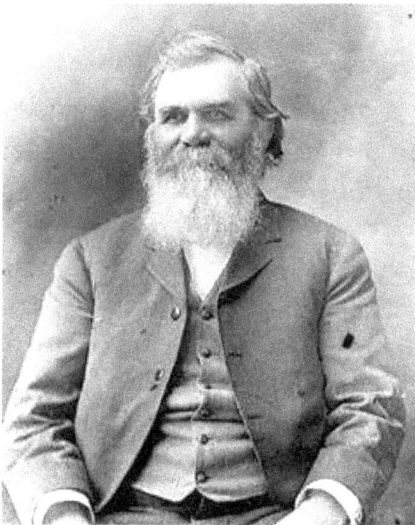

Dr. Daniel David Palmer

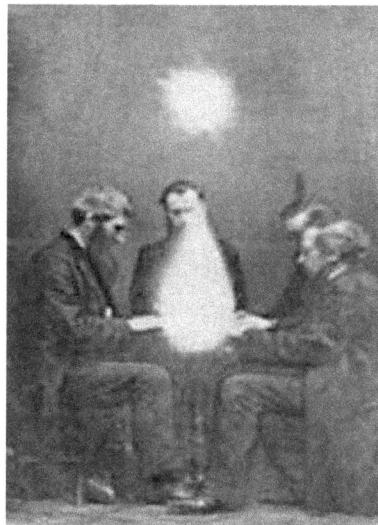

White table séance

I believe that a Higher Universal Force takes us in a direction and path in life and later in time we find the reason. We all have a mission to accomplish in life and when we find what it is, it's very rewarding. However, sometimes the answer to that higher purpose comes many years later. During the time that I was attending Dr. Sprieser's and Dr. Goodheart's seminars, I was also singing professionally, doing concert presentations and recording a Pop CD with a famous recording company. I remember one Sunday after finishing the seminar with Dr. Sprieser and Dr. Goodheart, I was invited to have dinner with Dr. Sprieser, Dr. Goodheart and their wives and they played my CD. Dr. Goodheart complimented me on the sound of my voice and singing style. My love for music and singing opened the path to dedicate my life to investigate and to experiment with **"The Healing Forces of Harmonic Sounds and Vibrations" and "Healing Through the Power of the Voice and the Mind,"** and its effects on the natural healing process of the body, mind and spirit. I've always been convinced that harmonic music and the power of the voice can help activate transformational healing effects in humans and in all beings.

Dr. Sprieser knew I was a singer and had been experimenting with Alchemist Crystal Singing Bowls' frequencies in combination with specific vowel sounds and their effects on the human body. In some A.K. tests we did in his workshops, we were able to bring high blood pressure to normal in about 3 to 5 minutes after exposing a person to specific sound frequencies. I have also been able to help alleviate joint and muscle pain on people after 10 to 15 minutes of sound healing therapy.

In 2004 Dr. Sprieser performed kinesiology tests with Tuning Fork sounds for **Dr. June Leslie Wieder,** who did research about the effect of sound frequencies in the central nerve system and wrote the book **"Song of the Spine."** Dr. Wieder's book is well-documented with her research on the resonance of the spine. Dr. Daniel David Palmer's concept "when the spine loses its **original tone** it results in a dislocation or subluxation of the vertebrae" was strongly supported by Dr. Wieder's investigations. She revealed that **"each bone of the spine has its own tone and frequency"** and when the vertebrae are exposed to specific sound frequencies, the vertebrae generate a response that can help correct **misaligned spinal vertebrae. Her research and work has been of great importance in the area of music therapy for the spine.**

I have also been testing people's spines, abdomens and meridians with Tuning Forks and have observed good results. I have also obtained amazing results by doing the same test but using Alchemist Crystal Singing Bowls. The sound volume and frequency generated by Alchemist singing bowls is louder and is naturally sustained for about 3 minutes, which is longer than the sound produced by tuning forks. Alchemist Crystal Singing Bowls are made with pure 99.99% Crystal Quartz and the ones that I use in my practice **"Magnetic Harmonic Vibrational Therapy"** are made from pure gold, platinum, emerald, diamond, ruby and moldavite.

These Crystal Bowls have been manufactured by William Jones and Paul Utz from **Crystal Tones,** which whom I have been working for over 20 years. I have done presentations and conferences for them about the therapeutic and natural healing effects produced by Crystal Alchemist Singing Bowls when used in combination with the power of the voice. I have presented at conferences for Crystal Tones at Health Life Expos in the U.S.A., Europe, Mexico, Canada, Japan, Colombia, Ecuador, Peru, Costa Rica and other countries for the past 20 years.

Our spine and bone mass consists of calcium, magnesium, silica, folic acid, collagen and carbon. In fact, **"we are crystal beings by nature,"** and our bones are made of the same mineral combination as quartz. Alchemist Singing Bowls resonate with the spine, bones and body meridians. Sound healing therapy is very effective in treating many conditions including alleviating pain, lowering blood pressure, calming anxiety, reducing stress and other conditions. I have also experimented with placing the Tibetan singing bowls directly on a person's back, solar plexus and rib cage area. The results have been excellent, but with the alchemist pure crystal singing bowls the results have been even more powerful.

When I vocalize vowel sounds that resonate with specific chakras simultaneously with the alchemist singing bowls in the diatonic harmony cords 3, 6, 9 and also in 5th in the diatonic codes tonality 432 Hz and also 440 Hz, the sound produced has been very effective in activating the body's natural healing response.

The human spine can be visualized as a musical instrument. Vertebrae differ in size, shape, weigh and mineral deficiency, and trauma can contribute to vertebrae imbalance and cause the spine to lose its natural harmonic tone. **The Magnetic Harmonic Vibrational Therapy** can assist with specific frequencies and offer an alternative and natural method that can help restore the natural tone of the spine and regain its harmonic function.

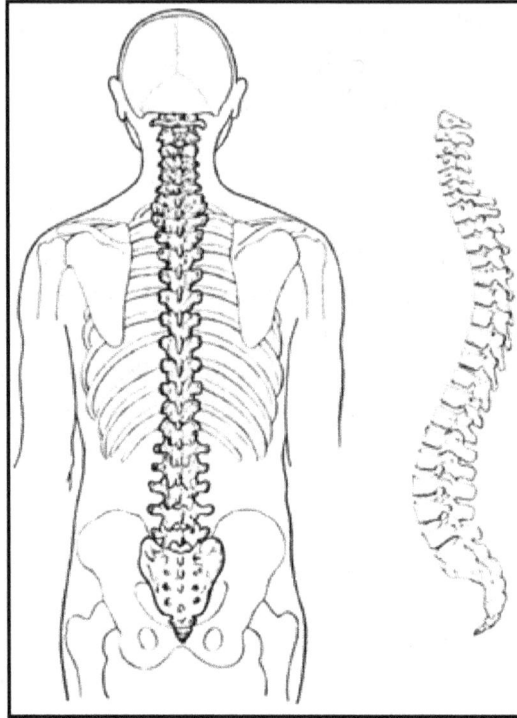

Illustration of the curvature of the human spine.

How do sound frequencies spread in the human body?

The epidermal tissue of human skin is connected to a network of nerves known as **"Dermatome or Skin Dermatosis Nerves."** When Pure Crystal Quartz Alchemy Singing Bowls or Tibetan Bowls are placed directly on a person's back and specific vocal sounds are made, a vibratory frequency is activated. This stimulates the nerves of the epidermal tissue, the central nervous system, and the crystalline substances in the blood stream, and the frequencies are transported to the organs.

Dr. Alfred A. Tomatis demonstrated that humans can perceive, and absorb sound frequencies and vibrations through the epidermal tissue, bones and nervous system more widely than through the ears.

A **dermatome** is an area of skin that is supplied primarily by a spinal nerve. There are **7 cervical vertebrae and 8 cervical nerves** (with the exception of C1- without dermatome), **12 vertebrae and thoracic nerves, 5 vertebrae and lumbar nerves and 5 sacral nerves.** Each of these nerves relays a sensation of a particular region of the skin to the brain including frequencies of sounds, pain, itch, and sensations of heat and cold, etc.

A spinal nerve is a mixed nerve, which carries motor, sensory, and autonomic signals between the spinal cord and the body. In the human body, there are 31 pairs of spinal nerves, one on each side of the spine. These are grouped into the corresponding cervical, thoracic, lumbar, sacral and coccygeal regions of the spine. The spinal nerves are part of the peripheral nervous system. Nerves on the skin (**Dermatome or Skin Dermatosis Nerves**) carry sensory information to and from the ventrolateral surface of the body, from the structures in the walls, the meningeal or sinuvertebral nerves, and from the branches of the nerves coming out of the vertebrae of the spine to the autonomic nerves. These carry visceral and sensory motor information to and from the tissues, organs and systems.

In my practice of **"Magnetic Harmonic Vibrational Therapy"** I have observed excellent results when I placed Pure Quartz Alchemy Crystal Singing Bowls on a person's back and in indifferent areas of the spine, while simultaneously using specific vowel sounds with the sound frequencies that resonate in those areas.

Therapeutic Method used with Alchemy Pure Quartz Crystals Singing Bowls and Vocal Sounds

To stimulate the root area: (Place the bowl between the sacrum and lumbar vertebrae area) (**Sacrum & L5 & L4**)
Sound: **U, U, UM** and use the Bowl with the note **Do = C, 396 Hz or 391.99 Hz** and stimulate with the sound frequencies for 4 to 5 minutes this area.

To stimulate the reproductive area: (Place the bowl between the lumbar vertebrae and the thoracic vertebrae) (**L3 to T12**)
Sound: **O, O, OM** and use the bowl with the note **RE = D, 417 Hz or 415.30 Hz,** and stimulate with the sound frequencies for 4 to 5 minutes.

To stimulate the solar plexus: (Place the bowl over the 11 thoracic vertebrae) (**T11 to T7**)

Sound: **O, O, OM** and use the bowl with the note **Mi = E, 528 Hz or 523.251 Hz** and stimulate with the sound frequencies for 4 to 5 minutes.

To stimulate the heart, lung, and thymus gland area: (Place the bowl over the 6' thoracic vertebrae) **(T6 to T2)**
Sound: **A, A, AM** and use the bowl with the note **FA = F, 417 Hz or 415.30 Hz** and stimulated with the sound frequencies for 4 to 5 minutes.

To stimulate the throat and face area: (Place the bowl between the cervical and neck area) **(T1 to C3)**
Sound: **E, E, EM** and use the bowl with the note **SOL = G, 741 Hz or 739.989 Hz** and it stimulates with the sound frequencies for 4 to 5 minutes.

To stimulate the third eye area: (Hold the bowl about **10 to 12 inches above or away from the head - the Crystal Bowl should not touch the head.**)
Sound: **I, I, IM** and use the bowl with the note **LA = A, 852 Hz or 830.609 Hz** and stimulate with the sound frequencies for 4 to 5 minutes.

To stimulate the crown area: (Hold the bowl about **10 to 12 inches away from or above the head - the Crystal bowl should not touch the head.**) Repeat the same Sound: **I, I, IM** and use the bowl with the note **Si (Ti) = B, 963 Hz or B5 987.77 Hz or A# 5 932.333 Hz** and stimulate the pituitary and pineal glands with the sound frequencies for 4 to 5 minutes.

"Magnetic Harmonic Vibrational Therapy" takes 35 to 40 minutes and the results are very favorable for people who receive this type of **"Vibrational Medicine"** therapy.

If you do not have the 7 Alchemist Crystal Singing Bowls Chakras Set for this therapy, I recommend that you use at least three of them in the musical notes: **Mi = (E), FA = (F), LA = (A)** and it is very effective when doing the vocal sounds for each area or chakra as indicated above.

I am not claiming that **Sound Vibrational Therapy** can cure a disease. Its use is merely experimental. The results may vary, but many people have achieved excellent therapeutic benefits which include relief from stress, anxiety, depression, and pain, and enjoying good energy and vitality.

25

The Healing Forces of Harmonic Sounds and Vibrations

Harmonization of meridians and chakras through the music of "The Healing Forces of Harmonic Sounds and Vibrations."

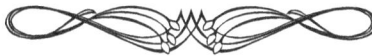

The music CD "The Healing Forces of Harmonic Sounds and Vibrations" has been programmed with specific sound frequencies to balance the chakras, meridians and body systems.

In 2004, I produced a music CD with specific vocal harmonic sounds that resonate with the chakras, using my voice, pure quartz crystal bowls and Tibetn bowls. I called this music production **"The Healing Forces of Harmonic Sounds and Vibrations."**

I also included the sounds of dolphins, whales, tropical birds, the coquí, and sounds produced by the five basic elements of Mother Earth. The CD is a new age musical production created with original arrangements and genuine music backgrounds. It is meant to be a revitalizing journey to the macro-cosmic and micro-cosmic universe that helps to harmonize all **energy centers or chakras of the listener.**

The harmonic sounds of the CD produce a relaxing feeling that helps balance the energy of the etheric, mental and physical bodies, and can improve health.

"The Healing Forces of Harmonic Sounds and Vibrations" CD is a sound therapy with many benefits.

Listening to the CD can revitalize and clean de-harmonizing energies, expand space, and harmonize energy fields (the holographic body and auric body.) It can also cleanse the mind and body from tension and stress, and balance thoughts, feelings and chakras. It stimulates intuition, increases optimism, encourages a good mood and activates higher perception. It also helps to activate the Delta, Theta, Alpha and Gamma brain waves.

The most effective way to listen to the CD is by sitting or lying in a quiet place for 15 to 30 minutes. Close the eyes, relax and listen to the album. Visualize and feel the sounds and vibrational frequencies moving inside the body, like waves or wind. Feel the chi or qi energy moving in harmony with the powerful sound frequencies, unblocking, regenerating and revitalizing all of the body's cells, organs and systems by stimulating the chakras.

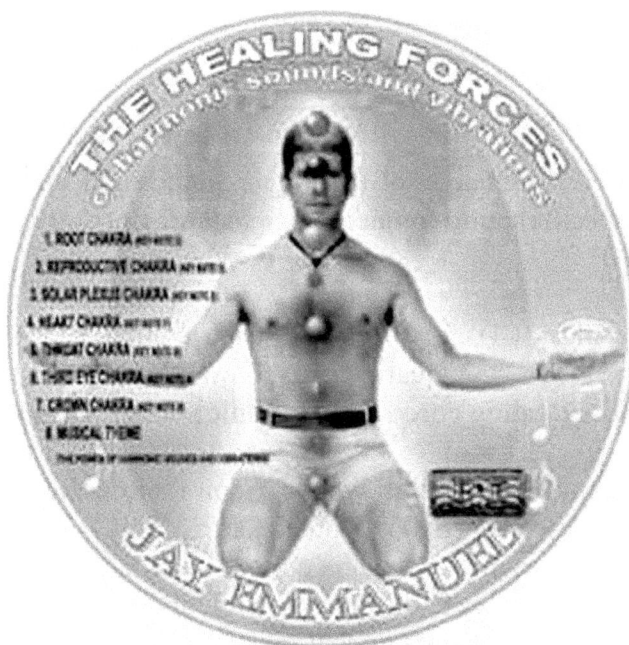

The music CD "The Healing Forces of Harmonic Sounds and Vibrations"

The macro and microcosmic universe is in a constant state of vibration. Harmonic sounds generated by this music will touch every fiber of your being, and stimulate the natural healing process of your body, mind and spirit. You will attain a state of harmony, peace and serenity.

Dr. Masaru Emoto is the author of ***The Hidden Messages in Water.*** In October 2004, Dr. Emoto and I participated in an event at the United Nations. The event was organized by Rev. Susana Bastarrica, president and coordinator of the United Nations Cultural Activities Department, Chapter Feng Shui.

The presentation was held to celebrate the **Vigil of World Peace**, and was followed by a concert in Central Park later that week. Dr. Emoto then took **"The Healing Forces of Harmonic Sounds and Vibrations"** CD to his native Japan and analyzed the CD in his laboratory to study the effect of sounds and vibrations on water.

On November 5, 2004, Dr. Emoto subjected 50 samples of distilled water in Petri dishes to **"The Healing Forces of Harmonic Sounds and Vibrations"** music CD. The 50 samples of frozen water were observed under an electron microscope and photographed. Twenty-four hexagonal patterns were formed. Dr. Emoto's analysis can be seen in the **healingpowerofharmony.com** page, under **"Sound Analysis."**

The purpose of this recording is expressed in song number 8 of the CD .

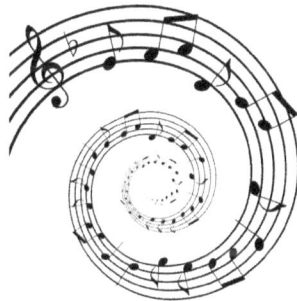

Harmonic Sounds and Vibrations

Open your heart to the power of the vibrations,
Open your mind to the power of harmonic sounds,
Everything in the universe is in a state of vibration,
Reflection of light counsciousness of God.

Open your eyes to the power of divine light,
Open your mind to the power of creative thoughts,
Every thought your mind creates,
It is in a state of vibration,
Reflection of the consciousness of your soul...

Harmonic frequencies turn into light,
And seven colors the rainbow form,
And all the spaces are filled with love,
The strongest force in all the universe.

(Music and lyrics: Jay Emmanuel Morales)

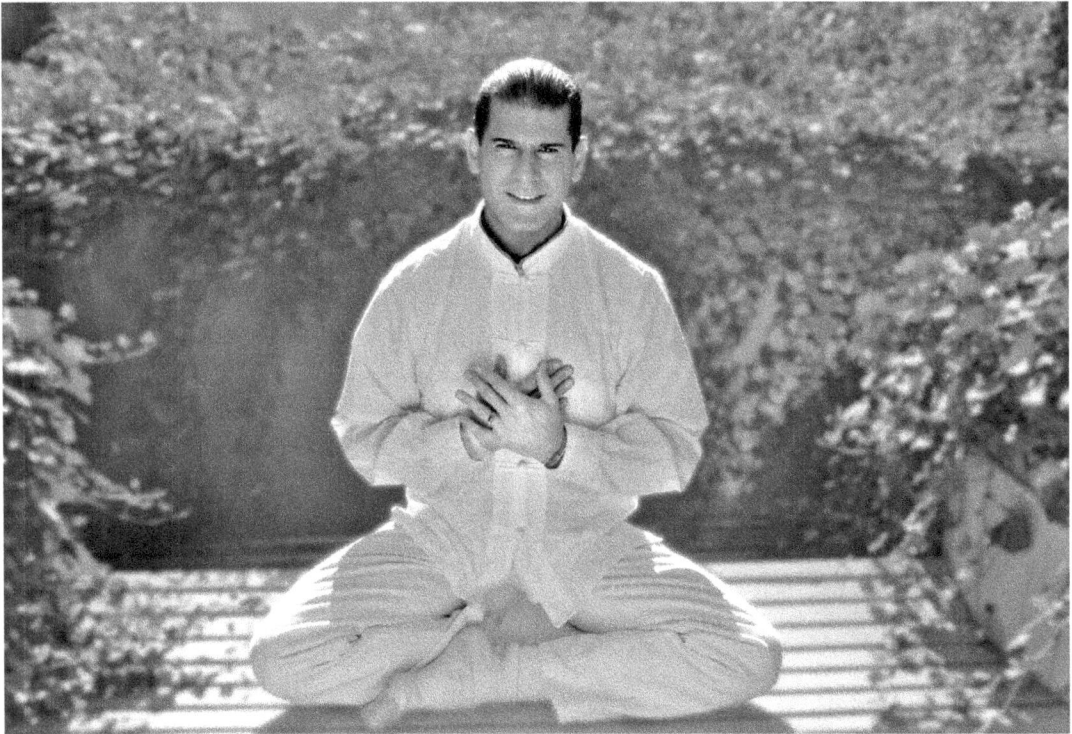

26

Analysis of Sounds and Music

Photographs of the analysis of sounds from the CD "The Healing Forces of Harmonic Sounds andn Vibrations." By Dr. Masaru Emoto's laboratory, in Japan, on November 5, 2004.

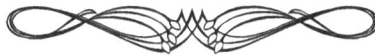

<hr/>

Photographs of the analysis of sounds from the CD "The Healing Forces of Harmonic Sounds and Vibrations."

The following photographs were obtained from the analysis of the harmonic sounds produced by the 8 songs on the CD **"The Healing Forces of Harmonic Sounds and Vibrations"** processed by the director of the I.H.M. Research Institute, Dr. Masaru Emoto, in Japan, on November 5, 2004.

Photograph taken in the laboratory of Dr. Masaru Emoto in Japan in 2004 of the music CD "The Healing Forces of Harmonic Sounds and Vibrations." **1st song: The Root Chakra, Musical Tone: C, Frequency: 396 Hz = 9.**

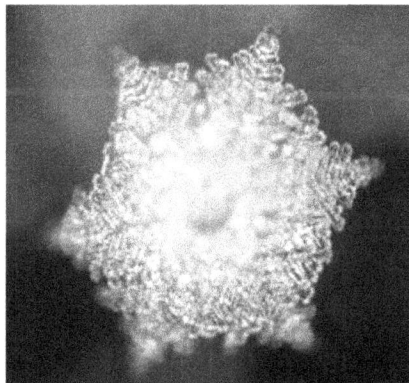

1ˢᵗ Chakra: MULADHARA

Photograph taken in the laboratory of Dr. Masaru Emoto in Japan in 2004 of the music CD "The Healing Forces of Harmonic Sounds and Vibrations." **2nd song: Reproductive Chakra, Musical Tone: D, Frequency: 417 Hz = 3.**

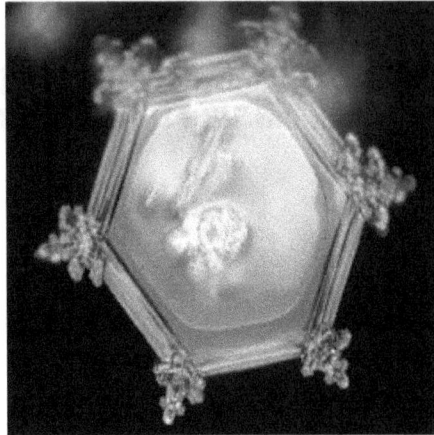

2ⁿᵈ Chakra: SVADHISTANA

Photograph taken in the laboratory of Dr. Masaru Emoto in Japan in 2004 of the music CD "The Healing Forces of Harmonic Sounds and Vibrations." **3rd song: Solar Plexus Chakra, Musical Tone: E, Frequency: 528 Hz = 6.**

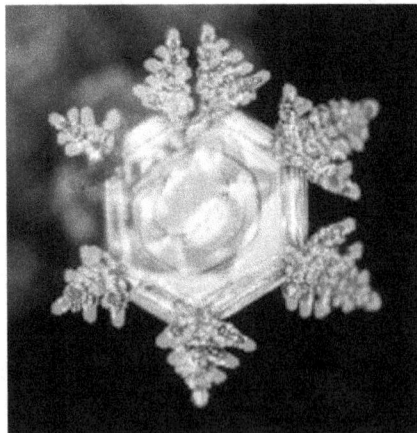

3ʳᵈ Chakra: MANIPURA

Photograph taken in the laboratory of Dr. Masaru Emoto in Japan in 2004 of the music CD "The Healing Forces of Harmonic Sounds and Vibrations." **4th song: Heart Chakra, Musical Tone: F, Frequency: 639 Hz = 9.**

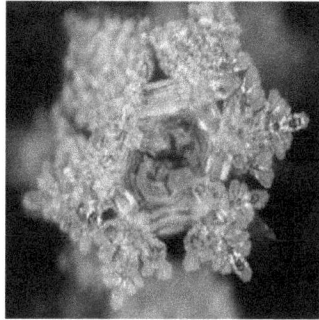

4th Chakra: ANAHATA

Photograph taken in the laboratory of Dr. Masaru Emoto in Japan in 2004 of the music CD "The Healing Forces of Harmonic Sounds and Vibrations." **5th song: Throat Chakra, Musical Tone: G, Frequency: 741 Hz = 3.**

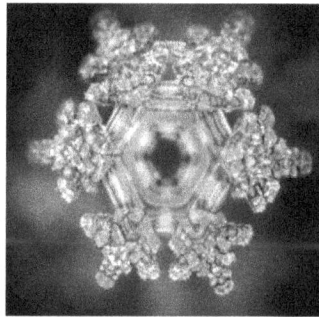

5th Chakra: VISHUDDHA

Photograph taken in the laboratory of Dr. Masaru Emoto in Japan in 2004 of the music CD "The Healing Forces of Harmonic Sounds and Vibrations." **6th song: Third Eye Chakra, Musical Tone: A, Frequency: 852 Hz = 6.**

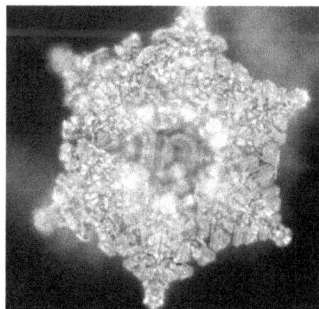

6th Chakra: AJNA

Photograph taken in the laboratory of Dr. Masaru Emoto in Japan in 2004 of the music CD "The Healing Forces of Harmonic Sounds and Vibrations." **7th song: Crown Chakra, Musical Tone: B, Frequency: 963 Hz = 9.**

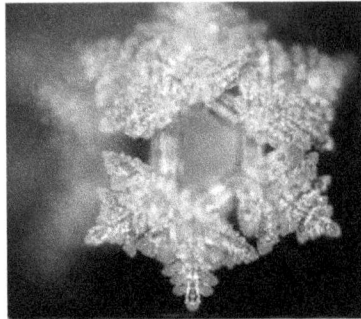

7ᵗʰ Chakra: SAHASRARA

Photograph taken in the laboratory of Dr. Masaru Emoto in Japan in 2004 of the music CD "The Healing Forces of Harmonic Sounds and Vibrations." **8th song: "Harmonic Sounds and Vibrations."**

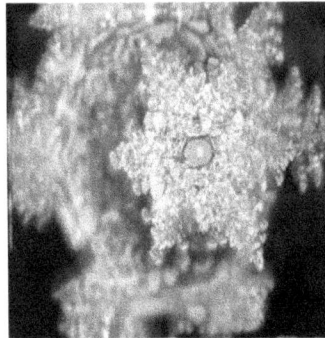

Harmonic Sounds and Vibrations
(Theme music CD)

Dr. Masaru Emoto, a Japanese scientist, discovered that water molecules can be altered by the frequencies of sounds and vibrations produced by our thoughts, words, songs and musical instruments. He titled his work **The Hidden Messages of Water.**

Dr. M. Emoto demonstrated that molecules of water reflect our emotions, feelings and words. Water is alive and responds to our emotions.

When water is exposed to melodious music and harmonic rhythm, as well as words like

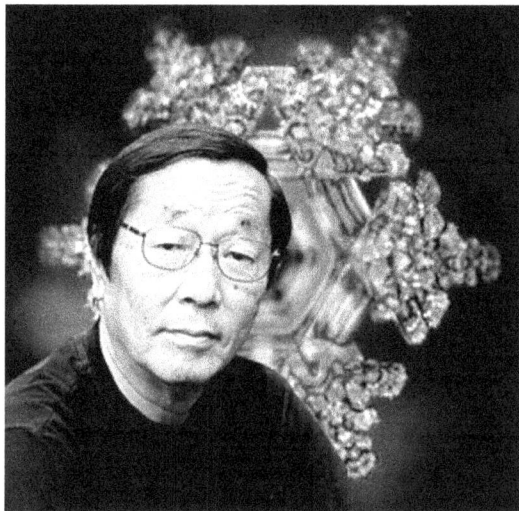

Dr. Masaru Emoto

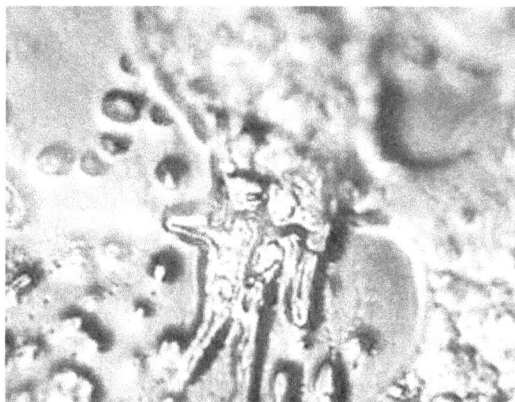

Photography of water that has been exposed to words with negative frequencies, "You make me sick, I'll kill you."

"love", "gratitude", "wisdom" and "divine order", water forms beautiful hexagonal crystals. The opposite happens when negative words are used such as "stupid", "hate", "anger", "fear", and "disease". The water becomes disorganized with deformed molecular agglomerations. Water also acquires a completely disorganized form when exposed to music with negative messages and not harmonic, such as hard rock, heavy metal, and rap.

Masaru Emoto's experiments have shown that when water is exposed to classical music and new age harmonic music, water molecules organize and form beautiful hexagonal shapes.

It has been scientifically proven that the spoken word can alter water's molecular structure. It is imperative to be careful when expressing our thoughts and emotions verbally. Words have the power to create and destroy.

Water is the most abundant element in our bodies and it facilitates the vast majority of our bodies' bio-chemical reactions at the cellular level. The brain is mostly water.

Thoughts generate an electromagnetic vibrational frequency that travels faster than the speed of light through specialized nervous cells. This stimulates the sensors of the larynx and tongue which produce sounds and words.

This sophisticated procedure is carried out through the conductive and universal solvent; water. Thus, when we create sound frequencies, they are recorded in the cell memory of our DNA, in our bodies and in our environment . Our words generate powerful sounds that activate vibrational frequencies that can alter the atomic structure of matter.

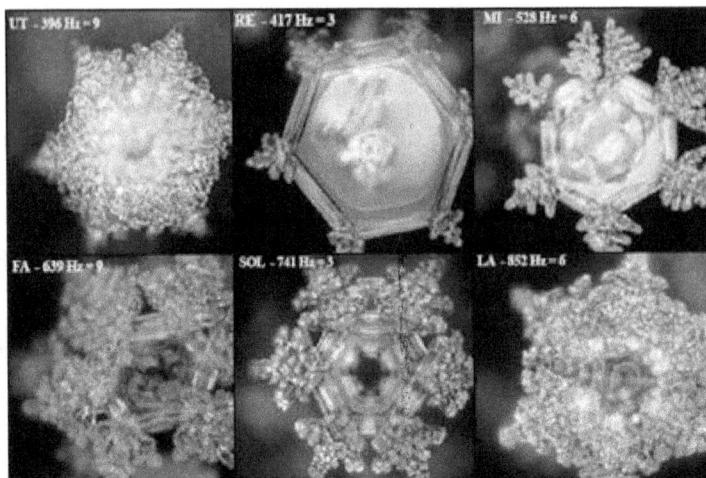

*Pictures taken in the laboratory of Dr. Masaru Emoto in Japan in 2004 of the
Music CD "The Healing Power of Harmonic Sounds and Vibrations."*

My theory is based on the following: The human body consists of 75% to 89% water. Sound frequencies have a direct effect on the water molecule.

When quartz crystal bowls are placed on a person's body or when they are played close to a person, the high frequencies of sound cause the body's molecules, lipids and mineral crystallizations to separate. This stimulates the natural healing process of the bio-physical systems at the cellular level.

When a person vocalizes specific vowel sounds and mantras in the Ancient Solfeggio Frecuencies they resonate with the chakras. The sound frequencies produce a separation of molecules and mineral crystallizations within the body at the cell plasma level. A balance between mind and body activates and contributes to good health.

Sounds produce vibrational frequencies and alter water and lipid molecules inside the body. When molecules get agglomerated inside the cell it is difficult for them to get out. Similarly, when molecules get agglomerated outside the cell it is difficult for them to get in.

Scientific studies have shown that specific harmonic sound frequencies can produce a vibrational energy that can prevent the agglomeration of molecules, allowing them to pass through the cell membrane and also facilitate better communication among cells.

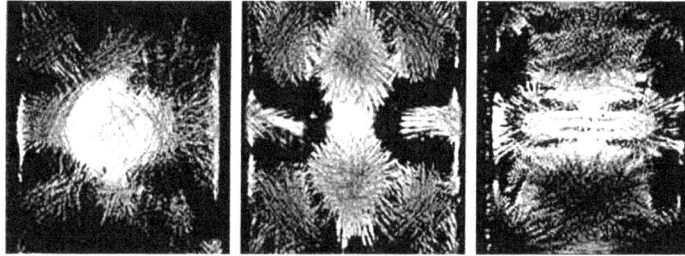

Image of water under vibrational sound frequencies.

Thus, the waste within a cell, can exit and nutrition products traveling in the bloodstream can enter the cell.

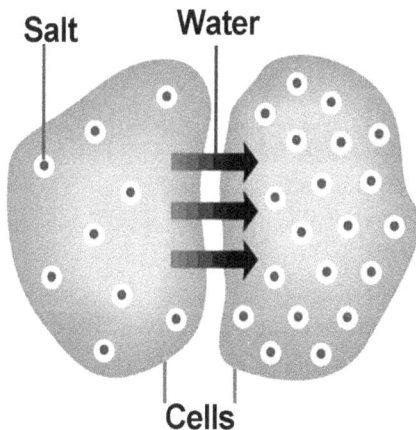

All this is due to harmonic sounds that produce vibrational frequencies that break the agglomeration of molecules, which allows them to move efficiently and quickly. Communication among cells increases, and detoxification and the body's natural healing process activates. This process is known as **electroporation.**

The effect of sound frequencies on water molecules.

Sounds produce vibrational frequencies that create geometric forms. Sounds and vibrations can alter the molecular and atomic structure of water, minerals and lipids and create a variety of geometric shapes.

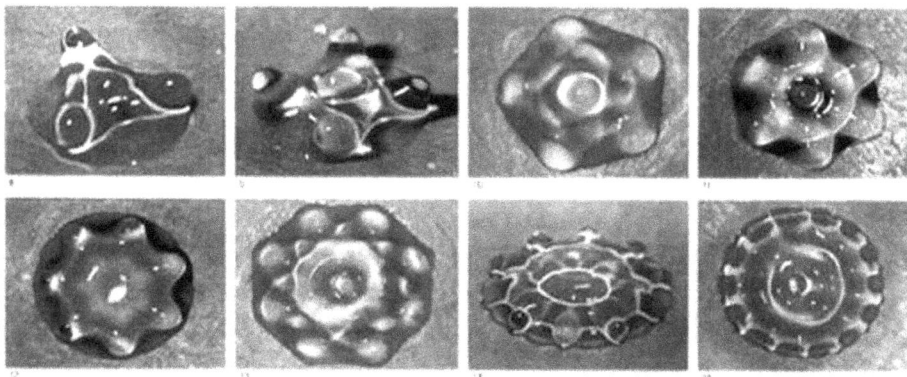

"Metamorphosis of water life energy"
Creative Words & Harmonic Vibrations,
Turn Life Energy of Water,
Into Hexagonalk Geometrical Diamonds formations,
Precious gifts jewels of positive mind creation... JEM

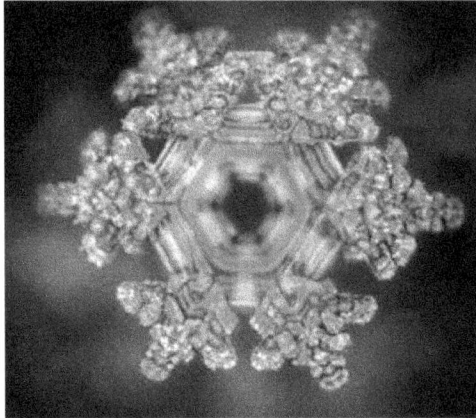

Hexagonal structure of the water molecule obtained from "The Healing Forces of Harmonic Sounds and Vibrations" CD.

Positive thinking can generate powerful vibrational frequency waves that create geometric shapes in water. Similarly, it can help to shape the world around us.

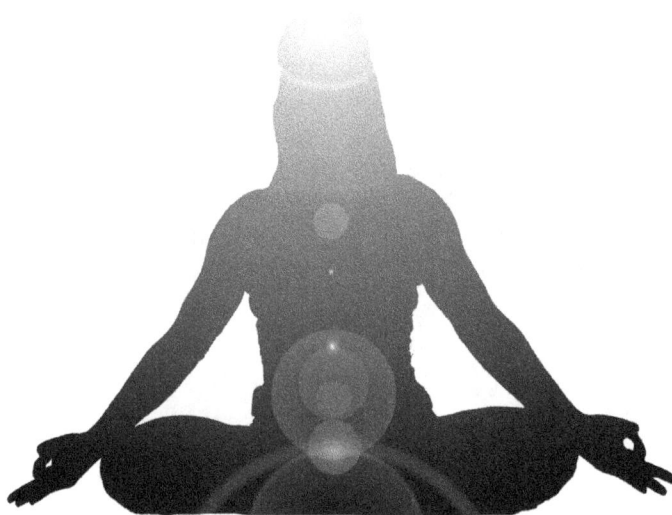

27

Effects of Sounds on Matter

Scientists Ernst Chladni, Hans Jenny, M.D. and the effect of Cymatics.

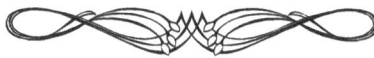

Scientific research of the effects of sounds on matter.

Sounds can alter the atomic structure of matter. More than two hundred years ago, German scientist **Ernst Chladni** (1756-1827), demonstrated that sand in a metal plate formed geometric patterns when a violin bow was played on the edge of the plate. Ernst Chladni is known as the father of acoustic research because of his work on the mathematics of sound waves.

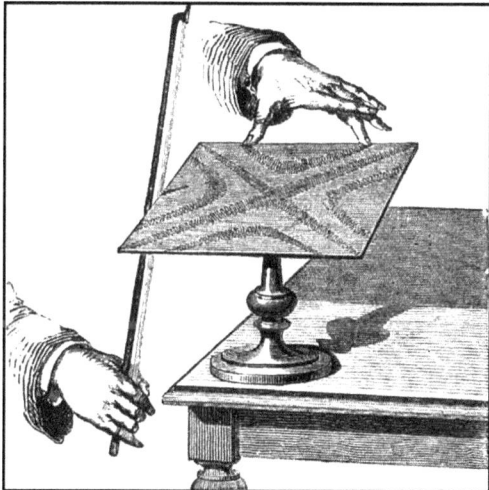

In the twentieth century, **Dr. Hans Jenny** (August 16, 1904 - June 23, 1972) was intrigued by Chladni patterns and spent fourteen years studying and doing experiments sculpting forms purely by sound.

Dr. Jenny's scientific experiments proved that geometric shapes were formed when particles of different elements were exposed to sound frequencies. He verified the effects by placing flour, rice, corn powder, liquid and fat on metal plates.

Intense sound frequencies cause these substances to dance and form shapes such as hexagons, pentagons, straight lines, curved lines, circles and other shapes. The geometric patterns seem to imitate astrophysical, geological, biological and atomic events.

Dr. Jenny photographed thousands of forms that were revealed in his investigation. Some shapes seemed like rotating spiral galaxies or solar flares, while others looked like flowers blooming or active amoebas. Dr. Jenny's work demonstrated that sound produces movement and gives rise to forms. Hans Jenny is known as the father of the **study of sound wave frequencies phenomena**. He called his scientific work **Cymatics.**

Hans Jenny published the first and second volumes of his scientific work on Cymatics, in 1967 and 1972.

Cymatics can influence the human body. When sound frequencies penetrate the human body, they stimulate water molecules, minerals and lipids, and can change their behavior.

When exposed to **"The Healing Forces of Harmonic Sounds and Vibrations"** individuals experience reduced tension in the connective tissue, pain relief, emotional stress relief and recovery from undesirable physical conditions. It also stimulates and balances the brain hemispheres, activates alpha relaxation and modifies thoughts and consciousness of the person.

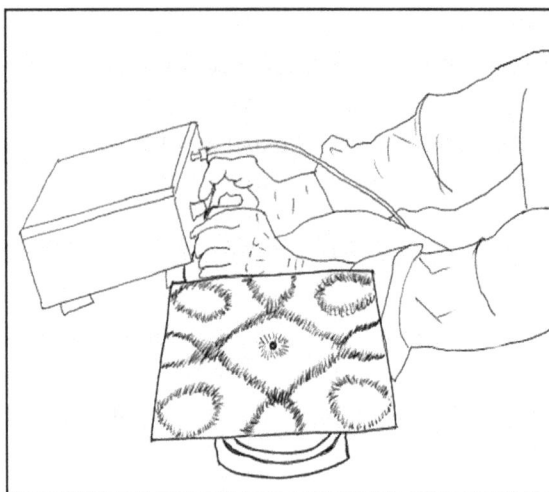

Formation of geometric forms through sound wave frequencies (Cymatics.)

Harmonic sounds produce vibrational frequencies that can modify the surface density of liquids which allows molecules, minerals and other substances to move more easily.

I have observed certain effects in my experiments with the vibrational frequencies on different elements. When I put water and oil in a pure quartz crystal bowl and begin to play it, I have observed that the intense vibrational frequencies produced by the bowl causes the oil to separate into small molecules and form tiny bubbles. The oil is fragmented and moves through the water causing it to have lower surface density.

The effect of sounds and harmonic vibrations on atoms, molecules, cells and the body

Sounds and harmonic vibrations can fix the atomic structure of our consciousness, magnetic body, energy body, sub-atoms, atoms, molecules and our body's cells.

In Buddhism and Hinduism, the repetition of sounds, mantras and the name of God, removes anger, hatred, selfishness, lust, etc. from our consciousness. A powerful magnetic vibrational healing force occurs, which harmonizes the spirit, mind and body.

Repeating mantras and affirmations with harmonic sounds purifies the mind, transports the person to the mental Alpha state of peace, serenity, inner joy and harmony. This mental alpha state effectively accelerates the natural healing process of the body, mind and spirit. In Eastern philosophy, this practice connects the person with the universal healing energy which is provided by the **Universal Cosmic Intelligence or God (the alpha state enhances the power of thought.)**

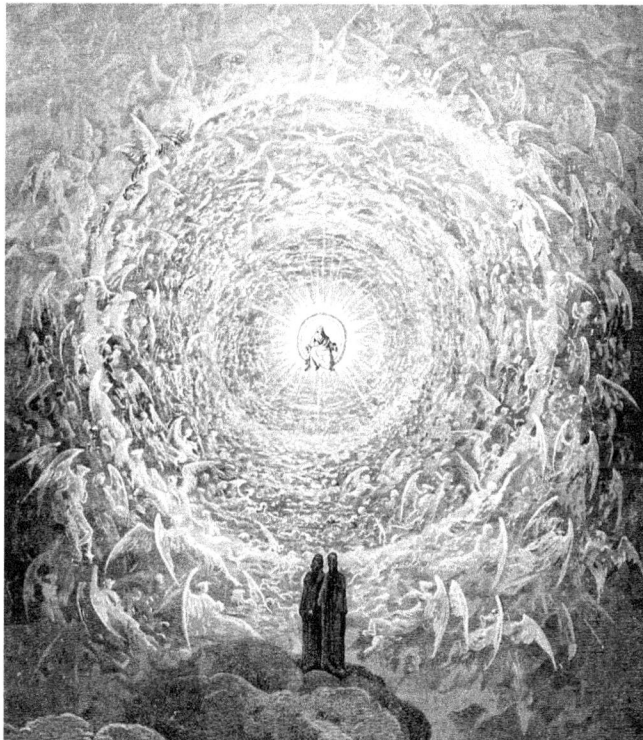

Illustration of the symbolic archetype of connection with the Universal Cosmic Intelligence.
(Cosmic Intelligence or God has no form, it is Pure Divine Energy.)

28

The Healing Effect of Meditation

**The healing effect of prayer and meditation, and
its connection to the matrix of creation.**

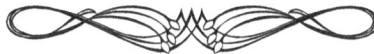

***

The healing effect of meditation

In 1993, members of the Transcendental Meditation group carried out scientific studies to determine whether mass meditation could reduce violence and crime. Approximately 4,000 meditators gathered from different cultures. The results showed that the meditation generated powerful vibrational frequency waves that reduced violence and crime almost to zero.

If a large number of people mantralize or sing songs with messages of peace, harmony and goodwill to all beings, a vibrational frequency could create positive changes. It transmits a collective vibrational frequency that activates a great energetic field or aura of protection that benefit all beings in our planet.

The healing effect of prayer

There is a spiritual axiom which says that what we establish into our minds and hearts will come true. That's why our thoughts, dreams, hopes and visions are important. What we think, and our focused intention while praying makes a big difference in the effectiveness of our prayers. It is the connection of mind and body. If our mind focuses on our Higher Self or the light that comes from our hearts as we pray, we can manifest and achieve peace, harmony, good health, creative situations and divine order.

When we pray, especially out loud, harmonic sounds are created and can manifest desired objectives such as self healing, healing a loved one, or peace, harmony and goodwill. These vibrational frequencies spread through the cosmos and help neutralize deharmonizing energy that can create chaos or destructive energy.

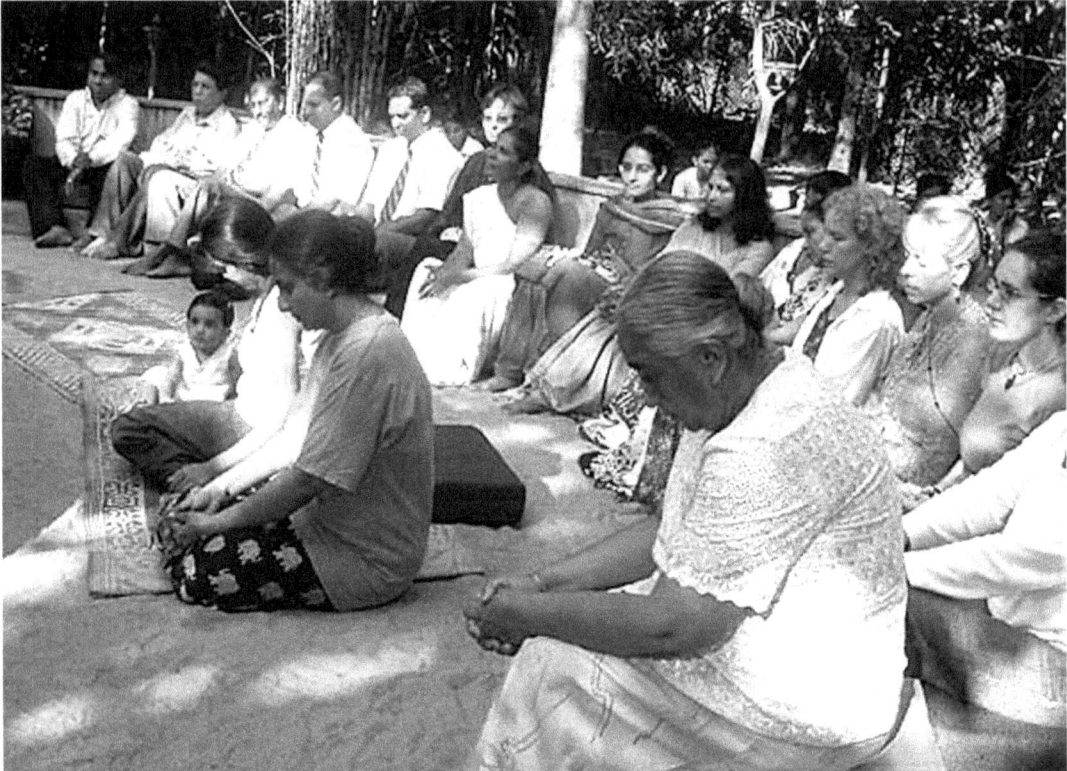

Group metitation for world peace.

The Universal Creative Force or Universal Infinite Intelligence responds to our prayers when they arise from the pure essence of our hearts.

Meditation through "The Healing Forces of Harmonic Sounds and Vibrations"

The meditation techniques described in **"The Healing Forces of Harmonic Sounds and Vibrations"** can help activate peace, harmony, and creative energy. It stimulates the natural healing power of our body and mind in order to neutralize negative energy from the environment.

By following **"The Healing Forces of Harmonic Sounds and Vibrations"** technique and the meditation, a powerful inner state of peace and balance can be achieved.

The practitioner's inner power is stimulated helping to transmute and eliminate negative energies, stress, fear, emotional traumas, diseases, hatred and resentment.

Meditation techniques described in "The Healing Forces of Harmonic Sounds and Vibrations" can produce physical and mental transformation.

A person's physical and mental constitution can change during meditation. People live with the energies of water and fire inside them. The energy of water lowers and the energy of fire rises. However, when the person meditates with **"The Healing Forces of Harmonic Sounds and Vibrations"** this tendency is reversed: The energy of water rises to the upper body and the fire energy moves to the lower body.

As time passes, this inversion accelerates. When the person's physical constitution is totally transformed, the fire energy descends to the bottom of the body to near extinction and water power rises strongly to the upper part of the body.

Water energy travels up along the spinal column of a person who sits and meditates for a long period. This movement feels like a thousand ants walking very subtly under your skin. The qi or chi energy of water produces an upward sensation from the cell level towards the bloodstream.

Inside the body moisture is extracted by the qi or chi energy. When qi or chi energy is activated, water energy moves upward. If this process continues long enough, your physical constitution changes completely. Another result of the transformation is cooling between the eyebrows, as if you had placed ice at that point.

In addition, a pure energy spreads upward toward the apex of the crown of the head. The vertex, which is also known as "the hole or mouse hole," is where the energy passes through. This meditation allows you to feel the movement of energy through the orifice or mouse hole. This opening is the vertex where pure energy extends to the sky and universe.

Through disciplined internal work and personal evolution, it is possible to activate enlightenment. When a person becomes enlightened, physical constitution transforms, the energy of fire descends, the energy of water ascends, and pure and clean energy extends towards the sky and universe. Human constitution can change radically in this case.

Using **"The Healing Forces of Harmonic Sounds and Vibrations"** techniques in combination with mantras during meditation, can create a balanced environment within our consciousness. The sounds and harmonic vibrations can have a profound effect on the mind, which can result in a new way of thinking. When we speak we produce sounds. Thoughts also produce inaudible ultrasonic sounds. Thus, to make important changes in our lives, we should make changes in the pattern of thoughts and the sounds that are created within our consciousness.

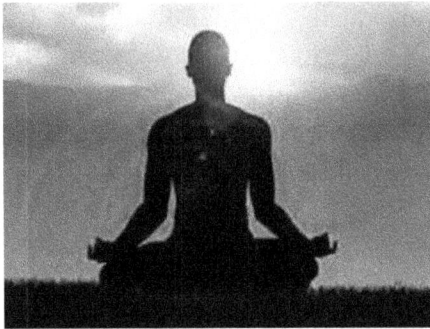

How should meditation be performed?

To meditate sit in the lotus position or in a chair with feet touching the ground and hands facing upwards, resting on the thighs. If you meditate on a chair make sure not to cross your feet. The spine must remain vertically aligned, without stiffness or tension.

Slowly inhale and exhale rhythmically four times, very relaxed. Visualize the energy of golden, silver white and violet rays, coming from the center of the universe to the crown chakra, third eye, cerebellum, throat, and thymus, directing them to the heart chakra.

From the center of Mother Earth, visualize golden, silver, white and blue rays up to the root, reproductive, solar plexus chakra and towards the heart chakra.

The 8 rays come together in the heart chakra and create a circumference that moves clockwise. As you inhale and exhale the circumference expands sunlight, leaves the heart and amplifies around the body, creating a protective oval field of sunlight energy (the auric egg).

The person becomes a sun-generating light and activates an internal powerful healing energy of peace, harmony and divine order. This can protect us from negative energies, connect us with regenerative harmonic sounds, with pure chi or qi energy coming from the universe, and help activate the natural healing process of mind and body.

Meditation and connection with the matrix of the collective consciousness of creation.

Many cultures, including the monasteries in Egypt, Tibet, India and indigenous cultures from the mountains of Bolivia and Peru, confirm a transforming bodily experience during meditation.

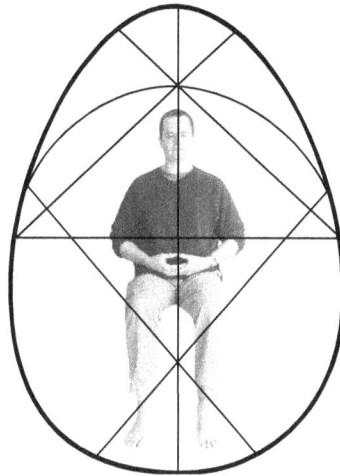

Activating the egg-shaped aura through meditation.

These cultures believe that meditation affects our cells and can affect the world. Initially, science did not recognize the power of meditation because they thought that when we meditate we enter space that is empty, but in reality is not empty. However, when we meditate we connect with **"the matrix of collective consciousness of creation"** (Universal Intelligence or Universal Mind) which has a great influence on us far beyond the capacities we have through our mind and body.

During meditation, we can access this matrix and manifest healing from any conditions, and experience miracles. Science is beginning to accept the power of the mind and meditation.

Western science is beginning to understand that the manifestation of healing and physical changes from the cellular level to the collective level around us, can be achieved through the mental power of intention, harmonic sounds and meditation.

Space is not empty, it is filled with a pulsating living essence that science has defined as "The Quantum Hologram."

Dr. Edgar Mitchell, a former astronaut from the Apollo mission, defines it as "Nature's Mind," Stephen Hawking called it "God's Mind" and other scientists called it "The Field." In 1944 the father of Quantum Physics, Max Planck, identified the existence of this field or space as the matrix and Edgar Cayce called it The Akashic Archives or "The Book of Life".

Max Planck said that everything we see around us, including our bodies is part of the matrix of collective consciousness of creation (Universal Mind or Intelligence). On March 31, 1999 the successful film **"The Matrix,"** was presented in the United States of America by an Australian company, written and directed by the Wachowski brothers. This movie was based on these ideas and concepts.

Max Planck said that each of us has the power to influence the collective consciousness or matrix. However, this must be achieved through the human heart. It is not a mental process. The great mystics of ancient civilizations knew this. They distinguished between thoughts, feelings and emotions.

In a previous chapter of this book I mentioned that there is an intrinsic relationship between mind and heart. Every thought in the human mind emits vibrational electromagnetic waves, which are generated from the base of the heart. Thought construction involves the biophysical operation of mind and heart. The heart is the strongest electromagnetic vibrational field generator in the human body. The deepest feelings in our heart give rise to the outward manifestation and is defined as coherent emotion.

When we feel love, compassion, and understanding, and when we forgive ourselves and others, our self-esteem changes. A biochemical electromagnetic reaction is triggered within our hearts, which creates an energy field that changes the energy in and around the body.

The heart generates the strongest magnetic field in the body, much stronger than the brain. When we generate positive thoughts, feelings, love, affirmations, mantras and meditation as described in **"The Healing Power of Sound and Harmonic Vibrations,"** we enter the matrix and miracles can be manifested. The altering of atomic structure is possible.

Western science is beginning to understand what ancient cultures and indigenous peoples knew thousands of years ago. They knew that everything is connected and we are all part of a network of collective consciousness and universal intelligence.

The feelings created in our hearts and minds can influence the **matrix** field, which is the collective energy field that connects us all. Science shows that we are made of atoms and when we produce changes, we produce changes in the atoms. We are literally altering the physical reality in a way that sounds miraculous to Western science.

Given this knowledge, it can be understood more clearly that the power to heal and to help heal others is within us. The human body has its own pharmacy of inner wisdom that responds to emotions and thoughts generated by our hearts and minds. When we create thoughts of love, compassion and creative positive energy, through the harmonic sound frequencies that are originated when we speak, when we sing, when we do affirmations and mantras, the internal pharmacy activates the natural healing process.

The healing process is naturally latent in each of us and the atomic structure of our cells is affected by our emotions and thoughts. Similarly, when we join our thoughts and hearts, and when we pray and meditate, we can help to heal our loved ones, plants, and animals. We can also help change the collective conscience of humanity to one of peace, harmony, love and goodwill. This practice has the power to neutralize fear, insecurity, disease, chaos or any deharmonizing energy.

How can we manifest healing for conditions and diseases?

When one has a condition or disease, do not judge the disease or condition as bad or good. You must say that it is a quantum possibility and there are many possibilities and of course this is only one of them.

You must invite the manifestation of a new possibility rather than make a change in what is there. In the case of a tumor or cancer you have to feel that somehow you have to manipulate or cut that condition or change the physical reality that activates submission to the condition or illness.

What is being done at that moment, is recognizing the change in the quantum model. In this case, healing is made by the union of several people who combine their energy to help the sick. These people are feeling that there is another possibility, and in doing so, allow the new possibility to replace what exists without judging the condition or illness.

The thoughts and words are very important. Mantras, prayers, affirmations, techniques described in **"The Healing Froces of Harmonic Sounds and Vibrations"** and creative visualization have the ability to manifest healing and positive changes.

Ancient civilizations speak about this in the Sanskrit texts. They say that thought is the image of quantum possibility. In other words, in the field of all possibilities, all that exists is already manifested. To manifest or materialize what we want, we must feel deeply in our hearts. Our self-esteem is important.

When we feel what we say and when what we say comes from the depths of our heart, the affirmations, mantras, prayers and harmonic sounds generated by our consciousness, mind, heart, and voice, all of these provide the energy to manifest our desires.

In scientific terms one could say that; "**The Divine Matrix**" is a mirror and bridge between our inner and outer world that can give us what we create through our thoughts, feelings, mind and heart.

Thoughts, emotions and feelings

The Sanskrit tradition speaks of seven energy centers or **chakras**. Upper centers: the crown, the third eye, and throat chakras are related to thinking and logical process. Lower centers: the root, reproductive, and solar plexus chakras are related to emotions and creative energy.

To make a picture in our minds of something perfect, like peace and perfect relations among nations, we must breathe deeply and carry that emotion into our mind and heart. This way you activate the thought and energy, which enable the power to manifest and transform. The emotion comes from the three creative lower centers of our body, from the bottom of our body to our mind.

Science defines the heart as a liquid crystal oscillator. The heart pumps the flow of life or blood throughout the body. Blood contains crystalline substances that resonate with sound frequencies produced by our mind and emotions when we talk, sing and chant mantras. Crystalline substances in the blood are also affected by sounds in our environment.

Through our emotions and thoughts, in combination with rhythmic breathing, the vibrational frequency is transported through the blood and nervous system. This happens faster than the speed of light, activates the heart, and manifests changes in our environment.

The heart is the most powerful liquid crystal oscillator of the body. It activates palpitations, rhythm, sound and vibrational frequencies that produce feelings, emotions and the thoughts of the goals we wish to manifest.

The power of faith

The Gospel of Thomas says that when thought and emotion become one, we can undergo amazing transformations and miracles. **Jesus said, metaphorically, that faith moves mountains.**

Feeling is the language that communicates with the body. Sometimes people complain that affirmations, prayers and chanting mantras do not provide results. **However, to obtain results one must feel deeply from the heart the emotion that what we asked for, has already been manifested.**

The connection between feeling and emotion is important. Furthermore, be sure to consider the right time to say affirmations, prayers and mantras in order to manifest the desired objective.

Human emotion, feeling and belief is not a verbal language. Therefore, we must be very specific about what we want to manifest in our lives. If we do not have a clear and specific picture of what we want to achieve, then it will be difficult to achieve the goal.

Meditation for recharging and healing the body and the mind

It has been scientifically proven that people who recite affirmations, mantras, or prayers, and also meditate at least 20 minutes a day, enjoy better health and increase their happiness and mind focus. These practices show increased activity in the brain's prefrontal cortex, harmonize the two hemispheres of the brain and fortify the immune and endocrine systems. Many corporations, hospitals and universities are utilizing these practices and have observed very positive results with employees, patients and students.

Learn to do affirmations, prayers, mantras and vocal sounds for at least 10 or 15 minutes, followed by a 20 minute mediation. Find a quiet place, and sit in a comfortable position with the spine vertically aligned and without tension. Close your eyes and breathe four inhalations and four exhalations rhythmically and slowly. Feel the entire body relaxing from head to toe and imagine or visualize yourself in a quiet, peaceful or beautiful place in nature such as by an ocean, on top of a mountain, in front of a stream or any other place you can transport your higher self that works for you. Contemplate deep within your mind and focus your attention on a specific point, such as in the movement of the ocean waves, the light coming from the sunrise or sunset, or the movement of a tree by the wind blowing or floating in the space. Find the visualization that works best for you. Feel an inner powerful sense of peace and harmony inside you and around your body and mind. Feel that at this moment of meditation you are traveling beyond space and time. You are floating in the matrix of creation. It's Nirvana. Nirvana in Buddhism is defined as a transcendental state in which there is neither suffering, desire, nor sense of self or ego. It is the state of perfect happiness.

Our mind, body and spirit need recharging in the same way that we recharge a laptop computer, cellphone or flashlight. People often get so involved with their work and daily routines that they forget to dedicate time to themselves. This can cause a drop in their internal energy and result in more tension and stress, and development of hypertension, mental imbalance, digestive system disorders, emotional problems, immune system deficiencies and cancer. We need to learn to take care of our mental, emotional, spiritual and physical health in order to be at our best in our daily work, to meet our responsibilities and accomplish our goals. Reciting affirmations, mantras or prayers for 10 or 15 minutes a day and a 20 to 30 minute meditation at least 4 times a week, can result in greater happiness, better energy, vitality and well being. Maintain a healthy diet by consuming fresh greens, fruits, seeds, legumes and organic non-GMO protein. A healthy organic natural diet helps to elevate the vibratory frequency since food is also one of the main sources of energy.

29

The Vibrational Nature of Matter

The vibrational nature of essential oils and frequencies generated by thought, body and food.

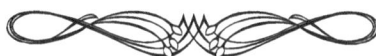

❧❦

Meaning of frequency measurements in Hertz (Hz)

Frequency is the number of occurrences of a repeating event per unit time. Everything has energy and produces a frequency.

Neutrinos, sub-atoms and atoms are constantly moving, producing vibrational frequencies and sounds. Each periodic motion has a frequency. The number of oscillations per second is what determines the measurement in Hertz.

1 hertz (Hz) = 1 oscillation per second (ops)
1 kilohertz (KHz) = 1,000 oscillations per second (ops)
1 megahertz (MHz) = 1,000,000 oscillations per second (ops)
1 terahertz (THz) = 1,000,000,000,000 oscillations per second (ops)

Essential oils and their natural vibrational energy

The frequencies of essential oils are measured in megahertz (MHz.)

Vibrational frequencies produced by therapeutic essential oils and their effects on the human body

Therapeutic essential oils contain high molecular concentrations that generate frequencies vibrating from 52 MHz to 320 MHz, and are able to increase the body's frequency. These can also help the immune system and to fight bacterial, viral, and fungal invasions which can result in disease. Microorganisms that cause disease cannot survive in the presence of therapeutic essential oils. Some essential oils have higher frequencies than herbs, food and the human body.

Each essential oil has a vibrational frequency which is measured in MHz. Each of our body's organs also has a specific frequency that is measurable. The frequencies of essential oils have frequencies that resonate with the systems of the human body. Lower frequencies absorb negative energy.

When the oil is inhaled or placed topically, the frequency remains in the body for a long time. Lower frequencies produce physical changes in the body. Average frequencies stimulate emotional changes in the body. Higher frequencies stimulate spiritual changes. The spiritual frequencies range from 92 MHz to 360 MHz.

Inhaling essential oils is beneficial. The oil's molecules travel through the nose and are trapped by the olfactory membrane. The nerve cells of the olfactory membrane send electrical impulses to the olfactory bulb in the brain and transmit electrical impulses to the body's systems. Essential oils can have a profound effect on the physiological, psychological and spiritual domains.

Essential oils and their frequencies in MHz

Essential Oil	Frequency (MHz)	Essential Oil	Frequency (MHz)
Basil	52	Juniper	98
Mint	78	Chamomile	105
Orange	90	Myrrh	108
Lemon	90	Lavender	118
Sandalwood	96	Incense	147
Aloe Vera	96	Rose	320

The human body generates vibrational frequencies

The human body generates an electric vibrational frequency which can determine a person's health.

Dr. Robert O. Becker, M.D., in his book **The Body Electric,** explains that a person's health can be determined according to the frequency generated by the body. For example, the frequency of bones ranges from 38-43 Hz; from the neck down the frequency is 62-68 Hz. All matter, as well as the human body, generates an electromagnetic frequency.

Nicolas Tesla (1856-1943) was one of the pioneers of electrical technology. He said that if you could eliminate certain external frequencies, we would have a greater resistance to disease.

Dr. Royal Rife demonstrated that every health disorder has a vibrational frequency that in turn responds or resonates with an optimal specific frequency. This can help eliminate the disorder and stimulate the body's natural healing process. Rife discovered that certain frequencies can destroy microorganisms, thus preventing the spread of disease.

Vibrational Medicine is being implemented as one of the revolutionary methods in the future of health science

Using electrical energy to reverse or eliminate disease led to the investigation and discovery of electrical frequencies that produce vibrational frequencies which can help recover, maintain and improve health.

In recent decades, Europe, Japan, China, Korea and the United States have been investigating the treatment of disease by electrical signals and vibrational frequencies. Implementing radio frequencies and electric impulses instead of chemicals may be the next wave in medicine.

In 1920 Georges Lakhovsky discovered that all living cells (plants, people, bacteria, parasites, virus, etc.) have attributes normally associated with electronic circuits. Dr. Royal R. Rife discovered that every disease has a specific frequency, and certain frequencies can prevent disease.

Dr. Harold Saxton Burr discovered that all beings, from men to mice, from trees to seeds, are molded and controlled by electromagnetic fields that are measurable. He defined his scientific work in terms such as **"life fields or fields L, which is the original basic level of life on this planet."** Measuring electrodynamic fields in people reveals their physical and mental conditions.

L-fields and electrodynamic fields can be used to predict diseases by observing their variations. Based on this research, doctors could diagnose their patients' conditions before they are expressed and thus would offer preventive treatments that would benefit them.

Dr. Reinhold Voll identified correlations between disease states and changes in electrical resistance of acupuncture points on the human body. The German biophysicist Fritz Albert Popp found that diseased cells radiate photonic patterns differently than healthy cells of the same type.

Dr. Robert O. Becker found that the human body generates an electrical frequency which can determine and influence a person's health.

Ancient civilizations used sounds to generate harmonic frequencies to heal their sick. Currently, recent technological developments based on the aforementioned scientists' studies have yielded precise, viable and effective instruments that generate electrical frequencies. The output of sounds and vibrations address disease and restore balance in the body.

Our thoughts create vibrational frequencies

Our thoughts influence the vibrational frequencies that are generated by the organs and body systems. **Negative thoughts** decrease the vibrational frequency to **10 MHz** and **positive thoughts** increase the frequency measured to **12 MHz**. It has been observed that **prayer and meditation** increase the vibrational frequencies to **15 MHz.**

People who maintain optimal and positive frequency benefit their immune systems and in turn can prevent the development of symptoms and illnesses associated with common colds and other conditions and diseases.

Stress, negative thoughts and emotional problems tend to lower the body's frequency and can make a person vulnerable to infection, disease and cancer.

Therefore, we must increase our body's frequency daily, through positive thinking, affirmations, mantras, **"The Healing Forces of Harmonic Sounds and Vibrations,"** classical or new age music, prayer and meditation. Also, pure essential oils are compatible with our cellular frequency and can increase the cells' vibrational frequency to activate good health.

The human body is a sophisticated biophysical system that is constantly generating vibrational electric frequencies

The human body generates an electrical and vibrational frequency which can determine one's health.

In 1992, Bruce Tainio of Tainio Technology, an independent division of the Eastern Washington University, in Cheney, Washington, built the first frequency monitor in the world and called it the **Frequency Counter BT2.**

Bruce Tainio's research determined that the human **body's normal frequency** during the day ranges from **62 to 68 MHz**. The frequency of a **healthy body** is from **62 to 72 MHz.** When the frequency decreases, the immune system suffers and the person becomes vulnerable to pathogens that can affect health.

The following are the frequencies of the human body in MHz:

The normal frequency of the **human brain and head** from 6:00 am to 6:00 pm ranges from **70-78 to 90 MHz.** The range of the **brain of a genius is 80-82 MHz.** The **range of a normal brain** is **72 MHz.**

The frequencies of the **human body from the neck up** have a range of **70-72 to 78 MHz.** The frequencies of the healthy **human body from the neck down** from 6:00 am to 6:00 pm range from **62-68 to 72 MHz.**

The frequencies of the **thyroid and parathyroid** glands have a range of **62-68 MHz.** The **thymus gland** has a range of **65-68 MHz. The heart** has a range of **67 to 70 MHz. The lungs** have a range of **58 to 65 MHz. The liver** has a range of **55 to 60 MHz. The pancreas** has a range of **60 to 80 MHz. The stomach** has a range of **58 to 65 MHz. The ascending colon** has a range of **58 to 60 MHz. The descending colon** has a range of **58-63 MHz. The bones** have a range of **38-43 MHz.**

Human cells begin to **mutate** when frequencies fall below **62 MHz.** The frequency of **colds and flu** have a range of **57-60 MHz. Pneumonia and Epstein-Barr** start at **52 MHz. Diseases in general, including headaches,** begin at **58 MHz.** The growth of **candida** is generated at **58 MHz**; **viral diseases** at **55 MHz**. The Epstein-Barr frequencies start at **52 MHz, tissue damage** due to illness starts at **48 MHz.** Receptivity of body cells with **cancer** begins at **42 MHz. Death** starts from **20 to 25 MHz.**

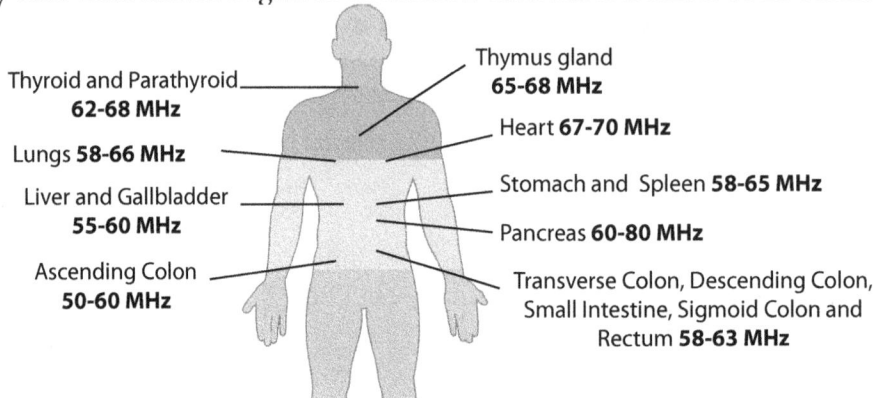

Thyroid and Parathyroid
62-68 MHz

Lungs **58-66 MHz**

Liver and Gallbladder
55-60 MHz

Ascending Colon
50-60 MHz

Thymus gland
65-68 MHz

Heart **67-70 MHz**

Stomach and Spleen **58-65 MHz**

Pancreas **60-80 MHz**

Transverse Colon, Descending Colon, Small Intestine, Sigmoid Colon and Rectum **58-63 MHz**

Disease frequencies in MHz.

When frequencies of human cells fall below **62 MHz** cellular processes begin to induce mutations. Low frequencies also indicate an imbalance in pH. When there is an acid environment in the body, pathogens that produce low vibrational frequencies harm the body and contribute to the spread of disease.

Friendly bacteria, which are part of the body's intestinal flora and produced by probiotics, generate high frequencies that help the body and strengthen the immune system. These beneficial bacteria improve the assimilation of nutrients at the cellular level and contribute to the pH balance in the body. **pH from 4.0 to 6.0** is acidic, **pH of 7.0** is neutral, **pH from 8.0 to 10** is alkaline.

Frequencies of food in Hz

Fresh food and herbs have high frequencies when grown organically **without** the use of preservatives, artificial additives and chemical pesticides. **Organic food and fresh herbs** have a range of **20-27 Hz. Dried food and dried herbs** have a range of **12-15 to 22 Hz. Processed, frozen and canned foods,** which are foods that most people consume daily, have frequencies of **0 Hz.**

The information of frequencies of essential oils, foods, the human body and the frequencies of diseases was obtained through Bruce Tainio Technology.

Electromagnetic Frequencies of mind and body are not perceived by the senses

The mind and body produce electromagnetic frequencies that cannot be seen. They are similar to the vibrational frequencies waves produced by radio sounds. Computers also generate vibrational frequencies that are not perceived by the senses.

Prayer, affirmations, mantras and spiritual songs also produce powerful, transformative, vibrational frequencies that are not apparent to the senses. The fact that you cannot see or perceive something at first glance does not mean it does not exist. The effects of vibrational frequencies and sounds not perceived by the human ear and other senses, are so obvious that they challenge current knowledge and understanding.

30

Homeopathy and Vibrational Medicine

Homeopathy – a form of vibrational medicine. History of homeopathy and Samuel Hahnemann, the creator of Homeopathy.

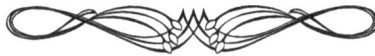

Homeopathy and Vibrational Medicine

Christian Friedrich Samuel Hahnemann is the father of **alternative medicine and homeopathy.** He was born in Meissen, Saxony, Germany near Dresden, on April 10, 1755 and died in Paris on July 2, 1843. He is buried in a mausoleum in the Père Lachaise de Paris cemetery.

Hahnemann studied medicine for two years in Leipzig and due to the lack of clinical services in Leipzig, moved to Vienna, where he studied for 10 months. After a period of further study, he graduated with the highest honors at the University of Erlangen on August 10, 1779.

In 1781, Hahnemann took the position of a village doctor in the copper mining area of Mansfeld, Saxony. Soon after, he married Johanna Henriette Kuchler and had 11 children. After leaving the medical practice, he worked as a translator of scientific and medical texts. Hahnemann traveled around Saxony for many years, staying in different cities and towns through different periods of his life.

Hahnemann was not satisfied with the protocols of medicine at the time, and particularly opposed blood draws. He claimed that medical drugs did more harm than good. Hahnemann gave up his practice in 1784 and then made his living primarily as a writer and translator, while researching causes of alleged medical errors. While

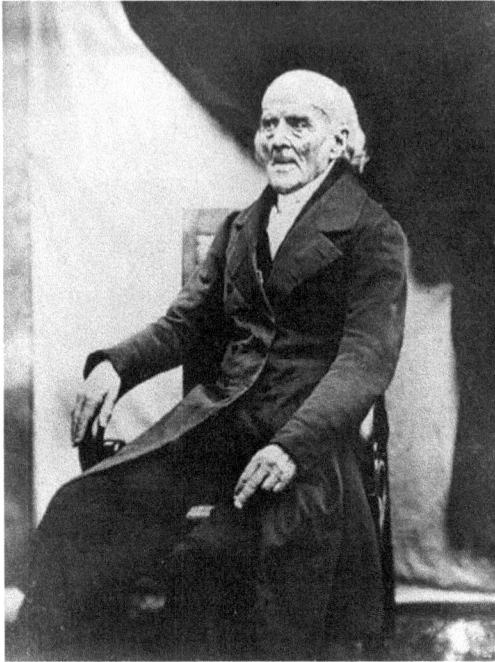

Samuel Hahnemann

Hahnemann was translating **"Treatise on Medical Matter,"** by William Cullen, he found a plant called Cinchona on the bark of a Peruvian tree which was effective in treating malaria due to its high astringents content.

Hahnemann did not believe that other substances containing astringents were effective against malaria and began to investigate the effect of Cinchona on the human body through self-application. He found that it induced similar symptoms of malaria, and concluded that it could do the same in a healthy individual.

This led him to postulate a healing principle: what can produce a set of symptoms in a healthy person, can be used to treat an ill patient who is manifesting a similar set of symptoms. This principle, (like cures like) became the basis of what he called **homeopathy.**

Homeopathy is a system of alternative medicine where elixirs, substances and pills, are programmed through the vibrational frequencies obtained from extracts, herbs, flower essences, minerals and other substances. **Homeopathic remedies contain only specific vibrational frequencies of the substances of which they are made.** There is nothing physically present in the essences. When a person ingests the homeopathic remedy, its programmed energy signature or vibrational frequency is disseminated in the patient's electromagnetic field. No side effects result from the fact that is non-material subatomic energy medicine.

There are two processes within homeopathic remedies:

1. The first action will cancel the problematic vibration or frequency, such as aluminum or mercury. Homeopathic remedies act as a "magnet" that attracts or draws vibrations that can cause imbalances.

2. The second action will produce a positive effect, such as a mineral, amino acid or

remedy made to impart a favorable vibration in the patient's electromagnetic field.

Currently, homeopathy is considered a form of alternative medicine. The idea is that substances that cause symptoms in healthy people, such as raw onions that cause irritation and watery eyes, can be used in a diluted form to treat diseases that cause the same symptoms. In this example, raw onion extract can be used as an ingredient (very diluted) in a remedy to treat cold or the flu or allergies which have eye symptoms such as irritation and watery eyes.

Hahnemann believed that life depends on a **vital force**, invisible and undetectable, (prana or qi) that passes through the body (vitalism.) If this force is disturbed or imbalanced, illness or disease will follow. He believed that his remedies restored balance in the perturbed vital force and allowed the body to heal itself.

The theory of homeopathy is that each person is subject to a universal **vital energy** that must be balanced to stimulate self-healing . When this energy is interrupted or imbalanced, health problems can develop. Homeopathic remedies aim to restore the balance of this vital energy, often referred to as the vital force, and send vibrational frequencies to stimulate the body's natural healing response.

The vibrational frequencies of herbology's elements and supplements are similar to homeopathy

In **"Magnetic Harmonic Vibrational Therapy,"** I use recorded sounds of **The Healing Forces of Harmonic Sounds and Vibrations**, Vedic mantras, Gregorian chants, Tibetan mantras and classical music to recharge and increase the vibrational frequency of Ayurvedic remedies, herbal supplements, and programmed water to activate holistic healing. This is similar to the principles used in homeopathy.

Ayurvedic supplements, water and other natural supplements are placed inside a pyramid, which contains sacred geometric figures. Through a sound amplification system and colored light frequencies, the supplements are programmed with such frequencies. This process amplifies the healing vibrational frequencies of herbology supplements, water, minerals and topically-applied substances.

Elements, water, liquids, herbs and minerals can store information. The vibrational harmonic frequency of sounds, mantras, harmonic music and colors are recorded in all these elements and increase their therapeutic potential.

I often recommend supplements of Ayurvedic herbology, natural herb supplements, water, minerals and substances for topical use. These supplements have been programmed with the **Healing Forces of Sounds and Harmonic Vibrations,** mantras, Vedic, Tibetan and Gregorian chants within a pyramid, in conjunction with other sacro-geometric forms. The individuals experience greater mental clarity, emotional well-being and find that their bodies recover naturally in a very short time.

Homeopathy uses electromagnetic vibrational frequencies stored in water molecules and mostly in compounds of oxygen bonded to hydrogen. That water is responsible for over 90 percent of the active functions of DNA. Homeopathy takes the specific frequency to the area that requires healing.

This healing system tries to heal people by using small doses of substances that have been programmed with specific homeopathic frequencies. Homeopathy is one of the more subtle methods of powerful vibrational medicine that stimulate the natural process of healing in a fast and effective way without side effects. This is achieved through the vibrational frequency or natural signature encoded in the herbs, flowers, plants and minerals used in the treatments.

31

Healing Bones with Ultrasound

Healing bones with ultrasound and tuning forks, and the effects of sound pulsations on bones.

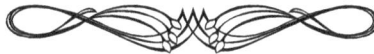

Ultrasound is used for healing bones

Ultrasound generates a vibrational frequency in a range that is not audible by the human ear. Ultrasound waves are generated into the body by a machine that has electrodes which are applied to the skin.

Ultrasound has many medical applications, including viewing the fetus in the womb, and locating calcifications and kidney stones.

Ultrasound is also used to accelerate the healing of fractures. When ultrasound frequencies are applied, the deep tissue's temperature increases and activate heat in the affected area.

There is evidence to show that certain fractures, specifically bone fractures where there is no fragmentation, (pseudo-arthrosis) can heal faster by using ultrasound vibrational frequencies. There is also evidence that ultrasound may help patients who have poor healing potential, including diabetics, smokers and patients taking steroids.

Australian aboriginals have healed fractures, muscle tears and different type of diseases by using sound frequencies produced by their enigmatic instrument; the didgeridoo (yidaki.) The didgeridoo is the oldest wind instrument that produces a deep and

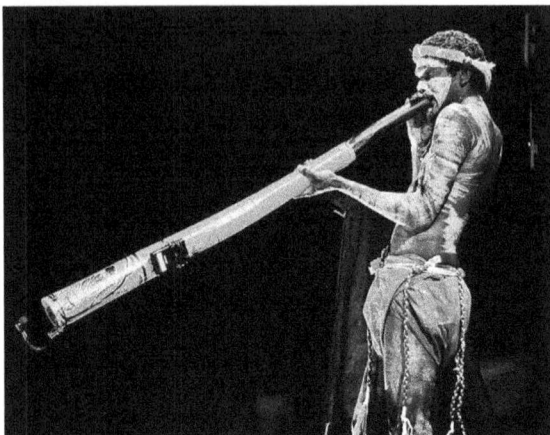

Australian native playing the didgeridoo (yidaki).

powerful bass sound that penetrates into the body and resonates with the bones and organs.

The sound frequencies produced by the didgeridoo are in alignment with modern sound healing technologies. Our ancestors knew that certain sounds produced by Mother Nature's instruments had healing effects.

Tuning forks

Tuning forks are a set of 15 tuned forks that generate specific sound frequencies and resonate directly with the organs in the human body.

Tuning forks are tuned to frequencies of healthy tissues and organs. In the 1980s, Barbara Hero, founder of The International Lambdoma Research, used tuning forks

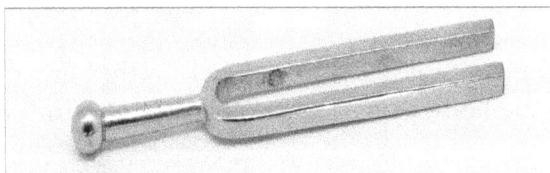

to study their direct resonance with the organs.

The sound waves pass through healthy organs and their frequencies travel at the speed of sound. The 15 tuning forks that resonate and stimulate the organs are calibrated in Hertz (Hz) and are:

Personality = C+ 264 Hz
Circulation, sex = C# 586 Hz
Blood = E 321.9 Hz
Adrenals = B 492.8 Hz
Kidneys = Eb 319.88 Hz
Liver = Eb 317.83 Hz
Bladder = F 352 Hz
Intestines = C# 281 Hz
Lungs = A 220 Hz
Colon = F 176 Hz
Gallbladder = E 164.3 Hz
Pancreas = C# 117.3 Hz
Stomach = A 110 Hz

Brain = Eb 315.8 Hz
Fatty tissue cells = C# 295.8 Hz
Muscles = E 324 Hz
Bones = Ab 418.3 Hz

32

Sound Therapy Instruments

A brief history of instruments and techniques used in sound frequency therapy including crystal quartz bowls and tuning forks.

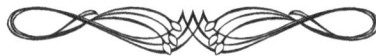

A brief history of instruments and techniques used in sound frequency therapy including crystal quartz bowls and tuning forks.

In 1550, in Pavia, Italy, Gerolamo Cardano, physician, mathematician and astrologer, noticed that sound can be perceived through the skin.

In 1553, in Padua, Italy, H. Capivacci, a physician, realized that if sound is perceived through the skin, then it could be used as a diagnostic tool to differentiate between disorders in the middle ear or acoustic nerve.

In 1684, German physician G. C. Schelhammer tried to use a common fork to improve Cardano and Capivacci's experiments.

In 1711, in England, trumpeter Royal John Shore, created the first tuning fork. At the time he jokingly called it a pitch fork. The tuning fork was made of steel and was calibrated with the A423.5 tone.

In 1800, German physicist E.F.F. Chladni and others, built a complete musical instrument based on tuning forks.

In 1834, J. H. Scheibler presented a set of 54 tuning forks with ranges of 220 Hz to 440 Hz.

Later, in Paris, J. Lissajous built a tuning fork with a resonance box.

Also in Paris, German physicist K. R. Koenig invented a tuning fork that produced continuous vibrations by using a clockwork mechanism.

In 1863, in Heidelberg, physiologist H. Helmholtz used sets of electro-magnetically charged tuning forks in his experiments.

Tuning forks are essential tools for producing defined sinusoidal vibrations and they are used as diagnostic tools in otology.

The tone of A440 Hz is the standard tone used currently by musicians and symphonic orchestras to determine the twelve notes in an octave.

Mr. Hipkins was the best known piano tuner in 1846 and was instructed by Walter Broadwood. All piano tuners of that time fine-tuned pianos based on the notes A433.5 and A436. They used tuning forks for that purpose.

In the 18th century, German physicist Ernst Chladni discovered that when a violin bow was frictioned vertically along the edge of a metal plate, it generated sound waves that produced geometric patterns in the sand dispersed on the plate. For each different musical tone, a different geometric pattern was formed.

In the 60s and 70s, Swiss scientist Hans Jenny discovered that low-frequency sounds formed simple geometric shapes and when the frequency was increased, more complex geometric shapes were formed. He also discovered that the sound "OH" produces a perfect circle and the sound "OOM" produces a pattern similar to the ancient Hindu mandala "OOM." He called his work Cymatics.

Although musicians were among the first to work with musical tones produced by tuning forks, scientists also used them in their research.

In 583 BC, Greek philosopher and mathematician Pythagoras built a musical instrument called the monochord and set it at the tone of 256 Hz. Egyptians and Greeks used the monochord to make complex mathematical calculations.

In or about 1834, a group of German physicists used a mechanical stroboscopic instrument to determine the tone of the tuning fork at A440 cps (A440 Hz).

The tone of the A note ranged from 373.3 Hz to 402.0 Hz in the 17th century. Then, on July 27, 1987, the International Society of Piano Builders and Technicians unanimously agreed that the A = 440 Hz note would be established as the international standard tone for piano manufacturers, modern pianos and tuning symphony orchestras.

In 1974, professional jazz musician Fabien Maman noticed that the audience filled with energy when he played certain musical notes. At the end of the 1970s, Fabien joined researcher Helen Grimal, from the National Center for Scientific Research in Paris, to study the effects of sounds in normal cells and malignant cells. The couple used all kinds of sound instruments, including flutes, drums and gongs.

They discovered that the sound between 30 and 40 decibels caused changes in cells. Higher musical notes produced vibrational frequencies that traveled from the center of the cell towards its outer membrane. However, the most surprising results occurred when sounds were made by the human voice.

At the cellular level Fabien Maman discovered that the C note caused cells to organize themselves into an elongated shape, and the D note produced a variety of colors in cells. The E note caused cells to be arranged in spherical shapes. The F note caused cells to organize themselves into balanced round shapes, generating colors of vibrant magenta and turquoise. The musical note A440 Hz has an effect on the energetic field of cells trfansforming the color from red to pink.

In the 1990s, Japanese scientist Masaru Emoto, discovered that water molecules respond to musical vibrations. The human body is comprised of 79% to 89% of water. Masaru Emoto's work demonstrates the importance of how the body's water is influenced by sounds and how the body's cells are affected by information stored in the water we drink.

In 1957, Dr. Alfred Tomatis experimented with using high frequency sounds (750 - 3,000/4,000 -20,000 Hz) to stimulate the brain. Such sounds can have a cognitive effect on thinking, perception and memory. Listening to these sounds can improve attention and concentration.

In the 1980s, Barbara Hero, founder of Lambdoma International Research Institute, in Kennebunk, Maine, was able to measure the optimal frequency of body organs using acoustic mathematical formulas. She used tuning forks to produce sounds that passed through the organs.

In 1997, William S. Jones and Paul Utz, founders of the company **Crystal Tones**, located in Salt Lake City, Utah, produced the first alchemic bowls. The bowls were made of pure crystal quartz with handles or sticks attached to the outer and central parts of the bowls. They named them Practitioner's Crystal Bowls. Crystal Tones produces a great variety of Practitioner's Crystal Bowls made from alchemical precious and semiprecious stones (diamond, ruby, emerald, citrine, amethyst, aquamarine, etc.) and metals (gold, platinum, silver, copper, etc.)

The Practitioner's Crystal Bowl has the ability to stimulate meridians and organs by using the glass handle as a tuning fork. The sound of the crystal quartz in combination with metals, precious and semiprecious stones, produces a more intense sound and its duration is longer than those produced by metal tuning forks. This is because quartz contains the same components as bone (calcium, magnesium, silica, folic acid and a collagen helix.)

In 1998, Crystal Tones also produced the first tuning forks made of pure crystal quartz in combination with precious and semiprecious stones. These tuning forks are larger than the metal ones and can create a more intense and longer sound.

In the same year, Crystal Tones increased the production of alchemic bowls making them in different dimensions, using a large variety of crystals and precious and semiprecious stones. These bowls are designed to be used on the body during vibrational therapy, or close to the person receiving treatment.

Both alchemy bowls and Practitioner's Crystal Bowls are used for group therapy and concerts. People perceive the powerful harmonic sounds through their ears, skin, bones and crystals in the blood . The vibrational frequencies produced by the harmonic sounds are therapeutic and can improve one's health.

33

The Color of Sound and the Energy Fields of the Human Body

Sound conversion to color. Representation of light colors, Dr. Valerie V. Hunt and research and scientific studies of the human energy field.

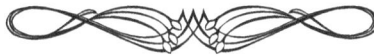

The Color of Sound and Light

Sound and light share the same nature; both produce vibrational frequencies. Although the sounds that we perceive through our ears, bones, epidermal tissue, and blood plasma crystalline substances have a lower frequency than light, there is a range of sound frequencies with corresponding colors.

Light's color resonance is 40 octaves above the F# tone. The standard tone, A = 440, has a frequency of 406.81 THz. Color has a wavelength of 736.93 nm. RGB colors near this light color are #750000 (hexadecimal value), based on a modified version of Dan Bruton's color approximation algorithm.

RGB = Red, Green, Blue
1 nm = 1 nanometer = 1×10^{-9} m
1 THz = 1 terahertz = 1×10^{12} Hz

F#4 frequency in standard pitch A4 = 440 Hz is 369.99 Hz. At a temperature of 72°F (22.22°C), the speed of sound is 1,132.91 ft/sec (341.31 m/sec). Under these conditions, the F# tone in standard pitch A4 = 440, has a wavelength of 36.74 inches (93.33 cm).

This calculation allows us to specify a note and observe the color in consonance with that note. Consonance means that color has a frequency which is a number of octaves above the harmonic sound frequencies.

Sound Conversion to Color

The previous code converts the sound frequency to a light frequency by duplicating the frequency of sound (up one octave each time) until it reaches a frequency in the range of 400-800 THz (400,000,000,000,000 - 800,000,000,000,000 Hz.)

Representation of Light's Colors

Light's colors are pure frequencies that our eyes perceive as one color. The RGB (Red, Green, Blue) color system that is used in web pages as HTML (Hyper Text Markup Language) are displayed in most color monitors using a mixture of three pure light sources (red, green and blue) to create the impression of a single color to our eyes.

In the RGB system, our eyes perceive some colors that are not pure, like pink and white. These colors are mixtures of various colors of the pure spectrum. The RGB color system is called "additive," because it is the addition of colors that make a perceivable color.

Chakras, Color, Frequency and Wavelength

Chakra	Color	Frequency(THz)	Wavelength (nm)
Crown	Violet	668 - 789	380 - 450
Third Eye	Blue	631 - 668	450 - 475
Throat	Cyan	606 - 630	476 - 495
Heart	Green	526 - 606	495 - 570
Solar Plexus	Yellow	508 - 526	570 - 590
Reproductive	Orange	484 - 508	590 - 620
Root	Red	400 - 484	620 - 750

Sound and light share the same nature, both produce vibrational frequencies, but the sounds we perceive have a frequency much lower than the light that is visible to us. In other words, light and color are the manifestation of sounds at extremely high frequencies.

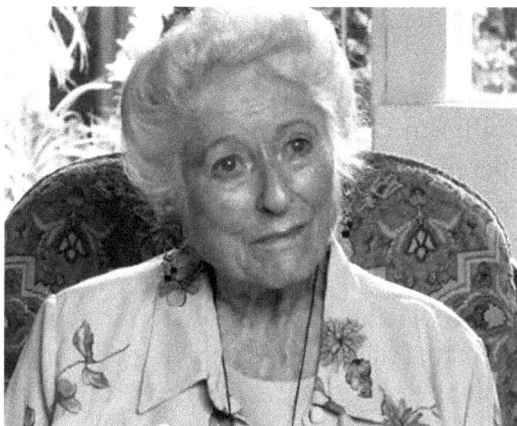

Dra. Valerie V. Hunt

Light was created with seven basic colors from which thousands of color combinations are created. **The stunning beauty of light energy was preceded by sound**. The seven musical notes form the basis for composing musical harmony. Extremely high musical chord frequencies give rise to the colors of the rainbow and to the colors associated with our energy centers or chakras, and they also manifest themselves in many ways in the universe.

Dr. Valerie V. Hunt is a pioneer in research about human energy fields (bioenergy), and is Emeritus Professor and researcher of Physiological Sciences at the University of California (UCLA.)

In her book *Infinite Mind* Dr. Hunt presents the science of the human vibrations of consciousness, based on 25 years of clinical research about energy generated by humans. She found that all cells, even subatomic particles contain small electrical components.

Dr. Hunt's studies have shown that the human energy field permeates the whole body and radiates outward from inches to feet beyond the body surface. This study of the human energy field and light emissions has been validated in laboratories using photometers and color filters.

During an investigation of complex waveforms and resonance that connects us to our source, Dr. Hunt found that the vibrations of the human energy field generate frequencies 1,000 times greater than the electrical signals produced by nerves and muscles.

These signals were recorded from the body's surface, by placing high frequency special sensors on selected points on the joints, abdomen, meridians and head.

To determine that the signals correlated with color, Dr. Hunt had eight different aura readers that registered the field around the subject's body while the instruments recorded signals.

The resulting data were subjected to Fourier's frequency analysis to determine each color's frequency spectrum.

She compared the different color waveforms and analyzed the voice spectrogram to accurately test the voice's purity.

The resulting vibrations were in the range of audible frequencies. When amplified they could be heard very easily and could also be differentiated. Despite low intensity, similar to a subliminal sound, you could feel the vibration in the soft body tissue, and in the hollow areas of the head, spine, thorax and abdomen.

The vibrations are believed to come from the molecular, atomic and subatomic activity of human cells. Quantum physics has described that all matter occupying space has atomic energy potential released in small amounts as electrons rotate in their orbits. One of the interesting features of any object energy emission is that it remains in organized fields, has its own integrity and is not dissipated at random.

Living substances emit higher frequencies with greater changes in dynamic patterns than those of inert substances. **The vibrations of the body are like music**. The human body is a transmitter and receiver of sounds that generate vibrational frequencies.

The sounds of the human energy field are signals emitted throughout the body and simultaneously the body also perceives and receives sounds from the outside world.

The vibrational energy field of a human does not have pure colors. The human energy field colors change rapidly and are affected by our will and needs. Thus, at any given time, it may have one color or multiple colors. When a person is in optimal health the color spectrum is observed clearly and distinctly.

During her research, Dr. Hunt designed many situations to understand the specific meaning of the five vibrational spectra generated by the human body, and their effects on a person's behavior, emotional and psychological state.

The Five Vibrational Spectra Generated by the Human Body

Red - Orange - Amber

The warm, vibrant and stimulating vibrational spectrum of red, orange and amber is more common in young people who are physically active. Red, orange and amber encourage athletic activity, and stimulate dances in primitive rituals. They can also express aggressiveness when a person is angry. The vibrational spectra of these three colors can also express joy and happiness.

Sadness, weakness, illness and depression do not have the color spectrum of red, orange and amber. This spectrum is the biological flux, material and sensitive, which flows into the realities of the universe and is encoded by the existence of life. Perceiving and hearing the vibrational frequencies of red, orange and amber can revitalize, excite and activate the body, stimulating and motivating it to reach new achievements.

Blue - Violet - Mauve

The spectrum of blue, violet and mauve is fresh, soothing and usually present during meditation, relaxation, and quiet thoughts, and when we are healthy. This spectrum stimulates well-being and is present when tasks are done slowly and repetitively, and when something is heard repeatedly.

This spectrum manifests in endurance athletes, when the body relaxes and when all systems operate at peak efficiency. The spectrum of blue, violet and mauve soothes emotions of the hyperactive body, clears the thought process and reduces hypertension. It also reduces inflammatory skin conditions. This color spectrum helps reduce stress, the nerve tension caused by the excess of work and amplifies the capabilities of the mind and body.

Natural and spa centers have used ultraviolet color in combination with heat, herbs and mineral-rich water as regenerative therapy for many centuries.

Yellow - Green - Amber

The spectrum of yellow, green and amber seems to be transitional; it helps people change from one state to another. It affects the neural harmonization of the senses, and supports creating, planning, handling relationships and interconnecting.

These colors stimulate a pure and elaborate awareness that helps encourage creative thinking, and facilitate learning. They stimulate feelings of hope, tranquility and anticipation towards changes when facing a problem.

Rainbow

This spectrum includes all white light color vibrations that are completely balanced without weaknesses or strengths. It permeates the environment with a coherent energy that helps offset confusing electromagnetic vibrations and sound pollution in big cities.

Blue - White - Gold

This is the spectrum of highest human vibration. If it were a stone, it would be a diamond. The vibrational frequency generated by blue, white and gold is similar to plasma oscillations around spaceships and sounds from outer space. This vibrational frequency seems to stimulate the will to find a home in another level or dimension.

As in music, higher frequencies seem to have the greatest recharging effects. Sound frequencies generated by the blue, white and gold spectrum activate vibrations that lead consciousness to a higher state of expansion, similar to sound frequencies of religious choral music, Gregorian chants and the Requiem Mass.

Choral music and the requiem, which is a mass music chorale for the dead has inspired generations of composers to write many works of profound beauty. It has been scientifically proven that choral music has therapeutic effects. It makes people feel better, because the music acts with neurochemicals rewards in the brain that is associated with feelings of pleasure and helps make them to be more alert. The people that sing in a Choir, and also the listeners benefit from the harmonic sounds produced by the harmonization of the voices of the singer and of the music of the choir. This music helps stimulate the production of endorphins, cortisol, serotonin and oxytocin hormones. Some of the most loved requiems interpretations have been by composers Mozart, Verdi, Dvorak, Berlioz, Faure, Durufle, and others.

Awareness that leads thought expands and rises from the material world to the spiritual world. These sounds can refresh and activate the regeneration process at mental, emotional, physical and spiritual levels.

The importance of sounds generated by a human's energy field is becoming widely known. Stimulation of the nervous system has effects mainly on the muscular and circulatory system, but has limited effects on emotional states and motivation. However, specific sound frequencies can stimulate the human energy field and generate vibrations that affect the entire body, including its abilities, and moods.

These sounds can be experienced when we listen to biofeedback recordings, classical music, Gregorian chants in the intonation of musical codes at 432 Hz, new age music recordings and in the CD **"The Healing Forces of Harmonic Sounds and Vibrations."** Biofeedback studies show that auditory feedback is accurate and effective because it provides a source of energy that goes directly to the brain.

234

Physical Therapy science has developed tools that produce ultrasound and heat waves to accelerate healing of deep connective tissue, and low vibrational frequencies of direct current (DC,12V 6A) to quickly heal fractures.

Biomagnetism therapists use magnets to accelerate the healing of burns, cuts, incisions, tissue inflammation and other conditions. Biomagnetism therapy is also used to remove tumors and fibroids, and to relieve muscle aches, headaches, migraines and spinal pain.

Magneto therapy, natural foods (organic vegetarian diet foods,) homeopathic medicine (substances programmed with vibrational frequencies) and the music therapy (harmonic sound frequencies) all stimulate the human energy field and assist in maintaining good health by activating the natural healing process.

"The Healing Forces of Harmonic Sounds and Vibrations" has sounds with specific harmonic frequencies that stimulate the human energy field and assist accelerating the natural healing process of the body, mind and spirit. These frequencies are detected by all body systems.

In previous chapters, it was mentioned that our bodies have the ability to absorb and detect sounds that go beyond our hearing capacity. We not only hear sounds and perceive vibrations through our ears, but also through our bodies. The bones, skull, skin, nervous system and crystalline substances in blood are particularly great conductors and receptors of sounds and vibrations.

The idea of basic biology, that life forms are complex energy exchange systems, is rapidly becoming the new frontier in medicine, psychology, education and communication. Physical science says that man exists, grows, works and interacts with all energies, including electromagnetic energy and the sounds and colors that generate vibrational frequencies.

As stated by Nicholas Tesla: "We have to think that we live in an ocean of energy, frequency and vibrations. We are aware that everything existing in the universe is in a constant state of vibration, it produces sound frequencies and high frequency sounds produce light and colors."

Based on this knowledge, we can help improve the health of humans and other life forms by incorporating methods of high and low vibrational frequencies.

We can expand the field of vibrational medicine by using classical harmonic music,

Gregorian chants , biofeedback recordings, Vedic and Tibetan mantras, chromotherapy, pure quartz alchemy crystals, **Magnetic Harmonic Vibrational Therapy, "The Healing Power of Sounds and Harmonic Vibrations"** CD, and the most powerful natural healing instruments of all, the sounds produced by the human voice, dolphins, whales, and the elements of nature.

34

The Voice Healing Power

The human voice has the greatest potential to activate the natural healing power of the body, mind and spirit.

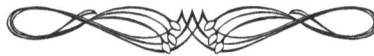

The voice healing power

The human voice is considered the most powerful natural healing instrument of all existing healing instruments on Earth.

The human voice has the most potential to activate the most powerful healing force

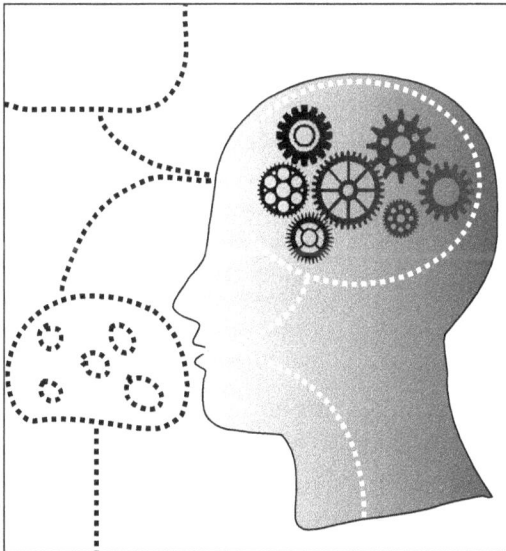

The human voice can produce sounds that stimulate mental and physical relaxation. It also helps in the area of personal growth, stimulates the capacity to create and helps balance the experiences of daily life. The human voice can produce very powerful sounds and vibrations that activate the natural healing process.

The human voice has the ability to produce sounds that release emotions of anger, fear, anxiety, jealousy, resentment, frustration, trauma and destructive emotions. It can also release negative energy from the environment.

Pythagoras recognized the significant therapeutic power of the human voice. He treated the diseases by reading poetry. He taught his students how to modulate the voice skillfully with beautiful words and with a pleasant tone of voice in order to restore balance to the body and soul. Belief in the healing ability of the human voice is common in many parts of the world.

Shamans, monks and saints of primitive societies used a harmonic language of sounds and songs to lift the spirits and to commune with higher intelligences, in order to extract information to heal the sick.

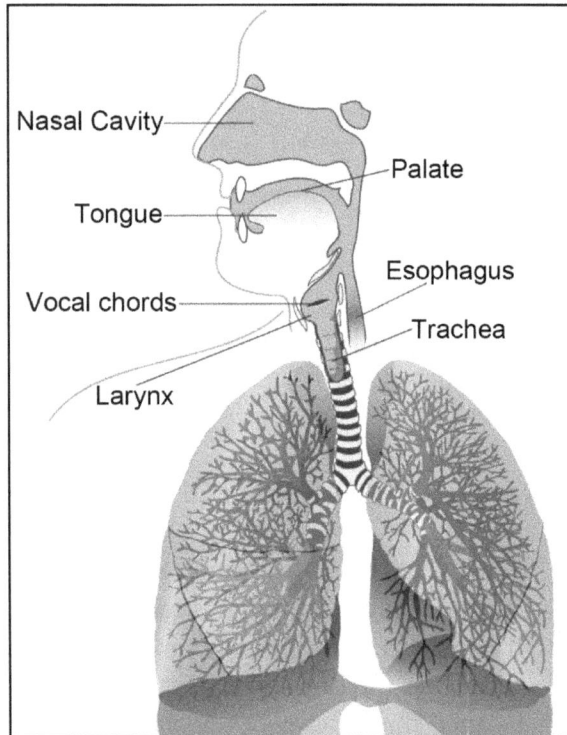

Illustration of the breathing process, expansion of the diaphragm and vowel sound production.

The mind can generate emotions that produce vibrational frequencies that unbalance the meridians and organs. Disturbances in the meridians and organs become blockages that generate disease and also affect the body's vital energy.

Through the voice we can produce harmonious sounds that elevate the mental, emotional and spiritual states. It is also possible to open our conscious to infinite possibilities and to enable mental relaxation. It helps eliminate stress, it helps in dealing with insomnia and invigorates all the biophysical systems.

The vowel sounds are the most dynamic aspect of the spoken sound; without them, the consonants would be silent. Early alphabets excluded vowels because they believed they were too stimulating and caused lots of energy.

The Tibetans believe that the most important musical instrument is the human voice. Tibetan monks are trained in projecting vocal sounds to create esoteric internal vibrations. They learn to use head and chest as resonance chambers for the whole body. The vocal tones and mantras are repeated creating a reverberation so that when the song is finished, the sounds continue to echo in the mind and in the body chambers.

When we sing harmonic sounds using vowels, we breathe profoundly and the diaphragm expands. This not only helps the body to take in more oxygen, it also opens the flow of life energy, **chi or prana**, which activates good health and long life.

According to numerous scientific studies, the mind, heart and body are not only connected but unified.

When we understand the connection between the heart, mind and body, we can recognize how the vibrations produced by the sounds have a direct effect on cells, organs, systems, in the brain and emotions. This union between the heart, mind and body also leads us to the next frontier through holistic vibrational healing medicine with high spiritual dimensions.

The sound of the voice reflects the emotional state, health condition, level of consciousness and the spiritual state of the person. Our breathing and the sounds we make through our voice are our life force, "Prana or Chi". The sounds produced by our voice affect atoms, molecules, cells, tissues, organs, systems and the whole body in general.

When we produce harmonious sounds with our voice we can restore our internal balance and manage to reach the alpha's mental state of peace and harmony. Alfa's mental state is the state between asleep and awake and is achieved when we have vibrations of **8-9 Hz to 14 Hz** in the electro encephalogram readings.

Alpha's mental state is the ideal state in order to activate the natural healing process of the body, mind and spirit. But it is important to consider that if the person is generating negative thoughts, they also can be amplified in the **alpha state of mind.**

The power of the human voice and singing

Sound therapists have come to the conclusion that the most powerful tool is the sound of the human voice. Through our voice we project our emotional, mental and physical state. The sound of the voice can project the area of the body that is unbalanced or ill. Through the proper use of the vocal sound or mantra that resonates with the affected area of the body, we can stimulate the balance of that area and restore its normal frequency.

Dr. John Beaulieu, in his book, **Human Intonation** (Human Tuning) says that the intonation of harmonic sounds stimulates the flow of Kundalini energy. Tibetan and Vedic mantras also have frequencies of vocal sounds that harmonize the chakras and contribute to achieve enlightenment.

Singing opens portals to healing vibrations. Singing is a very personal form of expression. It is like opening a door in our body that leaves out the deeper emotions stored in our hearts.

When we sing, we resonate from our diaphragm, chest, heart, lungs, throat, tongue, face and thus resonate all levels of our being. This connects us directly with our emotions, it helps us to open our heart and takes us to another level of consciousness, allowing the unification of the heart, body and mind.

Usually, when we sing songs with constructive and positive harmonic melodies, it is very difficult to remain in the emotional state of depression. Singing makes us breathe deeply. In this process the sounds and vibrations resonate with different parts of the body, allowing the person to express their emotions without limitations.

The more profound our breathing, the more vital energy, qi or prana, we have in and out of our body. In this way, hearing and perception of our mind and body are intensified. It is important to consider the selection of themes and songs, because if we use songs with themes of sadness, they can amplify negative emotions.

To open and expand the natural power of voice, no specific training is required. Most important is that the person hears himself or herself and makes a re-discovery of his or her internal capabilities. It is imperative that the person comes into direct contact with his or her stressful emotions and gradually release them.

It is essential to meditate and reach a state of relaxation, breathing slowly, expanding the diaphragm and also expanding the pelvic cavity. The diaphragm is the area where the support for producing voice sounds is located.

The throat, chest and rib cage must be free of tension so that the lungs can expand naturally to the fullest. You need to learn how to use the diaphragm correctly. When breathing correctly, the diaphragm expands when inhaling and contracts when exhale. The ribcage must remain filled with air and relaxed. The inhalation and exhalation should be slow, rhythmical and natural.

Applying this simple method the voice flows easily in a very natural way to release all our tensions and worries. The voice becomes a source of sounds and vibrations full of

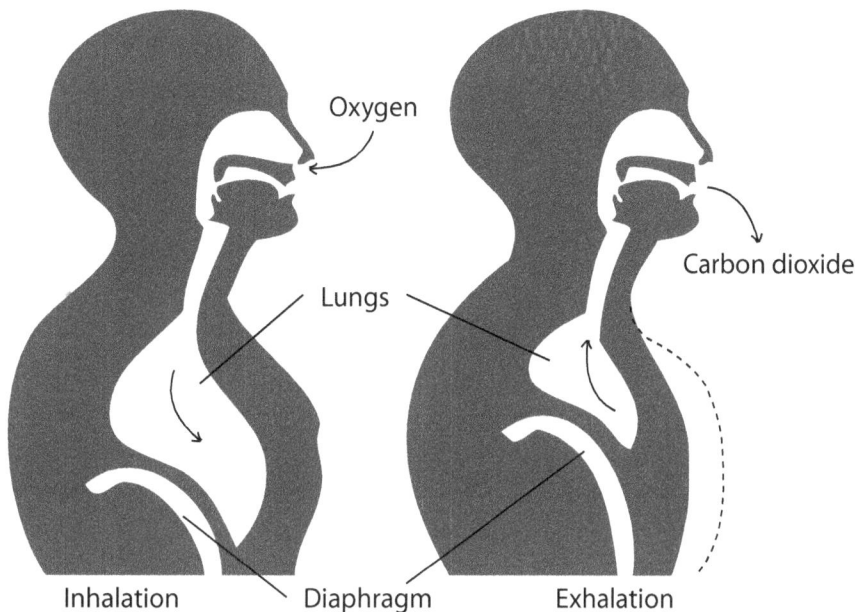

Oxygen

Carbon dioxide

Lungs

Inhalation   Diaphragm   Exhalation

life, very flexible energy and great power of resonance and expression.

Through singing, we can produce vibrations that stimulate our biophysical system. By this means we can also regulate blood pressure, blood circulation, and increase body oxygenation at the cellular level. At the same time, we harmonize the nervous system, the glands and the organs of your body.

As we develop these skills and we increase mental concentration, we release our problems and dissipate negative emotions, obtaining a high level of awareness.

The body produces sounds naturally. The sound of the heartbeat, the sound of blood flowing through arteries and veins. The sound of the movements of bones and muscles. The sound produced by the process of digestion. When we are tired, we yawn and create sounds. When we are happy we laugh and create sounds. When we are sad we cry and create sounds.

When we are physically hurt we moan and create sounds. When we are angry or shout, we raise our voice and create sounds. The body's sounds are produced spontaneously and often are not controlled by the mind.

35

Mantras

Activating the healing process through vocal sounds, mantras and their resonance with different areas of the body.

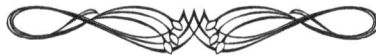

Activating the healing process through vocal sounds and mantras

Mantras and chants consist of vocal sounds which produce sound frequencies that resonate with the organs and stimulate areas of the body. To help heal a specific organ, when a vowel is spoken or sung during inhalation and exhalation, the organ should be visualized. This internal assessment is the key to many metaphysical teachings concerning therapeutic effects of sounds and mantras. When we produce the internal sound, we generate the external sound that amplifies the vibrational frequency, which in turn activates the body's healing process.

Singing involves two important aspects:

1) As we inhale, we concentrate on the body region associated with the vocal and make the vowel sound mentally or silently.

2) Then, as we exhale, we sing the vowel with our voice, making the sound audible.

When we inhale and visualize the vowel sound in our mind only, we penetrate deep into the region or organ we want to treat. The breath absorbs the energy of qi or prana and combines it with the vowel tones and together they open specific areas inside the body and consciousness.

Vowel's resonance with different areas of the body.

U - Pelvis, hips, legs, feet and lower body in general.

O - Abdomen and from the bottom of the solar plexus to groin, reproductive organs.

OU - The solar plexus, the whole area of the diaphragm, liver, pancreas, kidneys, adrenal glands, stomach, spleen, small intestine, large intestine.

A - Front chest cavity, heart, thymus, lungs and ribs.

E - EI - Throat, thyroid, parathyroid, larynx, salivary glands, tonsils.

I - The face, nostrils, cerebellar regions and head, front of the brain and back of the skull, third eye, pituitary gland, eyes, ears and nose.

I - MI - All the cranial cavity including the pineal gland.

Through our thoughts, creative imagination and the use of vowel sounds in diatonic harmony, we can restore balance to our chakras. Vowel sounds in different tones of the diatonic harmony produce music that can stimulate the natural healing process of the mind, body, and spirit.

Breathing is important in the process of vocal intonation. When we inhale, we activate the vital energy, qi or prana that carries our thoughts through vowel sound, towards the area we want to regenerate or heal. Breath is life. It is imperative that we have absolute control over our breathing patterns.

Rhythmic gradual and controlled inhalation and exhalation is essential to balance all of the body's systems. As we work with vocal sounds in diatonic harmony, our breathing becomes more fluid, our biological systems are harmonized, and good health is activated.

How to vocalize the vowel sounds in different harmonic tones

When we sing vowels in different tones of the diatonic harmony, we restore the vibrational pattern of the subtle body (holographic body and auric body) and the electromagnetic field of the physical body. Thus, our spiritual essence can manifest more fully through our physicality.

The voice creates sound through the physical body, and in turn is the most powerful instrument that expresses our spiritual energy. Because of the voice's immense power, we must use it with wisdom and conscience. The voice is a powerful tool that can create health and other transformations in our physical and spiritual lives.

To start the vocal exercises, take the vowel sound **A, A, A** which is the first sound we usually make when we enter physical life at birth. Chant slowly and gradually, in a natural tone, the sound **A, A, A** and continue until you remove all the air from your diaphragm. The sound of the vowel **A, A, A** should continue for about 12-16 seconds in the same pace, consistency and tonal level. Relax, take air slowly and wait about 30 seconds or a minute and start again to repeat the same process. Repeat this exercise three times and continue incorporating the vocals mentioned in this chapter. Make sure to visualize the body areas that resonate with the vocal sounds that you are singing. In this manner you can stimulate these areas, regenerating and unblocking them.

Once you feel familiar with the process of vocal intonation, start applying tones of the diatonic harmony in conjunction with vowels that have direct resonance with the organs and chakras of our body, as follows:

Root Chakra = C (frequency 396 Hz) Vowels: U, U, U
(Pelvis, hips, legs, feet and lower body in general).

Chakra Reproductive = D (frequency 417 Hz) Vowels: O, O, O
(Abdomen and from the bottom of the solar plexus to groin, reproductive organs).

Solar Plexus Chakra = E (frequency 528 Hz) Vowels: OU, OU, OU, (solar plexus, all the diaphragm, liver, pancreas, kidneys, adrenal glands, stomach, spleen, small intestine, large intestine).

Heart Chakra = F (frequency 639 Hz) Vowels: A, A, A
(Rib cage, heart, thymus, lungs and ribs).

Throat Chakra or neck = G (frequency 741 Hz) Vowels: E, E, E or EI, EI, EI. (Thyroid, parathyroid, larynx, salivary glands, tonsils).

Third Eye Chakra = A (frequency 852 Hz) Vowels: I, I, I (i, i, i)
(Face, nostrils, cerebellar regions and head, front of the brain and back of the skull, third eye, pituitary gland, eyes, ears and nose).

Coronal or Crown Chakra = B (frequency 963 Hz) Vowels: I, I, I, MI, MI, MI
(All cranial cavity including the pineal gland).

In my years of vocalizing I incorporated the use of the master key instrument pitch pipe, which is used to intone the voices of choral singers. Through the **master key pitch pipe** I intonate the musical notes that resonate with the chakras and once I hear the sound, I retain it in my mind. Then I start to vocalize the corresponding sounds for each chakra. In that way I get to work with all vowels and sounds that resonate with each chakra.

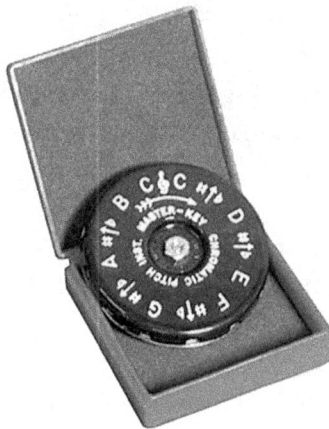

The master key chromatic pitch instrument.

When vocalizing, pay attention to the areas where the tone has difficulties or those points where the voice breaks or fluctuates. The voice often reflects what is happening inside the body.

This exercise in vocalization and intonation with vocal and musical notes corresponding to the chakras is very effective. Through the voice we can activate the natural healing process of the body and establish a high degree of consciousness.

Our voice transmits and identifies who we are through a combination of rhythm, melody, tone and dynamics. It not only reveals who we are, but it also reveals our level of consciousness. Our voice is the personal vehicle for spiritual and creative expression. According to the tone of our voice, the sound we produce and the vocabulary we use to express our emotions and thoughts, our voice creates an image of our being in the mind and conscience of the listeners.

Each voice represents a unique personality that defines the character of an individual. The voice of each person has two predominant levels: The level of natural tone and level of habitual tone. If both voice levels differ, it means that the voice is not being used properly. The misuse of the voice may be due to the vocal tone of voice being too high or too low. It is imperative that we learn to develop and improve the voice's natural frequency. We must learn to use the natural tone of our voice and extend it, expand it to its greater power and versatility.

I studied singing and music at the Conservatory of Music of Puerto Rico in the preparatory department of singing and music with a vocal range of a tenor. In my first audition the well-known and respected piano teacher Don Jesus Maria Sanromán accompanied me on the piano. At that time, Maestro Pablo Casals, composer, director and internationally recognized as one of the most important cellists of the twentieth century, was the director of the conservatory. I was honored to personally see Maestro Pablo Casals with the Casals Festival Orchestra of Puerto Rico. My teacher at the conservatory was Professor Raquel Gandia and she taught me the Italian Bel Canto method, which is also used in music conservatories in Spain and other parts of the world. Through the vocal exercises and singing Rachel taught me, and by incorporating the sounds of vowels and consonants, my vocal range increased in fewer than three months, and I became a lyric tenor.

In my first classes Professor Gandia helped me find the tone and the most comfortable octave for my voice. We used a piano to perform vocal exercises and singing. We started vocal exercises in 4-5 tones below middle C of the piano to locate lower vocal registers, and then climbed an octave to an acute C, to locate high registers. In a few months my voice very comfortably managed to achieve musical notes that exceeded the high C. As one continues vocalizing, voice registers expand and can reach grave and high-pitched tones more easily. The voice is a natural instrument that fortifies and expands by training with vocal exercises.

The average person should have a voice capacity registry of at least an octave and a half. The midpoint in that range of musical notes corresponds to the person's natural vocal tone.

We have to find the most comfortable tone and octave for us. With the help of a piano you can discover your natural tone. In connection with the middle C on the piano we must find the lowest and highest notes we can sing without losing the quality and consistency of our voice.

Vocal and singing exercises can make the voice more flexible and can increase the vocal registry and activate the ability to resonate with a broader spectrum of people and energies.

Everything in the world generates sounds, vibrations and music. All beings on Earth have the gift of music. Music can activate healing. It is important that we use and develop this virtue which has the power to regenerate, heal and transform our lives.

Music, rhythm and melody is life...do not let pass unnoticed the gift given to you from Universal and Creative Intelligence...begin to sing the vowel harmonic sounds for only 10 or 15 minutes a day, you'll notice that your innate natural power of healing is activated and your life will become health and happiness.

36

Sound is Paramount to Creation

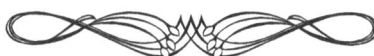

Sound is paramount to creation

The universe and Earth, from the sub-atoms, atoms, molecules, cells, tissues, organs, solid and gaseous systems are in a constant state of vibration and produce sound.

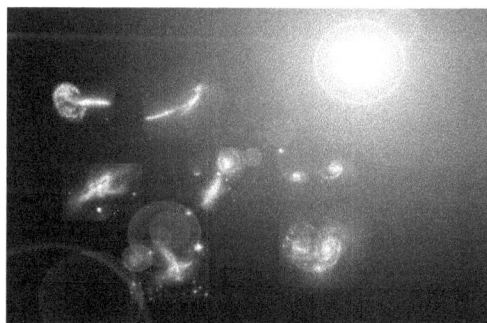

Thoughts give rise to the creation of vibrational frequencies which are manifested through verbs, words, actions, and behaviors.

Many sounds produced by the human body emerge from an unconscious level. Sounds can arise from our subconscious and conscious minds.

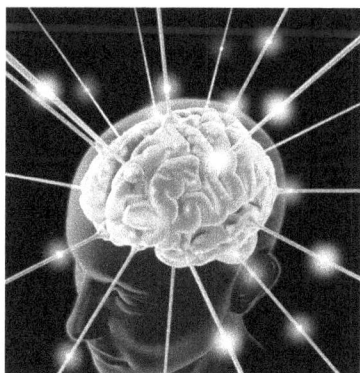

When we create a thought, a vibrational frequency is created in the subconscious and the conscious mind, which has not yet been manifested. When we speak or sing, that thought is manifested at a physical level. The process is sophisticated and involves many areas of the body's nervous system and other systems.

Creating a thought gives rise to a vibrational frequency in the brain that has not been manifested, but when

249

expressed verbally manifests itself physically. This sophisticated process takes place faster than the speed of light.

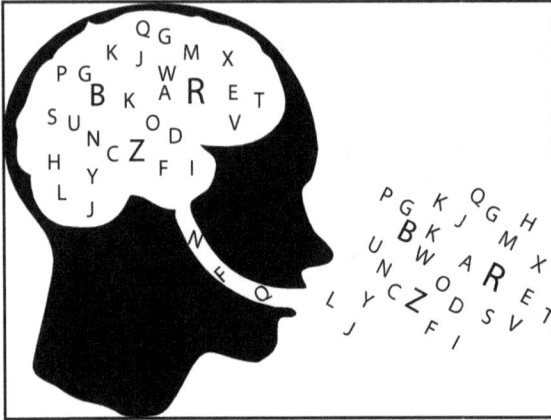

Once the sound is expressed verbally, it affects the atomic structure of matter, enters the body and gets recorded in DNA. In conclusion, the sound enters the body at the cellular level after it has been processed by the brain. Therefore, when we sing harmonic and positive songs, when we chant mantras or positive affirmations, we generate sound frequencies that create therapeutic vibrations. The sound produced by a person's voice indicates that person's emotional, spiritual and physical state.

The human body has great resonance potential. The human body is formed by millions of minerals and crystals. Much of our biophysical structure consists of water, minerals and bone matter. When we make vocal sounds, we create vibrational frequencies that resonate with mineral crystal substances which travel through the bloodstream, and resonate with the body's water and bones. This can affect the nervous system, mind and entire body.

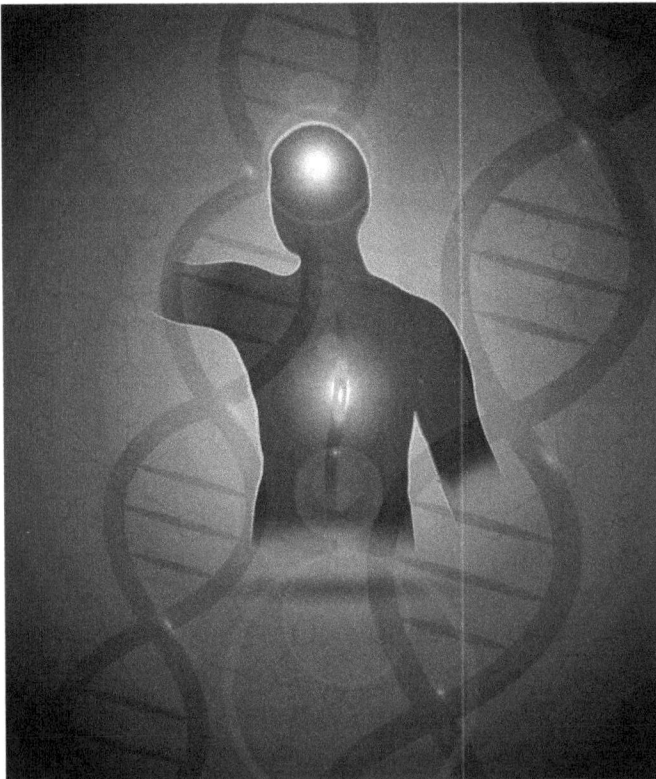

Sounds produce vibrations that can have a direct effect on the spine. The vibrations are distributed throughout the central nervous system, tissues, organs and body systems. These vibrational frequencies have a direct effect on the cells, blood, circulatory system, and endocrine system, and contribute to balancing the chakras.

By following the **"Healing Forces of Harmonic Sounds and Vibrations"** principles, one can achieve a mystical state of relaxation and achieve harmony with the pace and movement of space.

This could be likened to **the sound of sacred music of the spheres.** When one reaches a state of mental relaxation and connection with the macrocosmic and microcosmic universe, the natural healing process of the body, mind and spirit begins to activate. This relaxed state can be achieved through meditation.

37

The Vedas

The Vedas, India's holy book, contains powerful mantras and vocal sounds which resonate on the chakras.

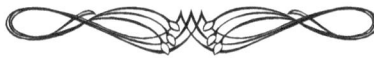

The sacred book of the Vedas

The sacred book of India called *The Vedas* contains writings that speak of powerful mantras and sounds that include the use of vocals, which resonate on the chakras and in turn help to balance and harmonize the body's energy centers.

The Vedas are four sacred books of ancient India. The Upanishads and all subsequent schools of Hindu philosophy are derived from them. It is said that Vedic wisdom and the books are 20.000 years old.

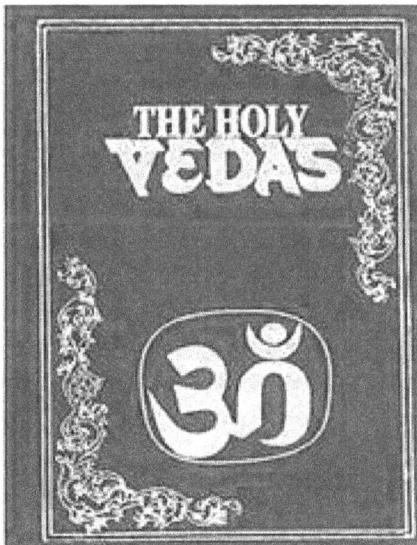

Hinduism has two very important words: **Veda and Rig-veda. Rig-veda** means divine word and **Veda** means knowledge of science and divine wisdom. **Rig-veda** is the science of the word. **The science of the word reveals the knowledge of the ancient sages and sound control.** The subtle levels of specific sounds produces knowledge, thought control and super-sensory planes.

The above discoveries are due to the masters of the ancient Vedic science, who applied control over the elements, and had the rishis' knowledge about the power of sound on matter, and the science of invocation and evocation. This was a forgotten science which is now recognized as one of the most powerful methods to transform the consciousness of those who practice the **Vedic sounds** and ancient knowledge.

The **Yajur Veda** is a collection of formulas sung in rituals and ceremonies. It is a collection of Vedic prayers for sacrifices. It contains approximately 30% of the verses of the Rig-Veda. The meaning of Yajur is the rhythm of sacrifice. The Sama Veda comes from the Rig-Veda and its main purpose is expressed through songs. The meaning of Sama is melody.

The **Atharvaveda** has been called the Brahma-Veda or Veda of prayer. It contains many charms and mystical poems from the **Upahnishads** and **Vedas**, having to do with life and beliefs. The Atharvaveda has about 16% of the verses of the **Rig-Veda** and it follows the **Upanishads.** Its name comes from the great sage **Atharva.**

The **Rig-veda** is, like the other three, a collection of over 1,000 Vedic hymns composed in Sanskrit. This is a much older form that became known as classical Sanskrit. The **Rig-veda** is considered the oldest scripture of Hinduism. Its hymns were written by early initiates of our fifth race. These scholars started their primary teachings through hymns. In short, the **Rig-veda** is the historical source which reveals primordial teachings and secret ancient doctrines found in the **Vedic** texts.

The Rig-veda is a mixture of enigmatic references which hide pearls of wisdom of the ancient secret doctrine. The Rig-veda has been sung in poetic, mystic, cryptic symbols, riddles and paradoxical form through language invocations expressing gratitude to various deities and **gods of nature.** The Vedic man, through invocations, identified himself with the **Surya,** which symbolizes the **Sun and the Agni,** which in turn symbolizes the **flame or fire.**

All collections of the Rig-veda's poetic language are expressed through songs which contain the mystical language of people who direct their thoughts toward an infinite path. The trail of the patriarchs, gods and mortals who originated from the divine energy, created life.

The whole concept of the evolution of this powerful ancient wisdom, metaphorically, is that the individual is like a seed of light which contains a universe of vast and deep philosophy with extensive teachings and secret doctrines.

The ancient wisdom of the Vedas leads to a multiplicity of gods, concepts, prayers, chants and mantras. However, there is a uniqueness that leads us to the core essence of

Vedic teachings, which is expressed in two verses:

"Burning in many places, fire is one.
Ruling over all, the sun is one.
The dawn illuminating all this, is one.
And certainly one is despite variations of all things."
(Rgv. VIII.58.2)

"He, with clean wings, but only One in nature,
Wise singers make many figures with songs. "
(X.114.5)

The ancient Vedic wisdom says that thought becomes sound, sound becomes word, and word becomes matter.

In the Sanskrit language of India and Vedic tradition, mantras are known as Bija Mantras and are recited aloud. Vedic mantras and sounds use vocals which resonate on the chakras and help to balance and harmonize the body's energy centers.

Vedic Mantras produce powerful sounds which are believed to have divine origins and in turn are emanated by the universal creative force.

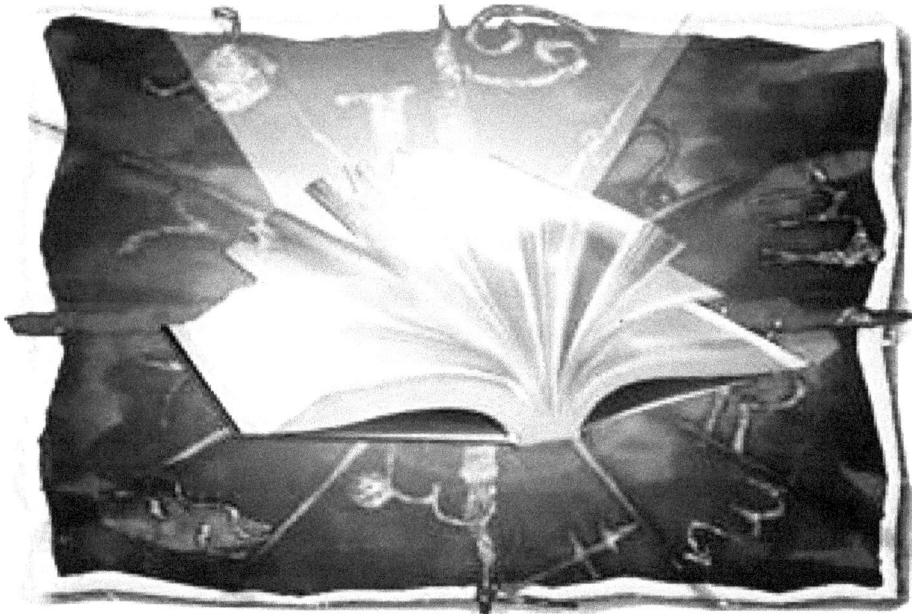

38

Activating the Chakras

Activating the chakras through vowel sounds in the diatonic and chromatic harmony in combination with the intention formula.

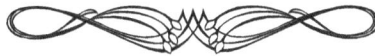

The diatonic and chromatic harmony

Many harmonic systems with resonating effects on the chakras have been used, but in our practice we use the **diatonic harmony** for the seven basic chakras and the **chromatic harmony** for the two additional chakras.

We will make exercises with vowel sounds to stimulate the chakras.

This system has been used in many spiritual traditions and has a musical scale of five complete tones, two semitones, higher tones, lower tones and other modalities. This leads to a total of seven musical notes: C, D, E, F, G, A, B.

Five semitones arise from the seven notes of the **diatonic harmony** which are: C, C#, D, D#, E, F, F#, G, G#, A, A#, B, C. We divide the distance between notes and refer to them as halftones.

Between the notes E and F and B and C we cannot halve the interval. This is due to the laws of acoustics and the ascending manner in which the brain translates sound. For the ascending mode we use the pound sign (#) which means that the sound of the note should be raised by a semitone or half tone and is defined as sharp. For the descending mode we use the letter (**b**) which means that the musical note should be lowered by a semitone or half tone and is defined as flat. There are only seven notes which, when divided, create five semitones and turn into twelve notes. The sharp (#) and the flat (b) symbols are used in front of the musical note to change the pitch by a semitone or half step.

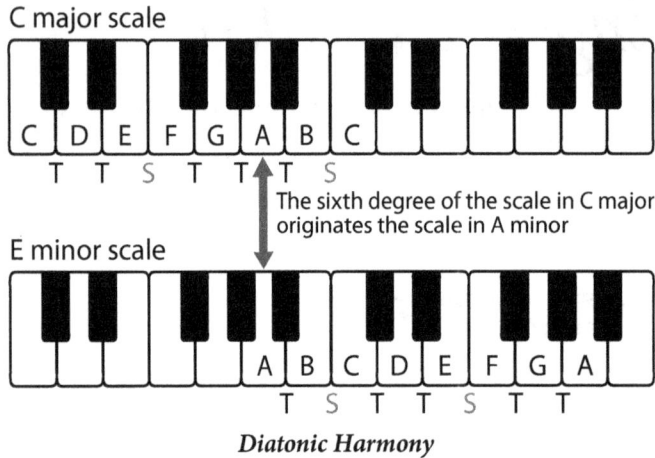

C major scale

T T S T T T S

The sixth degree of the scale in C major originates the scale in A minor

E minor scale

T S T T S T T

Diatonic Harmony

The **diatonic scale** has the basic notes from **C** to **B** and repeat the same cycle in **C**. There is also the **chromatic scale** when divided in five half tones or semitones creates twelve notes.

When activating the seven chakras we use the **Diatonic Harmony** for the following chakras: **C** = Root Chakra, **D** = Reproductive Chakra, **E** = Solar Plexus Chakra, **F** = Heart Chakra, **G** = Throat Chakra, **A** = Third Eye Chakra, **B** = Crown Chakra.

When activating the two additional chakras we use **Chromatic Harmony**: **F#** or **G b** = Thymus Chakra, **G#** or **A b** = Cerebellum Chakra.

B	493.88
Bb (A#)	466.16
A	440.00
Ab (G#)	415.30
G	392.00
Gb (F#)	369.99
F	349.23
E	329.63
Eb (D#)	311.13
D	293.66
Db (C#)	277.18
C	261.63

Illustration of the 7 diatonic tones and 5 chromatic semitones = 12 musical notes and frequency of the musical notes in Hertz.

Method to harmonize and heal the chakras with vocal sounds.

We start by sitting comfortably and very relaxed in a chair or in the lotus position on a cushion keeping the spine straight. When we keep the spine straight, the Chi or Prana energy, travels freely without blockages or interruptions through the central nervous system. In this way the vital energy is transported to the nine energy centers of the body or chakras.

We imagine that our head is suspended from a power cord that comes from the Center of the Universe and holds us from the center of the crown chakra.

In the execution of sounds and exercises to harmonize the chakras, we internally focus our attention and mental intent on the energy center that is being activated. The sound used must be the musical note and the correct vowel that corresponds to the chakra that is being harmonized. Example: In the root chakra, we apply the C note and make the sound UH.

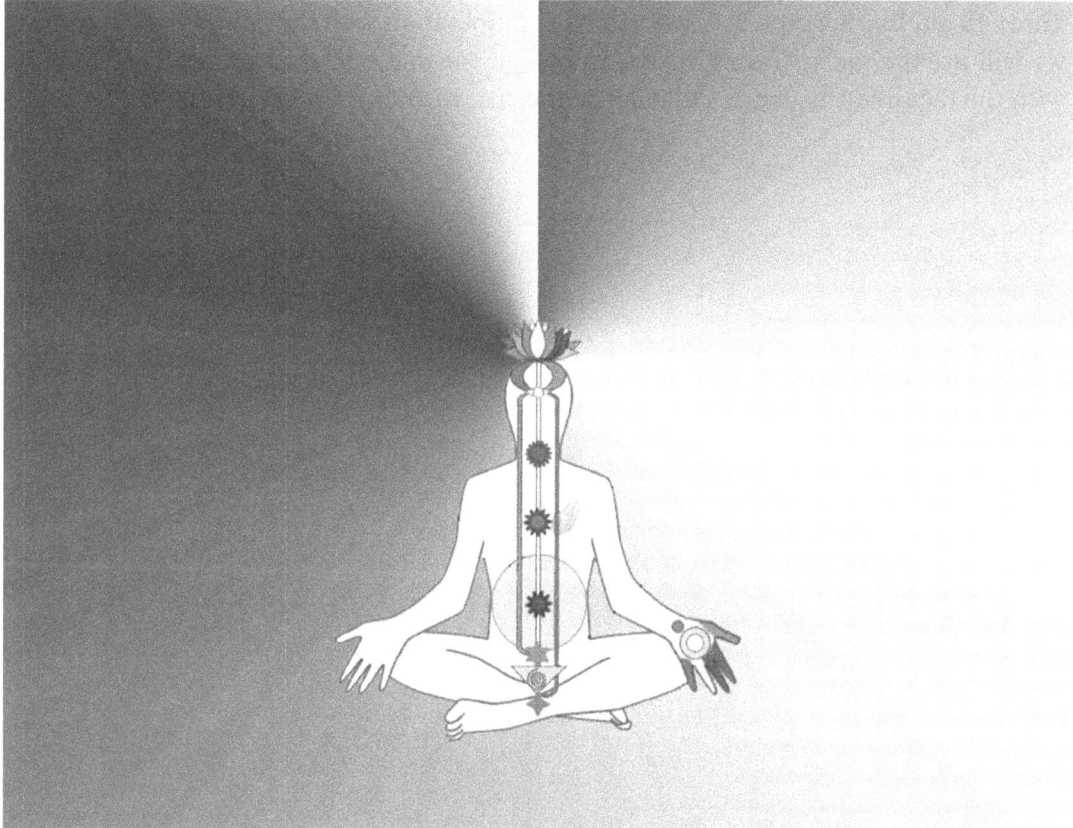

In activation and meditation we imagine that our head is suspended by a power cord coming from the center of the universe

We apply the intention formula:

Intention = visualization + (affirmations, mantras and sounds) + (have faith and believe) = manifestation

1st. We visualize the location of the chakra to be activated.
2nd. We apply the harmonic frequency, the note and the corresponding chakra vowel.

3rd. We visualize manifestations of peace, harmony, good health and regenerating energy in the chakra to be balanced. It is very important that when working on the chakra, you deeply feel the state of good health you want to manifest.

The sounds should be vocalized in a relaxed state without force or pressure in the voice.

Through our infinite power of intention, in combination with the power vocal harmony, we will use the music theory of seven notes in the diatonic and chromatic harmonies with the required frequencies to balance the chakra energy and activate healing.

39

The Chakras and Sounds

Description of the chakras and resonating vowel sounds.

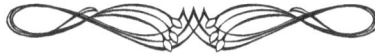

What are the chakras?

The word chakra in Sanskrit, the ancient language of India, means wheel. Chakras are vortexes of light energy turning in a spiral. They are like small revolving galaxies.

Many esoteric and mystical schools describe the chakras as energy centers. The concept of chakras has been adopted by many spiritual organizations but the existence of that concept **is not** based on religious principles. The original definition of the chakras is based on a concept of energy moving in a spiral.

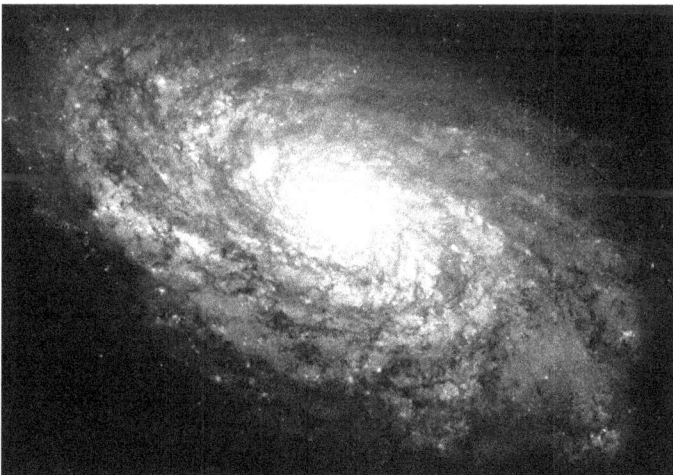

Chakras are like small galaxies moving in a spiral.

According to systems used in India, Tibet and China, we have seven energy centers. However, human beings have two additional energy centers, making a total of nine energy centers. They are called the root chakra, reproductive chakra, solar plexus chakra, heart chakra, thymus chakra, throat chakra, cerebellum chakra, third eye chakra and crown chakra. The chakras are

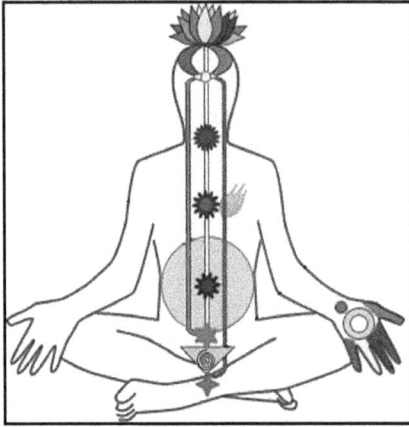

located on the front and back of the body.

Any imbalance of the physical body can be detected through the chakras. When the chakras are balanced, manifestation of adverse conditions, diseases and disorders in the body are prevented. There are also hundreds of energy centers throughout the body known as secondary chakras, which are related to the meridians and other body systems.

The process of healing the physical body of a person who has been injured is faster when the subtle body energy of the chakras has been balanced.

The Healing Forces of Harmonic Sounds and Vibrations, in combination with the mental power of creative visualization and intention, creates a powerful direct resonance that triggers balance of the chakras and stimulates the natural healing process of the body, mind and spirit.

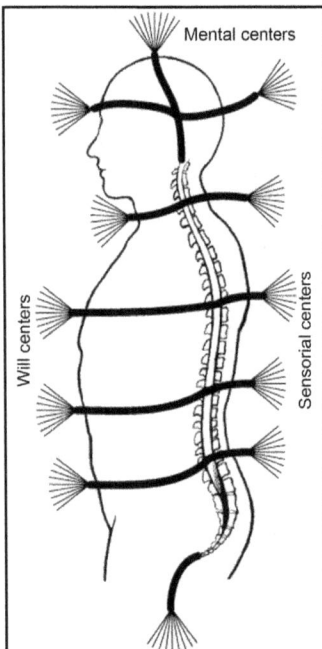

Frontal and posterior areas of the chakras in the body.

The chakras are in a constant state of spiral rotation and are affected by the frequencies and vibrations caused by sound. Various cultures speak of sounds that are generated by vocals which have effects on the chakras.

We have seven basic chakras and two additional. They are like small universes or energy circles which move in a spiral. The chakras are located on the front and back of our body.

One of the best ways to integrate the mind and body is through sounds and vocal intonations. The vocal tone is intended to balance the mind and body to connect the material and spiritual and achieve a balanced state of concentration. Scientific studies have shown that just 10 minutes a day of practice with vocal intonation is equivalent to 5 milligrams of the drug valium, which people use to relax.

Scientific studies show that vowel sounds can balance the chakras. **Vowel: UH, Vowel: OOO, Vowel: OH, Vowel: AH, Vowel: Aii, Vowel: EEi, Vowel: iii**

Description of the chakras and resonating vowel sounds

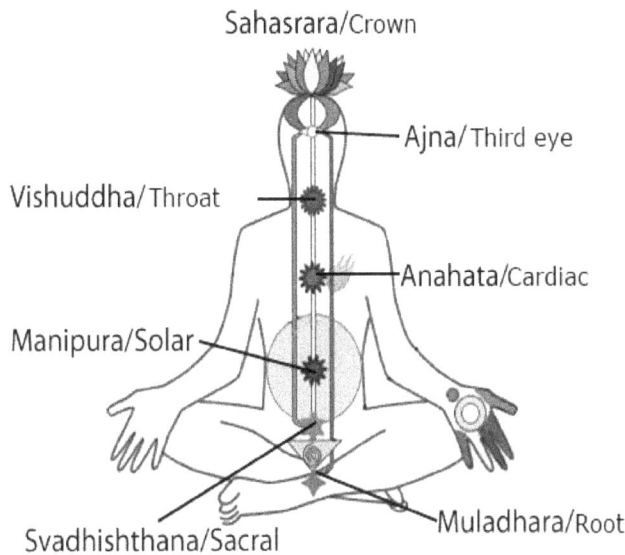

Sahasrara/Crown
Ajna/Third eye
Vishuddha/Throat
Anahata/Cardiac
Manipura/Solar
Svadhishthana/Sacral
Muladhara/Root

The correct pronunciation and enunciation of Vedic sound vowels or bijas, has a positive effect when resonating on the chakras. The sounds help to release blocked energy in the endocrine glands, organs and body systems. They can stimulate the natural healing process of the body, mind and spirit.

An intense practice by using harmonic vocal sounds, mantras and meditation, can result in a high spiritual level, and possibly reaching the state of enlightenment.

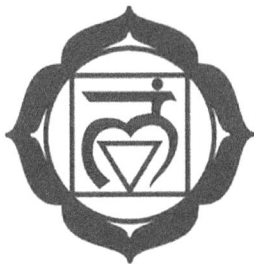

1st: Root Chakra (Muladhara), is located between the **anus and the genitals.** It is connected to the coccyx bone and opens downward. It relates to the physical process of elimination and the organs that work in those functions. **Color:** Fire Red, **Element:** Earth, **Sensory Function:** Smell. **Symbol:** Lotus with four petals. **Keywords:** Foundations, security and habits.

In the philosophy of Hinduism: The Root Chakra (Muladhara) is the basis of time and space and the chakra's memory. Is the memory's dwelling, the basis of all human knowledge. This center is also the seat of our basic survival instincts and sexuality, among others. **Deity:** Ganesha and Brahma.

The Root Chakra (Muladhara) Musical Tone: UT (DO), (C), **Frequency:** 396 Hz, **Vowel sound:** UH (We pronounce: **Cuu-uu-uu-uu-uu**). We release emotions of guilt

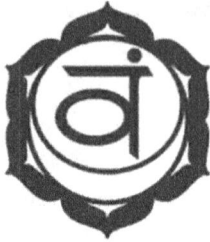

and fear. (Vedic Bija Sound: **Lam.**)

2nd: Reproductive Chakra also known as Sacral Chakra or Sacral Center (Svadhistana): Is located above the genitals and three inches below the navel. It is related to sexual energy, reproductive organs and much of the vital energy. Sexual energy is a divine energy used in the spiritual practice of Tantra. This chakra provides energy for reproductive purposes and creative energy; not only give rise to the creation of a baby, it is where we activate our projects, music, writings, paintings, designs, etc. **Color:** Orange, **Element:** Water, **Sensory Function:** Taste **Symbol:** Lotus of six petals. **Keywords:** Feel, wish, create.

In the philosophy of Hinduism: The Reproductive Chakra (Svadhistana,) is the heart of relationships and reason, home of intelligence. Educated people work through this center of logic and analysis. Great minds have mastery and control over this center. It is the abode of pragmatic shelter. Deity: Vishnu.

The Reproductive Chakra is also known as **Sacral Chakra or Sacral Center: (Svadhistana) Musical Tone:** RE, (D), **Frequency:** 417 Hz, **Vowel Sound: OOO (Ooo)** (We pronounce: **Yoo-oo-oo- oo-oo**). We create and initiate changes. (Vedic Bija Sound: **Vam.**)

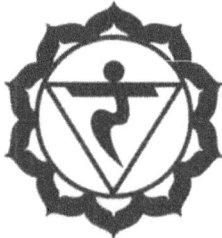

3rd: Solar Plexus Chakra, also known as the **Umbilical Center (Manipura).** It is about two fingers above the navel. It is related to the digestive organs and digestion. This chakra has the spleen, liver, pancreas, stomach, small and large intestines. It is also associated with human development. **Color:** Yellow or Gold **Element:** Fire, **Sensory Function:** Sight **Symbol:** 10 petal lotus. **Keywords:** The will of the spiritual warrior.

In the philosophy of Hinduism: The Solar Plexus Chakra (**Manipura**) is the center of willpower. Men and women achieve high mental and physical levels in this energy center. It is the center of discipline and endurance. **Deity:** Maharudra.

The Solar Plexus Chakra is also known as Umbilical Center (**Manipura**) **Musical Tone:** MI (E) **Frequency:** 528 Hz, **Vocal Sound: OH** (We pronounce: **gou-ou-ou-ou-ou.** In this energy center we manifest transformations and miracles. This frequency has the power to repair DNA and rejuvenate all the cells that shape our body (Vedic Bija Sound: **Ram.**)

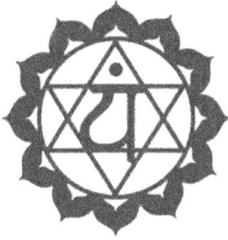

4th: Heart Chakra or Heart Center (Anahata) is at heart level in the center of the chest. Physically, it is associated with the functions of heart and lungs. Emotionally, it works with the energies of love and compassion. **Color:** Green, pink and gold, **Element:** Air, **Sensory Function:** Touch, **Symbol:** Lotus of 12 petals. **Keywords:** Love and awakening.

In the philosophy of Hinduism: The Heart Chakra, (**Anahata**) is the area of direct knowledge. Those who reach this level of evolution, with their penetrating and delicate vision, have influence in many areas of knowledge. They are the guides of humanity, counselors, mentors and they find solutions to problems. **Deity:** Ishvara.

The Heart Chakra is also known as the **Cardiac Center.** (**Anahata**) It is at heart level in the center of the chest. **Musical Tone:** FA (F), **Frequency:** 639 Hz, **Vocal Sound: AAA** (Pronounced: **Ma-a-a-a-a**). We activate connections and relationships with other beings. We activate the powerful energy of unconditional love. (Vedic Bija Sound: **Yam.**)

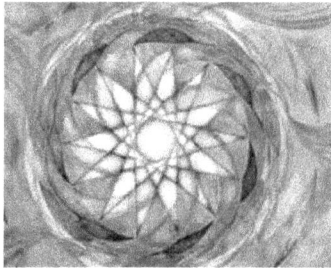

5th: Thymus Chakra. It is one of the first glands that develops in the fetal stage. It is located in the upper chest, just above the heart chakra, between the heart and throat. Physically, it is associated with the immune system and has our DNA pattern within. It has the design of our karma in this life, including information from past lives.

The thymus chakra is where intention originates; the link between the emotions of the heart and rational language. It is what makes us inhale before speaking, it is where words begin to form and where intention is behind the words we are about to speak. Emotionally works with the emotions of divine love, compassion, truth and forgiveness. **Color:** Turquoise, **Element:** Water, **Symbol:** 14 petal lotus. **Keywords:** I am, I am.

The Thymus Chakra is located in the upper chest just above the heart chakra, between heart and throat. **Musical Tone:** Fa# (F#) or Sol b, (Gb), **Frequency:** 690 Hz, **Vowel Sound:** We use the same vocal sound of the heart chakra, but in the tone of half (1/2) note higher. **Vocal Sound: AAA** (We pronounce: **Ma-a-a-a-a**). This is the area where intention originates and connects the emotions of divine love, compassion, truth and forgiveness with the area where language is originated. It is the area that can speak

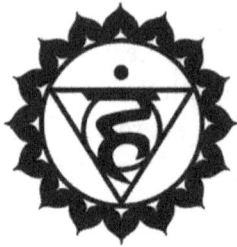

from the heart. We activate the powerful energy of divine love, compassion and forgiveness. (Vedic Bija Sound: **Yam.**)

6th: Throat Chakra or Neck Chakra. (Vishuddha) It is located at the base of the neck and larynx. It originates in the cervical spine and opens forward. This chakra is associated with communication, speech and audition. The ears are also associated with this chakra. In Hindu philosophy, is said that karma is accumulated in the area of the throat chakra. **Color:** Light blue, teal and silver. **Element:** Ether, **Sensory Function:** Ear, **Symbol:** 16 petal lotus. **Keywords:** Speak and create.

In the philosophy of Hinduism: The Throat Chakra or neck (**Vishuddha**) is the center of divine love, without limits. All beings are seen as brothers and sisters who are part of the sacred creation. It is where selfless souls, exceptional artists and mystical poets reside. **Deity:** Sadashiva.

The Throat Chakra or Neck Chakra (Vishuddha) is located at the base of the neck and larynx. **Musical Tone:** SOL (G), **Frequency:** 741 Hz, **Vowel Sound: E-e-e** (We pronounce: **Me-e-e-e**). Activates communication. (Vedic Bija Sound: **HAAM.**)

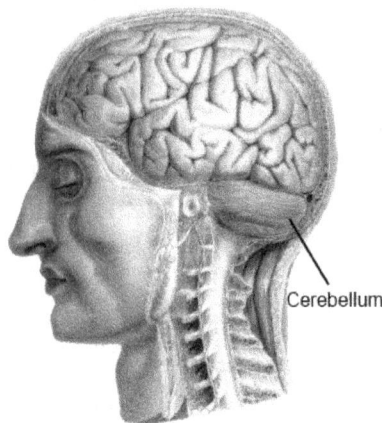

7th: Cerebellum Chakra. It is located behind the neck connected to the brain. It is in this center where our dreams take place. When this center opens we begin to see and remember our dreams. The cerebellum is also related to the causal chakra located above the crown chakra, left on the etheric body.

Cerebellum

The causal chakra is a small gray ball. It is usually said that to develop psychic abilities such as telepathy, telekinesis and remote viewing, we must exercise the 3rd eye, but it's really not the third eye that reaches these powers, it is the cerebellum chakra. Through meditation we can activate this chakra and our hidden abilities begin to manifest.

Color: Purple, Blue or Black. **Element:** Air/ether, **Function:** Spiritual lessons. It is the portal that leads to the universal akashic records and is through this chakra that we activate superior powers and communicate with the first source of creation or God. **Keywords:** I am, I am.

The Cerebellum Chakra is located behind the neck connected to the brain. **Musical Tone:** Sol#/LAb (G# or Bb), **Frequency:** 796.5 Hz, **Vowel Sound: E-e-e** (We pronounce: **Me-e-e-e-e**). **Another sound used to activate this chakra is: "Eh-Eh-Eh."** It activates communication with higher powers and the creative source of the universe or God. (Vedic Bija Sound: **HAAM**.)

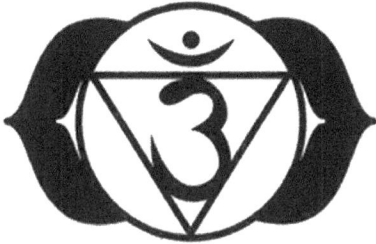

8th: Third Eye Chakra (Ajna) is also known as the **Inner Eye Chakra.** This chakra is located one finger above the base of the nose, in the center of the forehead. It opens forward. This chakra is associated with imagination, psychic powers, mental activity and brain function. **Color:** indigo, yellow and violet. **Sensory function:** All the senses, also in the form of extrasensory perception. **Symbol:** 96 petal lotus, twice 48 petals. **Keywords:** Intuition, being, vast, infinite.

In the philosophy of Hinduism: The Third Eye Chakra (**Ajna**) is the center of sensitivity and clairvoyance which opens portals to many higher levels of consciousness. It is where the internal words of light originate. **Deity:** Ardhanarishvara.

The Third Eye Chakra (**Ajna**) is also known as the **Inner Eye Chakra. Musical Tone:** LA(A), **Frequency:** 852 Hz, **Vowel Sound: EEI (Eei)** (We pronounce: **Sei-ei-ei, ei-ei**) We return to the spiritual order. Intuition. (Vedic Bija Sound: **Sham**.)

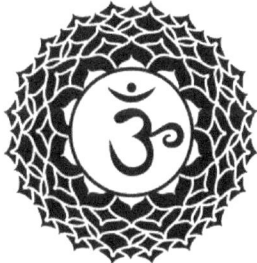

The 9th: Crown Chakra (Sahasrara). Also called **Crown Center**, 1,008 petal lotus or Tenth Gate. It is located on the highest point above the head in the center. It opens up above. This chakra controls all aspects of mind and body. It is associated with the process of enlightenment and union with God. This chakra is normally not fully open in most humans. Enlightened beings like ascended masters and saints are depicted with an energy circle of light over their heads. **Color:** Violet, white and gold. **Symbol:** 1,008 petal lotus. **Keywords:** Intuition, being, vast, infinite.

In the philosophy of Hinduism: The Crown Chakra (**Sahasrara**) is the center of enlightenment. It is the top of the mountain, the pinnacle of consciousness' light and energy. It is Aham Brahmasmi. "I am". This is where one remains in communion with oneself. **Deity:** Shiva.

Coronal Chakra (Sahasrara) is also called the **Crown Center**, 1,008 petal lotus or Tenth Gate. **Musical Tone:** TI (Si) (B), **Frequency:** 963 Hz, **Vocal Sound: iii (Iii)** (We pronounce **Mii-ii-ii-ii-ii**) We activate the higher state of consciousness. (This is the highest frequency of music theory). (Vedic Bija Sound: **OUM.**)

In Hindu philosophy there are 7 chakras below the root chakra (Muladhara.)

Like all the other chakras, people who are full of trauma, negative karmic energy and dark energy, have to work with the energy centers located below the root chakra in order to purify themselves. Negative energy is absorbed by the divine Mother Earth and is transmuted and transformed into energies of harmonic creativity and love. The chakras below the root chakra (**Muladhara**) have the following negative effects:

1) **Atala** = Fear and lust (indecisions that can block the ambitions.)
2) **Vitala** = Anger (instinctive fire that can hurt others.)
3) **Sutala** = Jealousy and retaliation (concern for wanting what others have. Envy.)
4) **Talatala** = Prolonged confusion (perversions that replace the natural joys, hardens the stream of consciousness creating negative karma.)
5) **Rasatala** = Selfishness (a veil of imprisonment which blinds the natural instincts and has no interest in helping others. All is "I" and "mine." Every action is for personal gain.)
6) **Mahatala** = No awareness (blindness where the prevailing feelings of guilt, remorse, even fear.)
7) **Patala** = Malice and criminal instinct (a virtual hell of hate, harm, these are those who kill for their own benefit without remorse. In rare circumstances some people can reach this level.)

In the Sanskrit philosophy of Hinduism there are infinite chakras above the crown chakra (Sahasrara)

There are countless chakras that are above the crown chakra. The chakras that are above the head are called **Antahkarana**. Agamic Hindu tradition delineates seven levels of Paranada dimensions. There are Tattvas or octaves containing seven chakras each, although God is infinite and there is actually an infinity of chakras. The first Tattva is the highest level of sound and the 7 chakras are called as follows: Vyapini, Vyomanga, Ananta, Anatha, Anashrita, Samana and Unmana.

The subtlest consciousness or the highest levels of manifestation, is organized as follows:

1) Iokas (3 worlds and 14 levels.) In Classic Agamic Vedic cosmology, there are 14 chakras above the head. In fact, there are infinite chakras ending in God, Atma, Purusha. The 14 levels correspond to the strength of the psychic center of the soul's internal organs. The 14 chakras are doors within man or woman that lead to each of the 14 planes of higher dimensions.

2) Kala (5 spheres.) The 5 Kalas are the great divide of consciousness or the mind's dimensions. Superconscious, sub-superconscious, conscious, subconscious and sub-subconscious.

3) Tattva (36 evolutions.) The 36 Tattvas are the blocks with which the universe is built.

4) Kosha & Sharira (3 bodies and five sheaths.) These are the body sheaths.

In addition, inside the body around the chakras are three primary streams which are like conduits of nerves transporting energy. They are: **Ida, pingala and sushumna.**

The main chakras mentioned in the previous chapter correspond to energy centers located in the glands and lymph nodes which secrete hormones and biochemical substances and regulate the body's metabolism.

Kundalini energy moves from the inferior chakras below the root chakra, up to the crown chakra and continues out of the crown chakra towards the higher chakras.

This practice helps eliminate energy blockages, disease, negative energies, karmic energies and gradually helps one reach enlightenment.

Synopsis of the powerful sounds and mantras mentioned in the sacred Hindu book "The Vedas," and the power of resonance that these sounds have on the chakras.

The sacred book of India called The Vedas talks about powerful Vedic mantras and sounds that incorporate the use of vocals. These mantras and sounds resonate on the chakras, balancing and harmonizing them.

Activation and harmonization of the chakras through vowel sounds and mantras

1st: Root Chakra (Muladhara) Musical Tone: UT (DO), (C), **Frequency:** 396 Hz, **Vocal Sound: UH** (Pronounced **Cuu-uu-uu-uu-uu**). We release emotions of guilt and fear. (Vedic Bija Sound: **Lam.**)

2nd: Reproductive Chakra or Sacral Center (Svadhistana) Musical Tone: RE, (D), **Frequency:** 417 Hz, **Vocal Sound: OOO** (Ooo) (Pronounced **Yoo-oo-oo-oo-oo**). We create and initiate changes. (Vedic Bija Sound: **Vam.**)

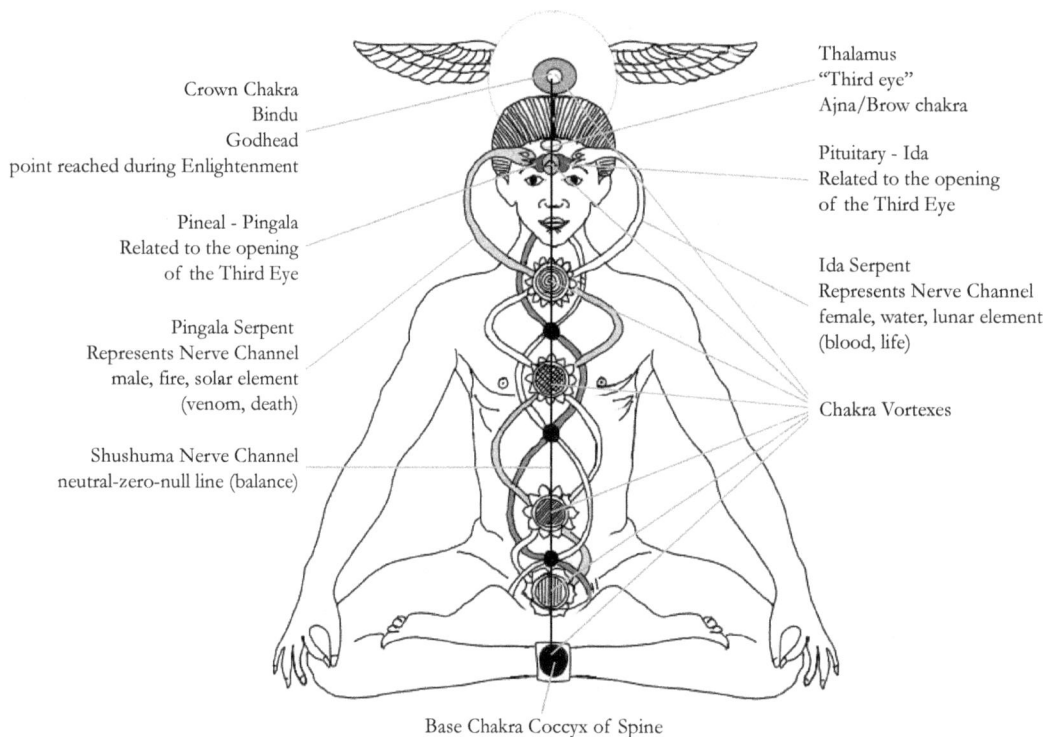

Crown Chakra
Bindu
Godhead
point reached during Enlightenment

Pineal - Pingala
Related to the opening
of the Third Eye

Pingala Serpent
Represents Nerve Channel
male, fire, solar element
(venom, death)

Shushuma Nerve Channel
neutral-zero-null line (balance)

Thalamus
"Third eye"
Ajna/Brow chakra

Pituitary - Ida
Related to the opening
of the Third Eye

Ida Serpent
Represents Nerve Channel
female, water, lunar element
(blood, life)

Chakra Vortexes

Base Chakra Coccyx of Spine

*Illustration of Kundalini's energy movement and
the conduits of energy, pingala and sushumna.*

3rd: Solar Plexus Chakra or Umbilical Center (Manipura) Tone Musical: MI, (E), **Frequency:** 528 Hz, **Vocal Sound: OOO** (Pronounced **Gou-ou-ou-ou-ou.**) We manifest transformations and miracles. (This frequency has the power to repair DNA). (Vedic Bija Sound: **Ram.**)

4th: Heart Chakra or Cardiac Center (Anahata) is at heart level in the center of the chest. **Musical Tone:** FA, (F), **Frequency:** 639 Hz, **Vocal Sound: AAA** (Pronounced **Ma-a-a-a-a**). We activate connections and relationships with other beings. (Vedic Bija Sound: **Yam.**)

5th: Thymus Chakra. It is located in the upper chest just above the heart chakra, between the heart and throat. **Musical Tone:** FA # (F#) or Sol b, (G b), **Frequency:** 690 Hz, **Chakra Sound:** We use the same vocal sound of the heart chakra but in a half (1/2) higher note. **Vocal Sound: AAA** (Pronounced **Ma-a-a-a-a**). It allows one to speak from the heart so we can activate the powerful energy of divine love, compassion and forgiveness. (Vedic Bija Sound: **Yam.**)

6th: Throat Chakra or Neck Chakra (Vishuddha) is located at the base of the neck and larynx. **Musical Tone:** SOL (G), **Frequency:** 741 Hz, **Vocal Sound: E-e-e** (Pronounced **Me-e-e-e-e**). We activate communication. (Vedic Bija Sound: **HAAM.**)

7th: Cerebellum Chakra. It is located behind the neck below the head connected to the brain. **Musical Tone:** G#/Lab (G # or Bb) **Frequency:** 796.5 Hz, **Vocal Sound: E-e-e** (Pronounced **Me-e-e-e-e**). Another sound used to activate this chakra is: "**Eh-Oh-Eh**" We activate higher powers and communication with the creative source of the universe or God. (Vedic Bija Sound: **HAAM.**)

8th: Third Eye Chakra (Ajna), also known as **Inner Eye Chakra**. **Musical Tone:** LA, (A), **Frequency:** 852 Hz, **Vocal Sound: EEI (Eei)** (Pronounced: **Sei-ei-ei-ei-ei**) We return to the spiritual order. Intuition. (Vedic Bija Sound: **Sham.**)

9th: Crown Chakra (Sahasrara), also known as **Crown Center**, 1,008 petal lotus or Tenth Gate. **Musical Tone:** TI, (SI), (B), **Frequency:** 963 Hz, **Vocal Sound: iii (iii)** (Pronounced **Mii-ii-ii-ii-ii**). We activate the highest state of consciousness. (This is the highest frequency of music theory). (Vedic Bija Sound: **OUM.**)

40

Dr. Alfred A. Tomatis

Studies on Harmonic Vocal Sounds That Resonate with the Chakras.

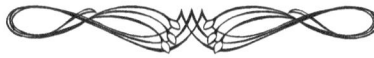

Dr. Alfred A. Tomatis spent his life researching the ear and the power of healing through sound. He showed that harmonic sounds of high frequencies boost the brain's energy. On the contrary, he also showed that low frequency sounds like the humming of computers, can drain the brain's vital energy and cause fatigue.

In 1957, Dr. Tomatis used high frequency sounds (750 to 3,000/4,000 to 20,000 Hz) to activate the brain and found that these sounds can have cognitive effects on thought, perception and memory. Hearing these sounds can increase attention, concentration, intuition, language interpretation and energy.

Tomatis' Zones

Body - Zone 1 (0-750Hz) balance, rhythm, coordination, muscle tone, reflexes, sense of direction, laterality, discrimination of right and left side.

Language - Zone 2 (750 to 3,000/4,000Hz) memory, concentration, attention, speech, language interpretation, vocal control.

Creativity - Zone 3 (3,000/4,000-20,000Hz) energy, intuition, ideas, ideals, verbal skills, the voice.

Harmonic vocals are important for healing. They generate powerful sounds that resonate with the chakras, organs and body systems.

We make vowel sounds automatically all the time. To create harmonic sounds that have a direct resonance with the chakras and organs, we must change the movement and position of the tongue, lips, and cheeks. It is also important to listen carefully. **"The voice can only duplicate the harmonic sounds that the ear can hear"** (Dr. Alfred Tomatis). In other words, the ear needs training to hear the harmonic tones, otherwise those energies cannot be expressed in speech.

First, breathe as deeply as possible by expanding the diaphragm as much as you can. Then place your lips making the sound **"MMMMM"**. You achieve the sound by puckering your lips. We will continue this exercise with vowel sounds in combination with the **"MMMMM"**. Some of these exercises work better than others. Most important is that you enjoy and benefit from this experiment.

Place one palm behind the ear while holding the other palm a few centimeters in front of the mouth. This will facilitate the ears hearing the harmonic sounds more clearly. Keep practicing. The bathroom is a good place to make these sounds because the solid walls reflect the sound back to you.

Continue the exercise by adding the following vowel sounds:

UUMMMUUU - With pursed lips you can emphasize the harmonic sounds.

OH MMMOH (OMMO)

AH MMMAAA (AMMAA)

EYE MMMIII (EYEMMII)

AY MMMAY (AIMMAI)

EEMMMEE (EMME)

Pursing your lips and placing the sound in front of your mouth continue by making a long sound: **MMMMOOOOOORRRRRR.** While pressing your lips and mouth, the tongue moves quickly to pronounce the sound **RRRR** (like the sound of a running engine). The tongue moves approximately a quarter of an inch (0.635 cm.) behind the teeth and you should hear a buzz above the basic tone.

Placing harmonic sounds in the nasal cavity can help to improve the conditions of the frontal sinuses and can relieve headaches. Nasal sounds also stimulate the pineal and pituitary glands in the brain.

It is believed that these sounds can stimulate the glands of the brain to produce biochemical substances and maintain its balance. The nasal sounds also balance the right and left hemispheres of the brain. This can improve mental clarity, concentration, memory and learning.

Nasal Harmonic Sounds

To begin with nasal sounds we use **"nnnn"** and add the following vocal sounds.

UUNNNUUU - Make the following sounds continuously:

OH NNNOH - As if pronouncing **GOU**

AH NNNAAA - As if pronouncing **AANNAA**

EYE NNNIII - As if pronouncing **EYENI**

AYNNAY - AINNAI

EENNNEEE - ENNE

NNNNUUUU-RRRR - When starting the nasal sound let the tip of the tongue move about a quarter inch (0.635 cm.) behind the teeth and you will achieve a buzzing sound.

Harmonic Sounds Produced in the Back of the Throat

GUNG GING GANG GONG - Repeat these sounds several times. These sounds open and close the glottis generating high frequency harmonic sounds.

Continue by combining the harmonic sounds using different techniques

MMMMMMOOOOORRRRRR - as if pronouncing **MMOORR.**

NNNNNUUUUUURRRRR - as if pronouncing **NNUURR.**

NNNNN-GONG-NNNNN-GANG-NNNNN-UUUUU-RRRRR-MMMMMM-OOOO-RRRRR, etc.

WWWWWOOOOOOWWWWW (GUUOOUU)

UUUUU-RRRRRR-EEEEEE (UURREE) - from the back of the throat to the front of the throat.

Make harmonic vocal sounds slowly passing from one vowel to another. Focus your attention on pronunciation when doing it loudly. Visualize that the sound is producing an energy that moves within your body in the areas where there is stiffness or a blockage. Let the resonance of the harmonics release energy blockages in organs, tissues, meridians and body systems. Remain silent after completing these exercises.

41

Vedic Mantras

Scientific research on the healing power of mantras, repetitive prayers and Vedic mantras that resonate with the chakras.

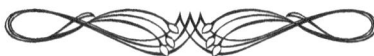

Scientific research shows the healing power of mantras and repetitive prayer

In the early 1970s, Dr. Herbert Benson, president and founder of the Institute for Mind Body Medicine at Harvard, documented a phenomenon called the **relaxation response,** which he says is the opposite of "fight or flight". Dr. Benson experimented with Sanskrit mantras. He told the participants to sit very quietly and repeat the mantras either mentally or verbally for ten to twenty minutes. He encouraged them to breathe easily, cast aside intrusive thoughts, and go deep into their minds.

Benson found that individuals who repeated the Sanskrit mantras for only ten minutes a day had remarkable physiological changes. This practice succeeded in slowing the heart rate, lowering stress and balancing the metabolism. Repeating mantras helped reduce the high oxygen consumption of individuals with high blood pressure. The individuals' bodies were in a state of relaxation and rest.

In subsequent studies Dr. Herbert Benson documented that the repetition of Sanskrit mantras can benefit the immune system, relieve insomnia, reduce doctor visits, and increase self-esteem.

Dr. Benson and his colleagues also experimented by having participants repeat phrases such as **"Lord Jesus Christ have mercy on me"** and "love and peace" and saw similar results. Dr. Benson and his colleagues found that repeating Sanskrit mantras, prayers and positive affirmations, can trigger relaxation and improve health.

What are mantras?

Mantras are sacred sounds that generate specific vibrations which purify, calm, create, energize, cleanse, modify, bind, raise and transform. Discipline, purity of heart, purity of intention, mental clarity and perseverance will ensure the effectiveness of mantras. To benefit from mantras it is necessary to know and understand the power of silence.

Mantras and songs have been used for thousands of years by civilizations in spiritual and religious healing traditions. Through the use of mantras the spirit rises, feelings of unity and love are expressed and a connection between man and the universe is established.

Mantras are composed of powerful words. To achieve maximum benefits, it is important to be consistent, and recite or sing continuously, with the intent of love and selflessness. When mantras are recited or sung in this way, internal and external harmony manifests. Cleansing can occur which can activate good health and happiness. Mantras can help us transcend the third dimension and free ourselves from the **Wheel of Samsara**, the wheel or the cycle of birth, life, death and incarnation.

According to Hinduism, Buddhism, Jainism and Gnosticism, Freemasonry, Rosicrucian and other ancient philosophies and religions of the world, during the development of every life, known under the term Karma, (actions done for good or ill) "the fate of each being, of evolution or devolution" is determined.

The **Wheel of Samsara** is derived from the Sanskrit samsari, meaning "to flow, pass through different states, wandering." **Samsara** is the root of the word Malay **Sengsara**, which means suffering. To be free from the **Wheel of Samsara** means **freedom from suffering and transcending to higher levels of consciousness and higher dimensions.**

What does the word mantra mean?

Mantras produce sounds that activate energy. Mantras activate a mystical power that allows us to connect with the cosmic energies of the highest levels that go beyond form, time and space. Mantras were originally conceived in the Vedas and the oldest and most revered spiritual texts of India.

The word **mantra** comes from two Sanskrit words, **manas**, meaning **mind**, and **trai**, meaning **freedom from**. So the word **mantra** literally means **freedom from the mind.** Scientific research has shown that properly chanted mantras, (with devotion and faith) activate production and dissemination of healing biochemicals in the brain. Mantras are effective in controlling blood pressure, regulating cholesterol levels and adrenaline and stabilizing heartbeats.

Mantras can eliminate negative feelings such as fear, anger and jealousy. Mantras can positively affect and enhance concentration, memory, emotions, blood circulation and the body's natural healing process. Mantras can calm an individual's nervous system which can eliminate stress and encourage relaxation. Mantras can be used to raise Kundalini energy and stimulate and balance the chakras.

Vedic mantra that resonates with the chakras

Gayatri Mantra: is a powerful mantra that helps to awaken intellectual powers . This mantra is in the book of the Vedas which is believed to be the repository of all divine knowledge and one of the oldest books known to mankind. Chanting this mantra can help an individual attract happiness and diminish difficulties. It helps to eliminate life's obstacles and achieve wisdom and spirituality.

Gayatri Mantra: The correct enunciation and pronunciation of the Gayatri Mantra can have a positive effect on the chakras. The Gayatri Mantra consists of twenty-four syllables which balance all energy centers of the human body, including the chakras. These sounds help release energy blockages in the endocrine glands, organs and body systems, and in turn stimulate the body's natural healing process and can raise spirits.

The maximum benefit of chanting the **Gayatri Mantra** is said to be obtained by chanting it 108 times. However, singing 9 or 18 times will also be beneficial. It is recommended to sing or repeat it at least three times in each of the following musical notes: E (MI) (Solar Plexus Chakra - Repeat 3 times), **F** (FA) (Heart-Chakra - Repeat 3 times), **G** (SOL) (Throat Chakra – Repeat 3 times) for a total of 9 times. It will take just few minutes to get positive results.

If you have time to sing it 108 times, it will be beneficial to sing it in the seven musical notes that have direct resonance with the seven energy centers or chakras, starting with the note C (DO) (root chakra) and ending with the note B (SI) (Crown chakra).

"ॐ भूर्भुवः स्वः ।
तत् सवितुर्वरेण्यं ।
भर्गो देवस्य धीमहि ।

धियो यो नः प्रचोदयात् "

"Om bhur, bhuvah, swaha (Oom Buu-Buvah-Sua-Ja)
that savithur varenyam (Tat-sa-vi-tur-va-reňyam)
bhargo devasya dhi mahi (Bar-go – de-va-sya-di-ma-ji)
dhiyo yo nah prachodayath (Di-yo-yo-nah-pra-cho-da-yath)

The meaning of the Gayatri Mantra in English

Oh God, You are the giver of life,
He Who removes the pain and sorrow,
The bestower of happiness;
Oh Creator of the Universe;
You are the most luminous, pure and adorable (or Supreme Divine Being, embodiment of knowledge and light)
We meditate on Thee;
Inspire, guide and enlighten our intellect,
So that we realize the supreme truth,
And dwell in righteousness...

OM: The oldest sound of the universe that represents Brahma. Who prevails in all worlds, Viz Bhulo-lok, Buba lok, and Swah-lok. He is omnipresent.
BHUR: The physical world that embodies the vital or spiritual energy.
BHUVAH: The mental world and the destroyer of all suffering.
SWAHA: The celestial and spiritual world that embodies happiness.
TATH: Tath or God, regarding the maximum Paramathma Transcendental Spirit.

SAVITHUR: The Creator or Divine Bright Sun (the ultimate light of wisdom) (not to be confused with the ordinary sun) and Preserver of the world.
VARENYAM: The best or most adorable, Supreme God who is the highest of the gods.
BHARGO: Destroyer of all sins. The light that gives wisdom, happiness and eternal life.
DESVASYA: Divine Deity or the Supreme Lord (The shining light of God).
DHEEMAHI: We meditate and take from.
DHIYO: The intellect,
YO: The light,
NAH: Ours, (Yo Naha: To be led by the Lord).
PRACHODAYATH: Inspired or illuminated or guided towards enlightenment.

India has the oldest tradition of thinkers and philosophers in their past and still continues its influence. **The Gayatri Mantra** is part of the Hindu philosophy and can be sung or recited by anyone regardless of religion.

The **Gayatri Mantra** transmits powerful vibrational frequencies which activate healing, wisdom, harmonization of chakras and the power of the senses.

How to use the mantras and what are its effects?

The mantras protect and purify the mind. In Sanskrit, mantras are implanted seeds in the mind. They are catalysts for the development of greater awareness.

The mantras sound repeatedly and with constant rhythm, either out loud or internally, allowing sound reproduction to work on the deepest levels. Many mantras have no logical meaning, so that the mind is not caught in analyzing them.

The internal repetition of the mantra can be started at anytime, anywhere. Sing for 5 to 15 minutes melting into silence as you direct your energy inside. Then remain silent during the time that you feel necessary. As in all work with sounds, you will feel the effect of silence afterwards.

It is recommended that the mantras are sung and repeated one to three times in each of the following musical notes: E (MI)(Solar Plexus Chakra - Repeat one to three times), F (FA) (Chakra of the heart - Repeat one to three times), G (SOL) (Throat Chakra - Repeat one to three times) totaling = 3 to 9 times. It should take only few minutes to see positive results.

If you have more time to sing, it will be beneficial to sing the seven musical notes that have direct resonance with the seven energy centers or chakras, starting with the note C (DO) (root chakra) and ending with the note B (SI) (crown chakra).

The meaning of the sound "OUM"

The sound **OUM** represents the light and sound of the whole creation of the universe. It symbolizes the divine Brahman and the entire universe. It means unity with the supreme, the combination of the physical and the spiritual. It is the sacred syllable, the first sound of the Almighty, the sound of which all other sounds emerge in music and language. Almost all mantras and songs are preceded by the pronunciation of OUM.

According to Hinduism, the Brahma (the name of the Creator of the Universe, or God) meditated on the three-letter mantra OUM and from there arose the three Vedas (Rig, Sama and Atharva.) The three words bhur (Earth) bhuva (Atmosphere) and suah (Heaven) also have the same origin. The OUM syllable also represents the Trimuti (three forms) Brahma, Vishnu and Shiva. In Hindu mythology it is said that Shiva made the sound of OUM with his drum and through svara came out the seven notes of the musical octave, sa, ri, ga, ma, pa, dha, ni. Through this sound Shiva creates and destroys the universe. The OUM is the sound form of Atman (soul or God).

The seven svaras are common to all musical systems. The way the notes or svaras are presented determines the style of music. The seven svaras are "Sa, ri, ga, ma, pa dha, ni," is the style of classical music in South India - Karnatic. In the West, they are called "Do, Re, Mi, Fa, Sol, La, Ti" (C, D, E, F, G, A, B).

When we invoke the sacred sound **OUM**, we expand, balance and harmonize the seven palaces or seven energy centers of the human body, the chakras, and these are activated with the unit of divine energy. The sound of the mantra OUM is universal and can be used as a powerful healing mantra. This sacred and powerful sound is built into most of the Vedic, Tibetan and Buddhists mantras.

Invocation in Sanskrit

The following is a powerful invocation sung in Sanskrit with the objective of manifesting the universal spirit of peace, love, harmony and light in all beings . May peace, love, harmony and light prevail in the hearts of all beings on Earth and the Universe...

It is recommended that this mantra is sung or repeated at least once in each one of the following musical notes: **E** (MI) (solar plexus chakra - repeat one time), **F** (FA) (Heart chakra - repeat one time), **G** (SOL) (throat chakra - repeat one time) for a total of three times. It should take fewer than five minutes to experience positive results.

Invocation of peace and harmony for all creation:

Asa-to-ma Sat-ga-ma-yia
Ta-ma-so ma youtir ga-ma-ya
Mi-trior ma-tan-ri-tan ga-ma-ya
Om Shanti, Shanti, Shanti
Lo-kah-sa-mas-tah Su-ki-no Ba-ban-tu
Yei shri sat-gu-ru mat-ja-ra-ki yei

Divine Universal Intelligence
Lead us from unreal to real
Lead us from the darkness to the light
Lead us from the fear of dead
to the knowledge of immortality
Oum Shanti, Shanti, Shanti

Made the entire universe
be filled with joy,
peace, love, harmony
Divine wisdom
divine guidance, create works
and divine light
Made the light of truth
overcome all darkness
Victory to the Divine Light
Victory to the Divine Light
Victory to the Divine Light
Oum Shanti, Oum Shanti, Oum Shanti

The basic meaning of **Oum Shanti** is peace, but it actually means to establish a deep level of peace where we can be protected from obstacles and delusions (such as lust, envy, anger, hatred and sadness.) The mantra **Oum Shanti** can help us focus deeply in meditation, and prevent negative energy from destroying our internal peace.

Om Namah Shivaya

ॐ नमः शिवाय

Illustration of the symbol Oum Namah Shivaya in Sanskrit.

Namah Shivaya is the holy name of God Shiva, recorded in the same center of the Vedas and elaborated in the Saiva Agamas.

Na is to hide the Lord's grace, **Ma** is the world, **Shi** stands for Shiva, **Va** is His Revealing Grace, **Ya** is the soul. The five elements are also incorporated in this old formula of invocation. **Na** is earth, **Ma** is water, **Shi** is fire, **Va** is air and **Ya** is ether or Akasha. It has many meanings.

Namah Shivaya has such power that the mere intonation of these syllables collects its own reward by saving the soul from the slavery of the treacherous instinctive mind and the steel bands of a perfected and externalized intellect.

The swamis Indian sages declare that this mantra is life, action, and love, and that repeating this mantra or japa brings out inner wisdom.

The Holy Natchintanai proclaims: **Namah Shivaya** is indeed both **Veda and Agama**. Namah Shivaya represents all mantras and tantras. Namah Shivaya represents our souls, our bodies and possessions. Namah Shivaya has become our safe protection. The meaning of the **Namah Shivaya mantra was explained by Satguru Shivaya Subramuniyaswami.**

The sound of the **Om Namah Shivaya** mantra is powerful when recited verbally at least nine times and is even more effective when sung 108 times incorporating shades of the diatonic scale. I incorporate the use of a mala, made with the seeds of the sacred and medicinal tree of India, **Tulsi**, in my right or left hand to count them correctly, while chanting the mantra 108 times. It usually takes me about three minutes to complete the repetition of this sacred mantra 108 times, and when I finish I feel very relaxed, with lots of vitality and also connected with the energies of the upper spheres.

Maha Mrityunjaya Mantra

The Mahamrityunjay Mantra, also known as the **Mahamoksha Mritasanjivani Mantra,** mantra of Lord Shiva. Shiva is one of the most revered gods in Hindu religion. Shiva is the god of destruction. Destruction executed by the god Shiva creates and transforms life and activates the energy for the welfare of the world. Shiva activates the technique that connects us to pure happiness and consciousness.

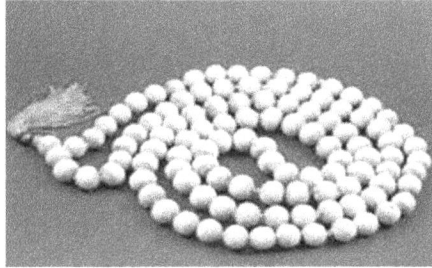

Image of the mala (Buddhist rosary), made with 108 seeds from the medicinal sacred tree Tulsi.

**"Om Tryam-bhakam Yaja-mahe
Sugan-dhim Pushtivar-dhanam
Urvaru-kamiva Ban-dhanan
Mrityor Mukshiya Maamritat"**

The **Maha Mrityunjaya Mantra** is a mantra that helps with rejuvenation, good health, prosperity, long life, peace, fulfilment, immortality and joy.

It is the mantra for protection that frees us from the fear of death and activates awareness of the immortality of our divine being. This mantra removes all negative vibrations and evil forces; it creates a powerful protective shield. It is said that singing this mantra protects people from accidents and misfortunes. It is also said to have the power to heal incurable diseases. This is the mantra for overcoming death and the connection with our own inner divinity.

The sound of the **Mrityunjaya Maha Mantra** is powerful when it is recited at least nine times and is even more effective when you recite it 108 times, while incorporating shades of the diatonic scale. I incorporate the use of a mala, made from the seeds of the sacred and medicinal tree of India "Tulsi," in my right or left hand, repeating the mantra 108 times.

42

Powerful Tibetan Mantras

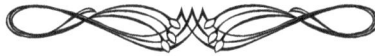

❧

Brief history of Tibet and mysticism

In 1950, Tibet was invaded by China and led to many years of turmoil. In 1959, the 14th Dalai Lama emigrated to India to seek asylum for himself and his people. The Sera Jey Monastery, located in Tibet, was bombed by the Chinese military. This caused the deaths of hundreds of monks, the destruction of many ancient texts, and the loss of priceless ancient works of art.

The monks and people who survived the invasion of the Chinese military fled to India under severe winter weather, walking across the Himalayan Mountains.

Following the mass exodus, hundreds of Sera Jey Lamas, monks and others established themselves in Bylakuppe near Mysore in the state of Karanataka, India. According to information from local sources, in 2011, the Tibetan community had about 3,000 monks and 5,000 Buddhists studying to become monks.

On my first trip to India in 1998 I was with my brothers, the Tibetan monks from the Sera Jey Monastery in Mysore, Karnataka State, India. I had the honor to meet and share every day of my stay in the Tibetan monastery in India with my brother of many past lives, the Geshi Lobsang Jamyang, the Lama Thupten Kunkhyer. Thupten taught me how to sing and vocalize the Tibetan mantras for harmonizing the chakras, how to activate that energy within and carry it with love, compassion and kindness to help all beings. There are so many lessons I learned from my brother Lama Thupten Kunkhyer, that I would have to write another book to include all of his teachings.

During my stay in the Tibetan Sera Je Monastery in Mysore I experienced an abundance of peace, harmony and happiness. It seemed as if I was in another dimension or on another planet. The monks and lamas devote their lives to spiritual mystical work. Through their practices of meditation, prayer, mantras, chants and different tones of vocal sounds they generate a powerful energy that is transmitted through the planet. This can open dimensional portals and allow more light into our planet, which helps the human race evolve and increase its collective vibrational frequency of peace, love, harmony and divine order.

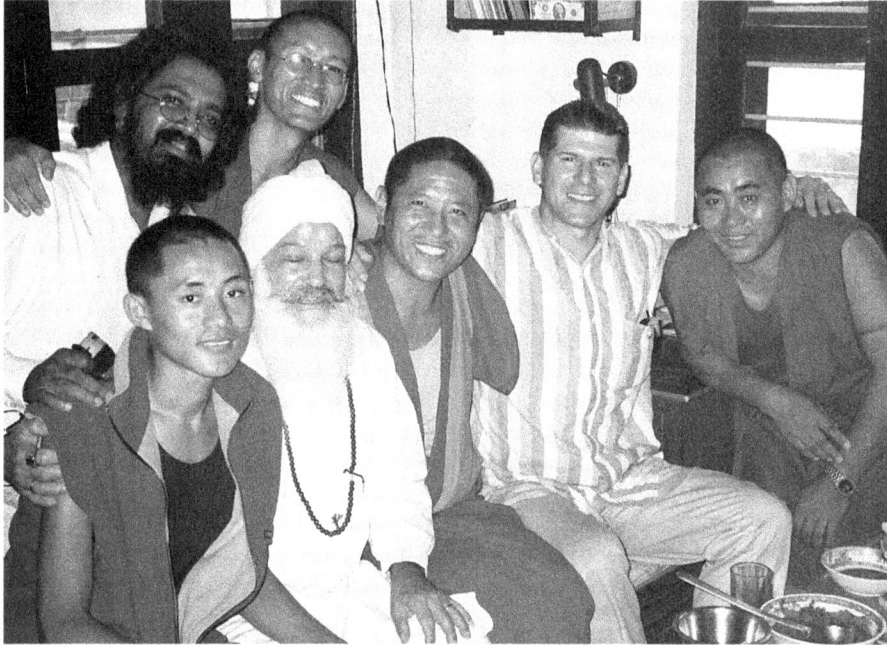

Photo of Lama Thupten Kunkhyer, Jay Emmanuel and his brothers Dharma in the Tibetan community in Mysore in the state of Karanataka, India.

Lama Thupten Kunkhyer and I frequently communicate by phone and through the Internet. He suggested that I share some stimulating and healing Tibetan mantras in this book.

Powerful Tibetan mantras

There are thousands of traditional mantras. **Om Ma Ni Pad Me Hum** is well known as the singing mantra, **Alokitesvars, the Buddha of Divine Compassion.** It is usually translated in the West as **"Hail the jewel in the center of the lotus,"** but it has multiple meanings and works on different levels. This mantra has been translated by great spiritual leaders.

The purpose of this mantra is to internally transform the body, speech and mind into a pure body, through the power of love and compassion that is inseparable from divine wisdom. This mantra is used in Tibetan Buddhism, and Chinese Buddhists include it in their rituals and ceremonies.

Repeating mantras in different tones of the **ancient Solfeggio** activates the regeneration process, and balances the chakras. The mantras can be done standing or sitting, and should be sung several times in one breath changing the sound gradually.

The meaning of the mantra "Om Mani Pad Me Hum"

Om = It refers to the Absolute Creator. OM is the universal sound. (In Latin, Omnes means all or everybody).
Mani = It is the jewel, the divine energy that dwells in the heart, also known as **Pad Me** = lotus flower.
Hum = It represents our self, which is a spark of the Universal Consciousness.

We could then say that **"Hum"** means perfect tone or sound, it is a full engagement of the **human individual being with the Infinite Divine Supreme being.**

A beautiful poetic version of the mantra **"Om Mani Pad Me Hum"** is: **"All nature is reflected in the jewel of my heart."**

Oum Aah Hum

Oum = The all-encompassing expression,
Aah = Love that blooms,
Hum = From the divine seed of my heart...

Oum Aaa Hum, Betgera Guru, Pat-Mat City Hum
(This mantra is for protection from any kind of negative energy. Recite or sing this mantra 9 times).

Oum Tare, Tu Tare, Tu Tare Soha
(This mantra is dedicated to the goddess Tara. It is a powerful mantra that can help free us from the Sansara wheel. It helps us to free ourselves from disease, accidents, disasters and hazards, and protects us from negative influences. Recite or sing this mantra 9 times).

Oum - Hara Patza - Na-di-di-di-di-di
(This mantra is dedicated to the Mandichuri deity, the goddess of wisdom. This mantra activates knowledge and divine wisdom. Recite or sing this mantra 9 times).

Ta Yia Ta Oum, Munie - Munie, Maha - Munie, Yee So Haa
(This mantra is dedicated to Buddha Saquiamuni. This mantra activates protection and divine wisdom of the Buddha within us. Recite or sing this mantra 9 times).

Ta Yia Ta Oum, Ve Can Ze, Ve Can Ze, Maha Ve Can Ze, Rat Zyia Yaa
(This mantra is dedicated to the Buddha that activates healing. This mantra is for the healing of any disease or condition. Recite or sing this mantra 9 times).

The mantras **"Om Mani Pad Me Hum" and "Oum Ah Hum" "Oum Aaa Hum, Betgera Guru, Pat-Mat City Hum"** are used in Buddhist philosophy and are beneficial regardless of religion. It is important to note that Buddhism is not a religion. It is a philosophy and way of life that connects a person with Universal Intelligence or God. It influences the essence of the individual, stimulating thoughts of peace, love, harmony, compassion and divine order.

43

Mantras, Prayers and Sacred Sounds

The mantras of the Emerald Tablets, names and sacred sounds in Hebrew and the Lord's Prayer in Aramaic.

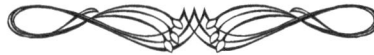

The Mantras of the Emerald Tablets

To understand the meaning of the powerful mantra in the book of the **Emerald Tablets**, it is necessary to get familiar with the mantra's origin and purpose .

The Book of the **Emerald Tablets** is an ancient book, which dates back 36,000 years BC, and was written by the **father of wisdom** Thoth, priest and king of Atlantis. The chapters in the Emerald Tablets are called tables.

The **ZIN-URU** mantra is mentioned in table ten (X) and the title of the table is the **key of time.**

These are the textual words of Thoth:

> *"The time came and I, Thoth, in the pursuit of wisdom, seek to the end of eternity and never turn back to the goal of what I want to achieve. Even the chief cycles know that they have not yet reached the goal, because with all their wisdom, they know that the truth never grows.*
>
> *Once, in the past I spoke to the Dweller. I asked a question that arose from the*

depths of my being, on the mystery of time and space. 'Oh Master, what is time?' -then the master told me: 'O Thoth, in the beginning was the void and nothingness, no space, no time, no nothing. And out of nowhere came a thought, purposeful, all-pervading and filled the void. Matter did not exist, only a force, a movement, a vortex, or vibration of intentional thought that filled the void.'

And I asked the Master: 'Was that the eternal thought?'

And he answered saying: 'In the beginning there was the eternal thought, and for thought to be eternal, time must exist. So the all-pervading thought grew the Law of Time. The time that exists through all space, floating in a smooth, rhythmic movement, is eternally in a fixation state.

Time does not change, but all things change in time. Time is the force that holds events separate, each in its proper place. Time is not moving, but moving through consciousness from one event to another. Time exists and it's definitely an eternal existence.

Although time and thinking are separate, yet they are one in every moment of existence.

Thoth: 'The voice of the Dweller ceased and I went to think about time. I knew that these words of wisdom are a way to explore the mysteries of time.

I meditated on the words of the Dweller and then sought to solve the mystery of time. I could find that time moves through strange angles. Yet only by the curves I could hope to attain the key that would give me access to space and time. Then I found that time only moves up, right and forward and through this movement I could be free from this movement in time.

Never let your heart be transformed into darkness. Your soul is light, a sun on the path. In the everlasting brightness, you will find the soul hidden in the light and you will never be chained and enslaved by darkness. Sunlight will always shine.

Light is life and without the great light nothing could exist. Throughout the formation of matter, the heart of light always exists. If, despite that, is tied to the darkness, inherent light always exists.

Although even the infinite is moving toward an unthinkable end. The cosmos is in

order and part of their movement extends to all space harmoniously.
I could see the wheel cycles as large circles in the sky. I knew then that everything
has to be, is growing to meet other being in a far grouping of space and time. I then
knew that words have the power to open the planes that have been hidden to man.
Yes, and even in the words is hidden the key that will open above and below.

Hear oh man, this word I leave. Use it and you shall find power in its sound. Say
the word "ZIN-URU" and you will find the power in its sound. However, one must
understand that man is of the light and light is of the man...

Listen, oh man, and hear a strange mystery than all that is 'beneath the sun and all
the space' is full of worlds within worlds, yes, one inside the other but separated by
the law."

The word **ZIN-URU** is a secret word connected to Egypt. It means **key**. It can help you open the doors of light. According to the esoteric book **The Emerald Tables** of Thoth, 32 mentors will be the founders of a sanctuary of light on Earth. It could be a reference to **Shambhala**. The **ZIN-URU** mantra can help to activate the pineal gland and connect with dimensional realities.

It is recommended to sing or repeat the **ZIN-URU** mantra at least nine times in each of the following musical notes: **E** (MI) (solar plexus chakra - repeat 9 times), **F** (FA) (heart chakra - repeat 9 times) **G** (SOL) (throat chakra - repeat 9 times) = a total of 27 times. If you dedicate a few minutes, you will experience positive results.

The names and sacred sounds in Hebrew

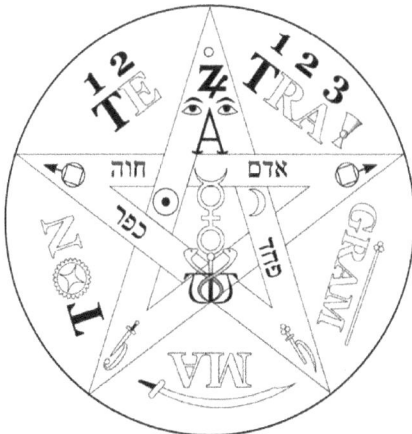

Tetragramaton

God's name in Hebrew consists of four words and appears in many Bibles as **LORD** in capital letters. The four Hebrew words of God's name **(YHWH)** also represent the **Tetragrammaton**. When Moses met with God on Mount Sinai he heard God's voice coming out of a tree that was lit with flames of divine fire.

God's name in most Bibles is presented as **"I Am"** and written **"Yud-Hed-Vav or Waw-Hed."** In old Hebrew it was pronounced **"Yud-Hed-Waw-Hed."**

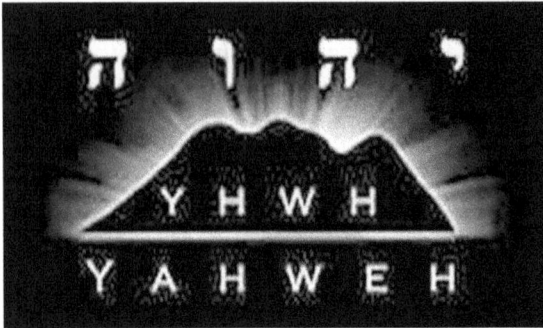

Generations of ancient Jews **did not** pronounce aloud the name of God "Yud-Hed-Waw-Hed" because it was forbidden by their religion. This contributed to the demise of the original pronunciation of God's name in Hebrew. Contemporary orthodox Jews refuse to utter the name of God aloud. Today's Christians write and pronounce it as **"Yahweh"**.

In ancient Hebrew language each word of God's name **"Yud-Hed-Waw-Hed"** has an ideographic meaning, translated as follows:

Yud = Hand.
Hed = A window or to gaze or to look.
Waw = Nail.

The translation of the four Hebrew words **"Yud-Hed-Waw-Hed"** would be **"Gazing at the hand with the nail."** According to the scriptures, God sent his son **"Yeshua,"** which in Latin is written **"Jesus,"** and in Hebrew means **"Yahweh"** "The Savior or Our Savior." Through **"Yahweh"** or **Jesus,** God the Father provided salvation to the human race.

The sound of the sacred Hebrew mantra can be powerful when it is vocalized . It is more effective when "Kodoish, Kodoish, Kodoish Adonai Tsebayoth" is recited nine times in different tones of the diatonic harmony, and pronouncing the name of God **"Yud-Hed-Waw-Hed"** three times in the tone of the heart **F** (FA) or the third eye **A** (LA), at the end.

Kodoish, Kodoish, Kodoish, Adonai, Tsebayoth (9 times)
Yud-Hed-Waw-Hed, Yud-Hed-Waw-Hed, Yud-Hed-Waw-Hed (3 times)

The sound of this Hebrew mantra activates the **sacred code** which sets a pattern of resonance in motion with **"The Throne of the Father, The Creator"** and prevents the manifestation of negative forces. It is used to disintegrate negative energies, invoke divine protection and create a vortex of power and connection with the **Universal Divine Intelligence.**

Sohar Hadash, Hadash Sohar, Sohar Hadash

Sohar Hadash is the Hebrew mantra used to neutralize natural phenomena such as hurricanes, earthquakes, storms, volcanic explosions, and tsunamis.

The sound of the Hebrew mantra **"Sohar Hadash"** is powerful when it is vocalized It is more effective when sung 9 times in different tones of the diatonic harmony.

The Lord's Prayer in Aramaic

The Lord's Prayer in Aramaic contains original words used by Jesus Christ when preaching to his disciples two thousand years ago. This transcript is from Dr. Neil Douglas-Klotz (The Awbwoon Resource Center.)

Abwoon d'bwashmaya
Father-Mother of the Cosmos who creates everything that moves in the light
Nethqadash shmakh
Focus your light within us – so that is useful: like the beams of a lighthouse showing the way
Teytey malkuthakh
Create now your kingdom of unity - through our willing hearts and hands
Nehwey sebyanach aykanna d'bwashmaya aph b'arha
Make your desire to always act with ours, as in all the light and in all forms
Habwlan lachma d'sunqanan yaomana
Grant us what we need each day in bread and vision: The survival of a progress towards a higher life
Washboqlan khaubayn (wakhtahayn) aykana daph khnan shbwoqan l'khayyabayn
Free us from the ropes of errors, as we have freed the chains of guilt with others
Wela tahlan l'nesyuna
Lead us not into oblivion
Ela patzan min bisha
But deliver us from immaturity
Metol dilakhie malkutha wahayla wateshbukhta l'ahlam almin
From You comes all the power, You renew the song that beautifies everything, from century to century
Amyn
Amen
I seal this in faith as the source that grows all my actions.

The sound of the **Lord's Prayer in Aramaic** is powerful when it is vocalized, and is more effective when done three times, each time in the 3 different tones of the diatonic harmony: 1st. **E** (Mi) (resonance with the solar plexus chakra) 2nd. **F or F#** (FA or FA#)

(resonance with the heart and thymus chakra) and 3rd. A (LA) (resonance with the third eye and crown chakra).

44

Activating the Pineal Gland

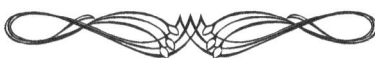

❧❧❧

Activating the Pineal Gland Through the Power of Sacred Sounds

The intonation of sacred sounds can help to eliminate unbalanced vibrations, and activate the pineal gland. For many centuries the pineal gland has been associated with the paranormal. Eastern cultures believe the pineal gland is a "chakra" that can generate important energy vortexes and expose the individual to psychic experiences and cosmic vision.

The ancient Greeks believed the pineal gland was the seat of the soul. This concept was further developed by Descartes, who philosophically suggested that it could help the soul exercise its somatic functions.

Spiritual activities such as praying, intoning sacred sounds, repeating mantras and meditating can stimulate the pineal gland. The pineal gland becomes more powerful when performing spiritual activities in groups. The frequency of 662 Hz also stimulates the functions of the pineal gland.

It has been scientifically proven that sounds can produce powerful energy vibrations which can break glass and activate electromagnetic energy in the body.

Most sound vibrations that are produced by speaking, commercial music, vehicles, and household utensils do not activate the pineal gland and therefore cannot produce spiritual experiences. However, the repetition of prayers, specific vocal tones and some mantras can activate spiritual energy in one's DNA, pineal gland and soul.

Some harmonic sound frequencies can stimulate the production of psychoactive substances in the pineal gland without the use of drugs. Individuals who have an active pineal gland seem to recall their dreams more vividly than others, and report having visions and paranormal experiences.

The Sun's wave vibrations cause the secretion of serotonin, beta-endorphin and dopamine, which make people feel good. When one looks at the Sun the endocrine glands secrete hormones that can raise one's energy level which can contribute to longevity and activate "samadhi" experiences of higher consciousness.

We constantly consume the Sun's vibrational frequencies and energy emitted by celestial bodies.

The third eye (pineal gland) is the most powerful source of ethereal energy available to humans, and is also important for clairvoyance, seeing auras, and other psychic powers. To activate the "third eye" and perceive higher dimensions, the pineal and pituitary should vibrate in unison. This can be achieved by practicing harmonic sounds, mantras, and meditation, and by looking at the Sun (Sun gazing.)

When one's personality is engaged by the pituitary gland, pineal gland and soul, a magnetic field is created. The pineal gland contains magnetite so it can generate its own magnetic field. This field can interact with the magnetic field of Earth. The charging of Earth's magnetic field activates the solar wind at dawn and the pineal gland is stimulated. This is why the best time to meditate and gaze at the Sun is between 4 a.m. and 6 a.m.

Be sure to drink a glass of purified or filtered water before and after looking at the Sun. Simultaneously looking at the Sun and ingesting water can stimulate the removal of toxins from the body. The Yin water helps balance the Yang energy from the Sun. It is also advisable to be barefoot when looking the Sun. Imagine that the Sun is the positive pole and Earth is the negative pole. We are the recharging battery and to achieve it we need a good connection.

Stand or sit with the spine erect and barefoot on sand, soil, concrete or pavement. Walking barefoot on the grass early in the morning is very similar to one of the techniques used in qigong to get a lot of energy. However, it is not recommendedd to look directly at the Sun when walking barefoot on the grass early in the morning because it drains your energy. You should also avoid walking barefoot on chemically treated lawns.

For beginners, it is recommended to look at the Sun for 10 seconds and gradually increase 10 seconds each day , up to 30 seconds. If you find it difficult at first, then increase gradually by 5 seconds. If the weather is cold look at the Sun through a window. If you live in a valley where there are mountains to the east and west, do not look at the Sun at the recommended hours. You can view the reflection of the Sun through a polished obsidian or through the Sun's reflection on water. This method will decrease the intensity, but make sure it is not salt water.

In Egypt, Cleopatra, known for her beauty, used a magnet as an amulet on her forehead to preserve her youth. We know today through science, that the pineal gland is located in back of the forehead and produces melatonin, known as the "youth hormone" due to its ability to regenerate and rejuvenate cells. There is a lot of anecdotal evidence in medical history regarding the power and benefits of sound frequencies and magnetic energy. In modern times we are rediscovering and incorporating scientific methods that were used by sages thousands of years ago.

Between 4:00 am and 6:00 am the pineal stimulates the secretion of the human growth hormone in the pituitary. Many people who use the aforementioned practice have experienced rapid hair growth with a restoration of its natural color, and the rejuvenation of other systems.

Many cultures and mystics have induced these experiences through the use of hallucinogens such as soma, mushrooms, mescaline and LSD. However, these methods tend to be short term and can result in adverse effects that can damage the pineal gland.

Most true mystics agree on implementing natural methods such as intense meditation, creative visualization, rhythmic deep breathing, singing, using harmonic vocal sounds, and watching the Sun from 4:00 a.m. to 6:00 a.m. All these methods are effective when combined with the purification of the body. These techniques have been known to activate the third eye and may have transformative effects.

In the industrialized world it is difficult for individuals to incorporate these practices into their lives. We all need a strong will, motivation and discipline to change our consciousness and implement changes in our lives to establish a healthier lifestyle and enhance our human potential.

All this is possible when we start and finish our days with prayers, positive affirmations, chanting mantras, harmonic vocal sounds, meditation and gratitude.

For thousands of years aboriginals and natives intuitively knew the power of sound. The expression of geometry and numbers is intrinsically connected with music of the highest levels in space, and is also connected with mathematical laws that are used in diatonic scales in the west.

Hawkin's theorems also produce these relationships. There is a link between crop circles and musical notes, both of which are products of frequencies generated by sounds.

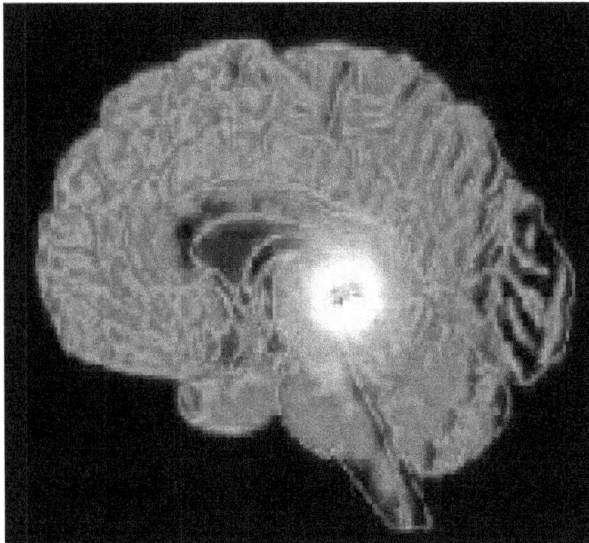

The Pineal Gland is a Crystal Radio Transmitter and Receiver

The pineal gland has finite and infinite properties. When the DNA of humans changed, the pineal gland's original role was no longer necessary. However, now it can activate a reconnection of the collective DNA in humans, and can enable the activation of the pineal gland as it originally occurred.

The crystallization of the pineal gland also has a function and a major role. For many years scientists have been saying that we are crystal beings. Medical experts are now using the term "bio-mineralization". One important discovery is that calcite crystals have piezoelectric properties. This means that they can send and receive electromagnetic frequencies (EMF). The piezoelectric crystals are the same crystals used in original radios, which send and receive radio frequencies.

When the crystals are activated, it is as if a new telecommunication antenna was installed, improving communication between individuals and improving an individual's communication with her/his higher self. It can also open awareness of a multidimensional reality.

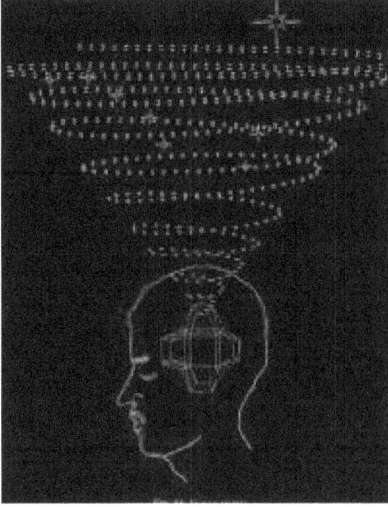

Since the 1970s quartz crystals have been used in clocks and watches to create a crystal oscillator circuit, which enables time measurement more accurately than high-quality mechanical watches. The invention of the crystal radio receiver gave birth to modern era electronics. All this gives rise to the thousands of millions of electromagnetic and radio waves traveling around and through us at any given moment with different amplitudes and frequencies.

The Universal Architect of Creation has given us a powerful and natural crystal radio receiver located in the center of the brain, the pineal gland. It is capable of sending waves of vibrational electromagnetic frequencies activated by sounds through words, music and frequencies through telepathic waves, allowing us to establish communication with other individuals and our multidimensional consciousness.

45

The Six Healing Sounds of Chi Kung (Tao's Qigong)

The Taoists and Shaolin Monks, the Five elements, their relationship with the organs and their frequency sounds.

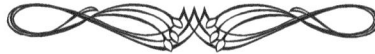

The Taoists and Shaolin Monks

The Taoist and Shaolin monks from China and other cultures have realized that specific harmonic sounds have the power to activate healing. They use singing to soothe themselves, attain clarity and greater mental control, and to boost various organs and body systems. They are aware that specific harmonic sounds contribute to good health and longevity.

Taoist and Chinese Shaolin monks observe the behavior, movements and sounds of animals. Chinese martial arts incorporate attributes of animals such as tigers, snakes, eagles and cranes into their practices.

Martial arts pioneers created their styles by watching animals fight for survival in their habitats. They observed that when the animals fought, each animal made a specific sound. They also observed that animals made sounds when they were sick or resting. The animals' sounds helped them while fighting , and also helped them recover faster from illnesses and injuries.

The Chinese discovered long ago that when a person is diagnosed with a disease, the origin of the disease has its roots in a particular organ. The sounds that people make when they have discomfort (groans/whining) are the same in all people regardless of language. From these observations, the Chinese created a system of sounds that have healing effects and called them **The Six Healing Sounds.**

The **Six Healing Sounds** are designed to help purge the body of excessive chi or fire that may accumulate daily in the organs. If two people had a weakness in a particular organ and only one practiced the healing sound for that organ, the person who practiced would recover more quickly than the person who did not practice the healing sound.

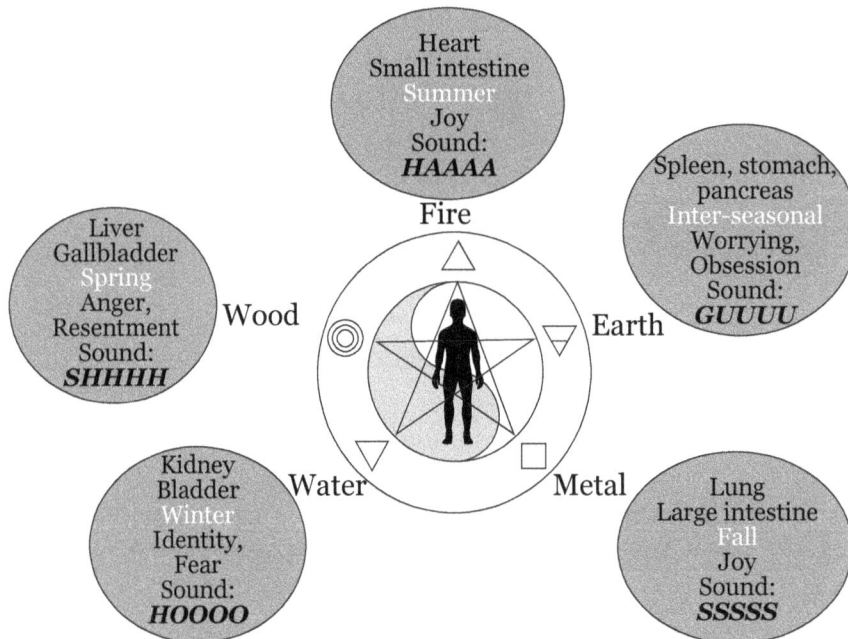

The Five Elements, the relationship with human organs and their frequency sounds.

The vital organs of the human body are always producing their own sound frequencies. The sound of the **heart** is like the sound of fire burning (Fire element), the sound of the **lungs** is like the sound of metal hitting metal (Metal element), the sound of the **liver** is like wood knocking on wood (Wood element), the sound of the **spleen** is like a stone hitting stone (Earth element), and the sound of the **kidneys** is like the sound of water flowing in a stream (Water element).

If we could record the sounds of the vital organs of our body, they would sound like a beautiful symphony that I would name **"The Music of Life."** These are the sounds and natural rhythms of the microcosmic universe in the human body.

When the human body is healthy, its sounds are strong, low, deep and reverberant in the vital organs. Its sounds are rhythmical and in harmony with the body's patterns.

The harmonic sounds of our vital organs change when we change our psychological or physiological state. I liken these sounds to a concert. As in a symphonic orchestra when instruments are out of tune, the harmonic music originally produced by the physical body will undergo changes in frequency, musicality and tone and unbalance will follow.

Specific harmonic sounds can cause the organs to resonate and generate vibrational frequencies which stimulate the natural healing process. The sounds act like a massage that soothes external symptoms such as pain, swelling, stiffness, tension, anxiety and worry. Specific harmonic sounds can soothe symptoms and heal internal diseases.

A disorder in the body's energy can cause an organ to lose its balance and may affect other organs.

Harmonic sounds produced by the voice are generated by deep breathing. The sounds activate the internal absorption of the energy of life (Prana, Chi) and have healing effects, balancing all the organs in the body.

According to the theory of the **Yin-Yang**, the **liver's** energy is ascending, the **heart** is descending, the **spleen** is accumulating, the **lung** is opening, and the **kidney** is spreading. With the practice of the Six Healing Sounds of Chi Kung (Tao's Qigong) the energy and functional activities of the vital organs are stimulated.

The Six Healing Sounds of Chi Kung (Tao's Qigong)

Diseases arise from the accumulation of negative incidents. When such incidents accumulate, imbalances occur in the body's biological systems, and can trigger diseases.

The Six Sounds of **Chi Kung (Tao's Qigong)** can help spiritual development, psychological balance and good health. The Six Sounds produce a powerful vibration that can stimulate calmness, serenity and peace, and soothe tension and stress.

The Six Sounds open energy blocks of the main organs of the body and stimulate the cleansing process. The Six Healing Sounds of Qigong have been practiced for hundreds of years and have recently become popular. When the sounds are practiced for 15 to 20 minutes daily, the body releases toxins, the natural regeneration and healing power is activated and the individual expands his/her spiritual capabilities.

When practicing, it is recommended that you make the sounds in order. You should sit very relaxed and comfortably in lotus flower position or on a chair. You should rest your hands on your thighs, with your palms facing up, your legs slightly apart and the soles of the feet resting on the floor.

When you begin, keep your spine straight. It is recommended to make each sound three, six, or nine times. Begin by making audible vocal sounds and then visualize the sound internally.

During the repetition of the sounds breathe gently and gradually three times. As you exhale, you should hear the sound internally even if you are not vocalizing the sound. With each exhalation, keep an inner smile in the back of your throat and keep a positive and radiant attitude. The intention is to release negative emotions and transmute them into positive, creative, and light energies.

1. Sound for the lungs:

Energy: Contraction of the back. **Associated organ:** Large intestine. **Element:** Metal. **Season:** Fall. **Color:** White. **Negative emotions:** When we exhale, we release the sadness, pain and depression of the lungs and other organs. **Positive Emotions:** When we inhale, we activate the energy of courage and good feelings in the lungs and other organs. **Sound:** Put your tongue behind your teeth and while exhaling slowly make the sound "SSSSS". Visualize a white light and much love filling the lungs and organs.

2. Sound for the kidneys:

Energy: Activation of your internal energy. **Associated organ:** Bladder. **Element:** Water. **Season:** Winter. **Color:** Visualize a navy blue or black light surrounding the kidneys. **Negative emotions:** When we exhale we release emotions of fear and insecurity. We release situations and people that created insecurity and fear in our lives. **Positive emotions:** We inhale while smiling internally and sending peace and kindness to the kidneys. **Sound:** The position of the lips forms a small circumference and the sound is like blowing a candle. The sound is **"HOOOO"**.

For this sound inhale and move your spine slightly forward forming a small curvature and place your hands on your knees. Exhale while making the sound **"HOOOO"** with the lips in the same position as if blowing a candle flame. This sound resonates with the kidneys. This movement is an excellent massage for the organs. When you inhale again straighten your spine and move your hands to the thighs. Rest for at least three breaths and put your hands upwards on the thighs. Continue doing the same exercise but this time only use your breathing. Do not make a sound with your mouth, but continue listening to the sound in your mind. Focus, do not get distracted, and mentally visualize the sound.

3. Sound for the liver:

Energy: Creating, productivity. **Associated Organ:** Gallbladder. **Element:** Wood. **Season:** Spring. **Color:** Green (envision a green bright light surrounding the liver.) **Negative Emotions:** When we exhale, we release emotions of anger, rage, and aggression. We release situations or persons who have caused us anger and aggression. **Positive Emotions:** We inhale with an inner smile, visualizing virtue, goodness, and kindness, and send the energy to the liver. **Sound:** Place the tongue on the palate and slowly exhale generating the sound **"SHHHH"**.

When you begin to make this sound, as you inhale, raise your hands and open them to the sides. Continue stretching your hands up until they are over your head, then join your hands and fingers pointing straight up. Lean a little to the left and exhale while internally making the sound **"SHHHH"** with the tongue pressing lightly on the palate. **Straighten your back as you inhale and open your hands and move them down and place them on your thighs.** Rest for about three breaths with the palms facing up. Repeat the exercise. Inhale, but this time do not make the sound, but continue to hear the sound. Focus during the exercise and do not get distracted.

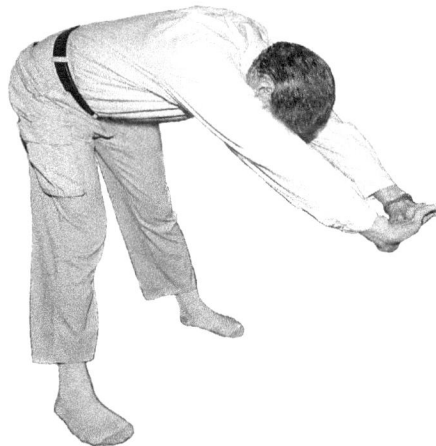

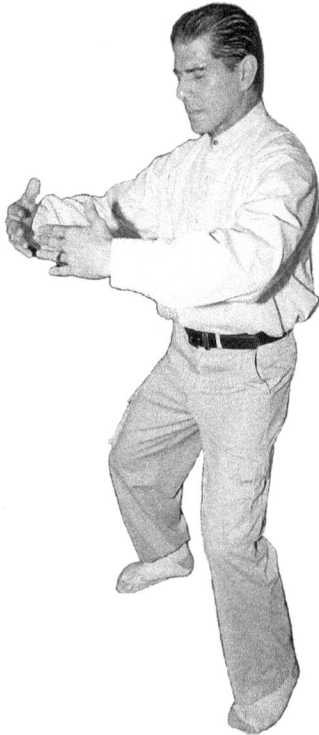

4. Sound for the heart:

Energy: Radiant. **Associated Organ:** Small intestine. **Element:** Fire. **Season:** Summer. **Color:** Red. **Negative Emotions:** While exhaling, emotions and situations of cruelty, arrogance, haughtiness, hatred, pride, haste and impatience are released. **Positive Emotions:** During the rest period breathe with an inner smile and send emotions of love, joy, honor, sincerity and respect for the heart. **Sound:** "HAAAAAA." Keep your mouth wide open and place the tip of your tongue behind your lower teeth, then exhale slowly and generate the sound "HAAAAAA."

5. Sound for the spleen:

Energy: Stabilizing. **Associated organs:** Pancreas, Stomach. **Element:** Earth. **Season:** Summer. **Color:** Visualize the spleen surrounded by a bright yellow light. **Negative emotions:** By exhaling we eliminate negative, worrying emotions. **Positive emotions:** While resting, we smile and breathe, sending energy of attraction, availability and beauty to the spleen. **Sound:** The sound is guttural. Roll your tongue and touch your palate, exhale slowly and make the sound "GUUUUUUU". The sound must be made from the deepest throat, as a groan.

6. The sound for the triple warmer: (It refers to the three energy centers of the body)

Upper: Brain, heart, lungs. It's warm and has yang energy.
Middle: Liver, kidneys, stomach, pancreas, and spleen. It's warm and has yang energy.
Lower: Large and small intestine, bladder and sexual organs. It's cold and has yin energy.

Sound: Keeping the mouth open and exhaling gradually "HIIIIIIIIIIIIII". It is recommended that the person lies down looking up, relaxed and with an internal smile. Visualize a flattening cylinder moving on your chest, stomach and abdomen, which is ejecting negative and disharmonizing emotions. By using this method, we can balance the body's energy.

On the practice of Qigong for the **Triple Warmer** we lie down with a relaxed body. The Dan Tien is the vital energy residing within us and moves through the whole body. **The upper Dan Tien is hot** (yang), **the middle one is warm** (yang) and **the lower Dan Tien is cold** (yin).

Begin breathing from the lower abdomen and then towards the thorax, expanding the chest. Visualize that you are moving the heat down while exhaling. Or visualize that you are moving the heat down from the brain, lungs and heart. In this way you are balancing the three centers of the **triple warmer**.

The Six Healing Sounds of **Chi Kung (Tao's Qigong)** eliminate negative energies from the meridians, organs and body systems. They activate a positive and creative mental state and eliminate feelings of sadness, insecurity, fear and depression. These sounds stimulate the body's natural healing process.

46

The Five Sounds of Tibetan Syllables

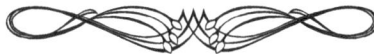

* **I express my infinite gratitude to the honorable Tenzin Wangyal Rinpoche for all the Tibetan wisdom he has shared publicly with the world about the healing power that it is activated through the five Tibetan syllables. The Tenzin Wangyal Rinpoche says "Through this simple and powerful Tibetan practice, you become a kinder and powerful being, clear in your thinking...wake up..."**

The Five sounds of Tibetan syllables are known as **The Five Warrior Syllables.** The practice of these five Tibetan sounds is believed to help eliminate harmful patterns of behavior and negative energies of the body and mind. These sounds stimulate a spontaneous, creative and authentic expression of being.

Practicing the sounds can help individuals experience mercy, compassion, joy and equanimity. Ultimately, the practice can lead to full self-recognition.

Learning these sounds can be compared to a child instantly recognizing his mother after being separated from her. He recognizes the connection to his home and roots which is defined as the natural and pure mind. In the natural mind all virtues are perfected spontaneously.

This practice can be done in different ways. It is imperative to connect with one's being by finding the key that will unlock the door that leads to one's happiness. Practicing the **Five sounds of Tibetan syllables** is a way to overcome the suffering one might experience when influenced by negative emotions. This practice can help to eliminate anger, attachment, jealousy, pride, ignorance and fear. It can help to overcome fear and achieve success in life.

The sounds of the Tibetan syllables are five: **A, OM, HUNG, RAM and DZA.** Each syllable represents a specific realization of the individual. They are known as the **seed syllables,** because they possess the essence of enlightenment. The five syllables represent the body, speech, mind, virtuous qualities and enlightenment of the individual. All five syllables represent the true nature and expression of self.

In this practice every syllable is sung in sequence, with a focus on a corresponding energy center or chakra. The sequence moves from the pure essence of the individual to the manifestation of virtue.

As you begin practicing, direct your attention to the conditions and patterns that you wish to clarify, transform and manifest. Make sure you include conditions of which you are aware, and also conditions that may be hidden inside you.

The first point to focus your attention on is the brow chakra (**chakra of the third eye**). A chakra is simply an energy center in the body, similar to a wheel or center where energy converges. These centers are not only on the body's surface, but also within the body along the spine. It is a light channel that extends from below the navel up through the center of the body and then opens in the crown.

The Five Tibetan syllable sounds are associated as follows:

A = brow chakra (third eye) and is associated with the unchanging body.
OM = throat chakra and the quality of the persistent voice.
HUNG = heart chakra and the pure mind.
RAM = solar plexus chakra or navel and the virtuous qualities.
DZA = secret chakra and the spontaneous action.

Pronunciation Guide:

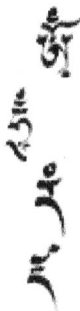

A ~ is pronounced like "A" in the word calm
This sound is used to eliminate anger from the mind. The sound focuses on the area of the **third eye chakra.**

OM ~ is pronounced as OUM
This sound is used to discover the qualities and power of light. It focuses on the **throat chakra.**

HUNG ~ is pronounced Joong
In this sound the power of space and light come together. It focuses on the **heart chakra.** We discover the energy of love with more intensity. The individual can deeply feel the union of space and love through the sound Hung.

RAM ~ is pronounced Raam

This sound is associated with the **Solar Plexus Chakra**. The element is fire. It is the continuation of the Five Sounds' work to eliminate anger and to cultivate love. In this stage the power of love is strengthened and bears its fruits. The individual can feel so full of love that he can give it unconditionally to others. It can be compared to seeing sunlight on a tree full of fruit, and then seeing the fruit ripen enough to feed others.

In the same way, the light can activate the energy of love until that energy is ripe and ready to be given. The light strengthens and ripens love within the self, feeds it and gives its fruits to others. After taking the energy of love from the heart to the solar plexus, the individual can have a clear and open mind to love. Avoid making an analysis, or judging the situation. Instead, focus your attention on your solar plexus with peace, harmony and love.

DZA ~ is pronounced DDZZZAA. The sound is produced by pressing the tongue against the front upper and lower teeth, then abruptly releasing the sound

This focuses on the **reproductive chakra**. We all want effortless love and happiness in our lives. We could manifest unconditional love towards our families, co-workers, and friends but this is not often the case. To help develop our reproductive centers we must focus on the reproductive chakra, making the DDZZAA sound, and visualize giving birth to a baby. In this way we can activate the energy of light and love from within ourselves.

Our fundamental nature is not manufactured or created- it exists already, and we can awaken it. In the same way that the sky is obscured by clouds, we too can be obscured by harmful patterns of behavior.

The practice of the **Five Tibetan syllables** can be effective in eliminating our negative patterns of behavior. By using these sounds we can create space for spontaneous, creative and authentic expression.

The **Mother Tantra** describes the practice of the **Five Tibetan sounds** as an effective way to treat physical ailments, such as headaches, chest pains and other problems.

These sounds create balance between the five elements: **earth, water, fire, air and ether**. These elements are present in nature and in us and play an important role in the internal balance of our mental and physical states.

Specific exercises with chants, sounds and syllables can activate and harmonize the elements. The sounds can have a powerful effect on our organs and mental states. "The shining sphere of light is born or arises from the essence of bodies of light, and from that sphere of light wisdom arises." This quote illustrates the wisdom from which the seed syllables arose and awakened enlightened beings to the power of the mantras. They then shared that knowledge for the benefit of all.

Enlightened beings developed complete cycles of teaching and practices related to mantras. In essence, each sound is generated by its own roots, which are deep and transcend time and space.

These sounds are seeds that contain elemental qualities that vibrate in different parts and chakras of the human body. The main goal of these sounds is the to activate **self-realization**.

The simple and powerful practice of the **Five Tibetan syllables** is based on the highest teachings of the Tibetan Buddhist tradition, by Buddhas, lamas, rinpoches, monks and Tibetan masters for the benefit of mankind.

47

The Origin of Music and the First Musical Instruments

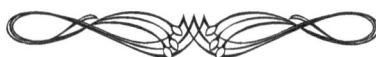

Some historians suggest that the origin of music comes from the sounds and rhythms of nature. Music can make use of the phenomena and patterns of the repetition of tonalities and the echo produced by nature's sounds. Even today, some cultures have certain examples of their music where they intentionally mimic the sounds produced by nature. In some cases, this is related to shamanic beliefs and practices. It can also serve as entertainment to attract animals in a hunt. Birds and monkeys have been seen hitting hollow logs. Although this can serve to establish territorialism, it suggests a certain degree of creativity and seems to incorporate a dialogue of call and response (zoomusicología). Explanations of the origin of music depends on how the music is defined. **If we assume that music is a form of intentional emotional manipulation, music as we know it was not possible until the beginning of intentionality:** the ability to reflect on the past and the future. Fifty-thousand (50,000) years ago humans began to create art in the form of paintings on walls of caves, jewelry and so on - a **"cultural explosion".** They also began to bury their dead with ceremonies. If we assume that these new forms of behavior reflect the emergence of intentionality, then music as we know it must also have emerged during that period.

From a psychological point of view, it is difficult to answer the question of the origin of music. **Music evokes strong emotions and changes in the state of consciousness of beings.** Generally, strong emotions are associated with evolution (sex and survival). But there is no clear link between music and sex, or between music and survival. As for sex, music can often be used to attract companions (such as when male birds use their plumage and sounds to attract females or when amphibians such as the coqui establish territory and call females to join in mating). However, that is just one of the many functions of sounds and music produced by animals and is one of many ways to attract partners. As for survival, societies with a musical culture may be better able to survive because the music that coordinates their emotions helps to communicate important messages within their groups and in their rituals. The music motivates them to identify with the group and to support other members within their group. However, it is difficult to demonstrate the effects of music to improve the survival of a group in competition with other groups. Once music exists, it can promote the effects of cultural development, but it is unclear whether the final source of the music can be explained.

The human voice was probably the first musical instrument, which can make a great variety of sounds, from singing, humming, communicating through the sound of words, mimicking the sounds of animals, whistling, coughing and yawning. The oldest Neanderthal hyoid bone known to the modern human form has been dated to 60,000 years old, before the flute made from the earliest known bone of the Paleolithic period about 20,000 years ago, but the true chronology can be traced far beyond.

The earliest rhythmic instruments or percussion instruments were likely to involve hand clapping, beating stones or other things and in fact there are examples of musical instruments dating to the Paleolithic Period. There is some ambiguity about archaeological findings that can be interpreted in various ways as musical or non-musical instruments or tools. **Examples of paleolithic objects that are considered unmistakably musical are the flutes or tubes of bones;** the Paleolithic findings that are open to interpretation are the perforated phalanges (usually interpreted as **"Falangian whistles"**), objects interpreted as roars or bull growls.

Music can be traced theoretically before the Paleolithic age. Anthropological and archaeological designation suggests that music first emerged among humans when stone tools began to be used by hominids. Noises produced by labor such as seed and stick roots in food are a likely source of rhythm created by early humans.

Prehistoric music is followed by ancient music in different parts of the world, but still exists in isolated areas. However, it is more common to refer to **"prehistoric music"** that still survives as folk, indigenous or traditional music. Prehistoric music is studied along with other periods within the archeology of music. Findings from sites of Paleolithic archeology suggest that prehistoric people used carving and drilling tools to create instruments. **Archaeologists have found paleolithic flutes carved into bones in which lateral holes have been drilled. It is believed that the Divje Babe (didgeridoo or yidaki) flute, carved from a cave bear femur, is at least 40,000 years old.** Instruments such as the **seven-hole flute** and various types of string instruments, such as Ravanahatha, have been found in the archaeological sites of Valley Civilization in India. **India has one of the oldest musical traditions in the world - references to Indian classical music (marl) are found in the Vedas, the ancient writings of the Hindu tradition.** The earliest and largest collection of prehistoric musical instruments was found in China and dates back to between 7000 and 6600 BC.

The **didgeridoo and hompak** according to historical records, are believed to be the oldest musical instruments in history and **date back approximately 40,000 years.** These instruments were used by Aboriginal Australians and there is evidence that many centuries later, an instrument very similar to didgeridoo was used by pre-Columbian cultures, the Mayan culture and they called it the Hompak. Crystal bowls and certain metal bowls are also believed to date back thousands of years to the Atlantic and Lemuria continents, but research is still under way to officially confirm the truth of the existence of these two continents.

Egypt is one of the oldest cultures in the Near East and had a highly developed musical culture dating back to around 3000 BC. The Egyptian sources include pictorial relics of some instruments and some literary records related to the use of musical instruments. **In various pieces of sculpture appear harp and flute players who participate in religious ceremonies and social entertainments.**

Several instruments have been identified in Egypt, including the **lira (a type of harp), an oboe-type instrument,** several Asian drums, the laud and the sistrum. Murals have also been found which show singers and instrumentalist performers. **According to music historian Homer Ulrich, it is likely that Egypt influenced the "educational and ethical aspects of Greek music."** Stephen Batuk also noted that the historical link of music was related to the celebration of creation week, where birds flying in the air make sounds that can be seen as music.

In Sumeria and Babylon, although records are minimal, it is known that between 3,000 and 2,300 BC groups of singers gathered to make music in the temples. In the excavations they have discovered several musical instruments, including **harps, lauds and double oboes.**

Music historian John Stainer points out that the relationship between Abraham and the Canaanites "most likely influenced future Hebrew music," and probably led to his posterity by bringing a certain amount of Assyrian music and musical instruments to Egypt. He adds that in a stay of four centuries "in a culture as civilized as Egypt must have greatly expanded its knowledge of art."

Music in religious rituals was first used by King David between 1010 - 1002 BC. David lived about 3,000 years ago and he used the lyre (a wooden harp) to sing the Psalms. According to the Larousse encyclopedia, he is credited with confirming that the men of the tribe of Levi are the "custodians of the music of divine service." Historian Irene Hesk points out that of the twenty-four books of the Old Testament, the 150 Psalms of the Book of Psalms attributed to King David have served as "the foundation of Judeo-Christian hymnology", concluding that "the song of poetry of the Psalms has been adapted to the music of today's Western civilization. "In fact, much of what we know about music comes from the biblical record of David's activities from the time he was a young shepherd to a king and a capable leader.

The Gong. Historians believe that gongs were made and used before the second millennium BC. It is an ancient instrument that dates back more than 3,000 years and has been used in different functions by ancient civilizations. The gong is one of the oldest and most authentic musical instruments in South East Asia, but they were not noticeable in Chinese history until about 500 A.D. Chinese history attributes the gong to the HSI YSI nation, located between Burma and Tibet. Historians believe that Java, Annam, Burma, and China were the main gong-producing centers. It is known that these centers produced at least seven forms of gongs and corresponding sound structures. Therefore gongs have long been at the center of sound systems and music. For centuries, a gong was a symbol of success, power and high standards among Asian families and still continues. There are many uses for the gong. Both in antiquity and today, gongs have been used essentially for the same purposes: to communicate, make announcements in the royal courts, to make music, to celebrate life events, and to meditate and to heal. Gongs are no longer in Asia alone. They have been traveling the world for centuries. In Europe, gongs have been used in orchestras since about 1790 since the time of Mozart. European orchestras often call the gong "Tam Tam" and "Gong". The gongs are a true and timeless percussion piece, similar to the drum.

The story of the creation of the first gong is lost in time. The gong may have appeared during the Bronze Age (around 3500 BC to 2000 BC), when the first bronze tools and weapons were created. The first gong may have been a bronze shield that was struck during a battle to signal an attack or retreat. Another possibility is that the first gong evolved from a bronze disk that was created to represent the sun, which was worshiped by ancient agricultural civilizations.

The gong has been used in rituals, ceremonies, prayer and meditation since the Bronze Age. **Its sound is relaxing and soothing, focusing and energizing, and transforms and stimulates the healing process. The gong's sounds have been used in meditation,**

and healing therapies since ancient times and are still used. According to the physicist David Bohm when it is played and when the metal is being "excited" by the frequency of sounds, the electrons are charged highly with electromagnetic energy and form an energetic field that is defined as Plasmon. A plasma energy field is created around the gong and the listener becomes part of that field of vibrational energy. Metal is the only known material where electrons release their atoms and join other atoms. When the activity of the gong ends, the electrons return to their original atoms. Once the gong is finished playing, the Plasmons and the energy field are neutralized. When the gong is played again the field of Plasmon expands and intensifies. Participants who receive the frequency of sounds are electromagnetically charged positively and holistically.

The gong is an acoustic instrument that opens the door to high states of consciousness. It is an ideal tool for stress reduction, to stimulate the glandular system, and to eliminate emotional blockages. When played harmoniously, the gong stimulates and resonates simultaneously with all cells of the human body and re-calibrates the parasympathetic nervous system, regulates heart rate and activates relaxation of muscles and joints during meditation. The gong generates powerful multidimensional ripples of sound that bathe the whole body in streams of sound. This instrument has been described as magical, rhythmic and purifying.

Magnetic Harmonic Vibrational Therapy with the Gong

I incorporate the use of the gong in my practice. I have two large gongs, one Tibetan made of 7 metals and one large Chinese gong with a thinner layer of bronze and other metals. Both gongs produce different shades of deep and powerful sounds. In addition to working with the Pure Quartz Alchemy Bowls and the Tibetans Bowls, I have also been experimenting with the sound frequencies of these two gongs in combination with the sound of my voice for over 20 years. The sound generated by both gongs is very powerful. However, I play them with a soft touch that helps to generate very pleasant sound vibrational frequencies. I have a solid wood frame of square mahogany, where I hang the gongs. It is 4 feet high and 5 feet wide. I ask the person receiving the sound therapy to sit in the Lotus posture on a yoga cushion or in a comfortable position in meditation with the body facing a distance of 6 to 8 inches from the gong. I ask the person to rest his or her hands on the knees, and I start playing the gong very gently and gradually increase the intensity of the sound. I also sing specific harmonic vowel sounds that resonate with the chakras during the vibrational therapy. I do this for about 8 to 10 minutes and if necessary, I also ask the person to sit in the lotus position or in a comfortable position with his or her back towards the direction of the gong and repeat the same procedure. I work in all chakras, but I dedicate more time on the chakras where I find more intense blockages.

The frequencies of sounds and vibrations are felt as electromagnetic waves of electricity traveling through the body of the person receiving the therapy and the therapist. People who have received this therapy have stated that they feel an energy moving in a circular spiral direction inside their body, vibrating and releasing blockages from many areas in the organs and muscle. In many cases muscular joint pain is completely released, and transports the person to a deep state of relaxation, peace, harmony and contemplation after finishing the section. They have also experienced an expansion in their etheric energy field and a sense of sharpened perception. Before beginning therapy, I concentrate on the intention of love that flows from my heart and I visualize golden, silver, white, blue and violet rays of light coming from the center of the universe and from the center of earth and illuminate the person who is receiving the Harmonic Sounds Therapy. I believe that when we establish intention with pure energy of love, the curative therapeutic frequency is amplified thousands of times and travels faster at the body's cellular level. It helps to activate the natural healing process of all the biological systems. I combine Gong Therapy with the sounds of Alchemy Singing Bowls made of Pure Crystal Quartz, but always use the most powerful instrument in the universe, **the voice and mental power of intention.** The power of mind, heart and voice can manifest miracles. **We are the power, the power is within us and around us. When we cultivate our inner power, there are no limits.**

48

Music Therapy

Music therapy and the healing power of classical music.

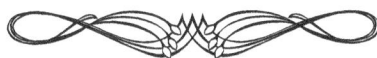

What is the purpose of music therapy?

Music therapy is a therapeutic method where the use of music is incorporated to reduce health problems. Music is believed to have a direct effect on a person's emotional state. When we listen to happy music we can be filled with energy and joy; however, the opposite can occur when we hear sad music. Sad music can lower our energy and bring us sadness. Individuals' moods can be affected by music.

Most diseases are believed to originate at the energy level or mental emotional level, and then manifest at the physical level. Many diseases are believed to be caused by mental energy and negative emotions. This can result in an imbalance in the organs and body systems. The negative mental energy can also affect the production of hormones secreted by the endocrine glands, and other biochemical components. When the body suffers imbalances, it can result in diseases. This usually occurs when the mind is confronted with emotions such as fear, sadness, resentment, hatred, doubt, and insecurity. This can happen after the loss of a loved one, either by separation, divorce or death, or when experiencing financial or work problems.

Music therapy can stimulate an individual's brain to establish a state of mental relaxation. This relaxation can change the frequency of negative thoughts, which can cause an imbalance in the biological system. **Music therapy** can reduce stress and pain, promote mental relaxation, and stimulate creative abilities. Music therapy also encourages and facilitates the learning process. **Music therapy** has been used throughout history by many ancient civilizations including those of Australia, North America, South America,

Africa, Europe, China, the Middle East, and Russia. The healers and shamans of these countries used repetitive chants and vowel sounds along with Mother Nature's sounds to heal the sick.

Music therapy has been implemented since 1940 as an alternative method for treating patients who have experienced emotional trauma, depression, anxiety, stress, mental imbalances and many other conditions. Research has shown that **music therapy** has beneficial effects, which include balancing emotional states, stimulating alpha mental states and contributing to psychophysical balance.

Music therapy has been used by people suffering from heart and lung conditions, drug and alcohol addiction, and immune system imbalances. People who have attempted suicide have also been known to benefit from music therapy. Music therapy has been known to create favorable changes in the emotional, mental and physical states of individuals.

Researchers of vibrational medicine continue to study **music therapy**. They seek to pinpoint music that will generate specific sound frequencies to activate the body's natural healing process. This therapy is non-invasive and help people recover from their illnesses.

The basic scheme of work in this discipline involves three aspects:

1) The positive interaction of the patient with others.
2) Self-esteem.
3) The use of rhythm and music as to generate energy and order.

Music therapy has been shown to develop self-esteem with techniques that encourage feelings of self-realization, self-confidence, and self-satisfaction. The rhythm and power of music is the guiding psychomotor process that promotes stimulus-controlled movements, which can raise awareness of space throughout the body.

The Healing Power of Classical Music

Classical music can stimulate relaxation, balance, good energy and natural healing. The scientist and musician Manfred Clynes has done extensive research on the effects of classical music on human emotions. He noted that many of the great classical composers' musical compositions, musical styles and unique techniques can elicit specific emotional responses from the listener.

Manfred Clynes concluded that a human's central nervous system is stimulated by vibrational frequencies produced by music.

Classical symphonies, harp and flute sounds, and many chants, have healing powers and can help strengthen the immune system and accelerate recovery from illness. In fact, sound systems are being installed in many recovery rooms to broadcast these sounds.

In hospitals, surgeons are being exposed to relaxing classical music before and while operating on patients. According to scientific studies, the soft and pleasant background music helps patients heal faster and helps surgeons relax while performing surgery.

Classical music can help eliminate stress and is also a natural remedy to alleviate and eliminate depression. A three-week scientific study demonstrated this by exposing a group of clinically depressed individuals to classical and meditation music for one hour before and after sleeping. Ninety percent (90%) of the patients showed recovery after the session. Patients suffering from high blood pressure, also showed improvements after three weeks.

In the business sector, many companies are incorporating classical and appropriate music in their workplaces. Recent studies show that employees work more efficiently and productively when listening to classical or soft background music. Human resources psychologists use classical or soft music to maintain a healthy working environment.

Classical music stimulates the natural frequencies of the brain. Depending on the format of the concert's intonation, rhythm, form and dynamics, this music can stimulate different brain states and brain frequencies of Delta, Theta, Alpha or Beta.

Symphonic music that stimulates brain wave frequencies: Delta, Theta, Alpha and Beta

Dr. Jeffrey Thompson, who is a faculty member of the Department of Clinical Research in the California Institute for Human Science, has performed twenty (20) years' worth of clinical studies about the effects of classical music in stimulating Delta, Theta, Alpha and Beta brain wave frequencies.

Dr. Thompson compiled four CDs of classical music which have been used in health centers in 26 countries. It is titled **Brainwave Symphony.**

The selection and sequencing of the music in Dr. Jeffrey Thompson's Brainwave Symphony was done by Dr. Pat Moffitt Cook. Dr. Cook is the founder and director of the **Open Ear Center for Music in Healthcare**, and is a pioneer in the use of alternative means for maintaining good health.

The classical music that stimulates **Delta** waves produces sound pulses that induce a state of deep relaxation, rejuvenation and restful sleep. The frequency of **Delta** brain waves achieves the deepest sleep and it was demonstrated that the physical body begins to recover at a very high level. The symphonies and composers are:

(1) The Planets Suite, Venus, Bringer of Peace = Gustav Holst
(2) The Planets Suite, Neptune, The Mystic = Gustav Holst
(3) Adagio for Strings = Samuel Barber
(4) Adagio in G Minor = Tomaso Albinoni
(5) Symphony No. 4 in C Minor, Andante = Felix Mendelssohn
(6) Symphony No. 5 in B-Flat Major, Andante = Felix Mendelssohn
(7) Violin Concerto in E minor, Andante) = Felix Mendelssohn
(8) Lady Radnor's Suite (Slow Minuet) = Hubert Parry
(9) Sighing Op. 70 (Sospiri, Op. 70) = Edward Elgar
(10) Suite for String Orchestra, Nocturne) = Frank Bridge
(11) Funeral March, Slow, Excerpt = Frederic Chopin
(12) Calm Sea & Prosperous Voyage, Op. 27 = Felix Mendelssohn

The symphonic music that stimulates the frequency of **Theta** brainwaves has sound pulses that induce a deep state of meditation, increased intuition and creativity. The Theta state is generally achieved when we are sleeping, dreaming or in a very deep state of relaxation. Theta is where ideas, visualizations and suggestions are more likely to enter the subconscious mind and we are less aware of what is happening around us. The symphonies and composers are:

(1) Fantasia on a Theme by Thomas Tallis = Ralph Vaughan Williams
(2) Lark Ascending = Ralph Vaughan Williams
(3) Ecloge for Piano & Strings = Gerald Finzi
(4) Clair de lune = Claude Debussy
(5) Clarinet Concerto, Adagio = Gerald Finzi
(6) Variations on a Theme of Frank Bridge, Op. 10, Adagio = Benjamin Britten

(7) Variations on a Theme of Frank Bridge, Op. 10. Chant = Benjamin Britten

The symphonic music that stimulates a frequency of **Alpha** waves induces an alert meditative state, calmness, and active relaxation. These symphonies are also effective at stimulating the mental process of learning and information retention, for example, when studying, relaxing, reading, or observing a landscape while traveling. The Alpha state is the most effective state to activate the natural healing process of the body, mind and spirit. The symphonies and composers are:

(1) Violin Concerto in A Minor, BWV 1041, Andante = Johann Sebastian Bach
(2) Concerto for 2 Violins in D Minor = Johann Sebastian Bach
(3) Sinfonia Decima a 7 for 2 Trumpets and Strings = Giovanni Bononcini
(4) Cello Concerto in C, Adagio = Joseph Haydn
(5) Cello Concerto in D Op. 101, Adagio = Joseph Haydn
(6) String Symphony No. 4, Andante = Felix Mendelsohn
(7) Capriol Suite Pieds-en-láir = Peter Warlock
(8) Violin Concerto No. 4 in D, K. 218, Andante Cantabile = Wolfgang Amadeus Mozart
(9) Concerto in F Major, F VII 2, RV. 455, Grave = Antonio Vivaldi
(10) Concerto in A Minor, F VII 5, RV. 461, Larghetto = Antonio Vivaldi
(11) Symphony No. 6 in F Major, Op.68 ('Pastoral'): II. Andante molto mosso: Szene am Bach (Scene by the brook) = Ludwig Van Beethoven

The symphonic music that stimulates a frequency of **Beta** produces sound pulses that induce focusing, orientation and energy efficiency during everyday life. When in the Beta state, we are aware of everything around us. The symphonies and composers are:

(1) Concerto in D for 2 Trumpets, Strings, and Continuo = Antonio Vivaldi
(2) Sonata in D for 2 Trumpets, Strings and Continuo = Giusseppe Matteo Alberti
(3) Violin Concerto in A minor, BWV 104, First Movement = Johann Sebastian Bach
(4) Cello Concerto in C, Moderato = Joseph Haydn
(5) Oboe Concerto in B flat, Op. 7, No. 3, Allegros I and II = Tommaso Albinoni
(6) Oboe Concerto in D major, Op. 7, No. 6 Allegros I and II = Tommaso Albinoni
(7) Oboe Concerto in D major, FVII 10 RV. 453, Allegro, Largo, Allegro = Antonio Vivaldi
(8) Symphony No. 40 in G minor, K. 550, Andante = Wolfgang Amadeus Mozart
(9) Basset Clarinet Concerto in A, K. 622, Allegro = Wolfgang Amadeus Mozart

Classical Music and its Effect on Adults and Children

The first rhythm we hear when we are in the womb, is our mother's heartbeat. At birth, the first music we hear is the melody produced by the comforting voice of our mother. Harmonic and soft classical music has relaxing vibrational frequencies, which can have a subtle effect that induces calm and leads to a peaceful state, as when we were babies.

NAXOS is a classical music record label that has collected the works of great classical composers and put them on a CD featuring an hour of classical music. This classical music has frequencies that attempt to stimulate the brains of infants and adults to reach a state of relaxation and restful sleep. NAXOS titled this CD, **"Listen, Learn and Grow Lullabies."**

The gentle melodies of classical music can help bring calmness and serenity to your home and office. This music also stimulates and inspires the mind to relax, assimilate and retain information when reading, studying, working on the computer, or doing artwork. This music can help infants and adults to sleep deeply.

(1) Twinkle, Twinkle, Little Star - excerpt, K.265 = Wolfgang Amadeus Mozart
(2) Lullaby (Wiegenlied), Op. 49, No. 4 = Johannes Brahms
(3) Dance (Pieds-en-l'air) = Peter Warlock
(4) Clarinet Concerto, K. 622: Adagio = Wolfgang Amadeus Mozart
(5) Lullaby (Berceuse), Op. 16 = Gabriel Faure
(6) Songs without Words No. 9, Op. 30, No. 3 = Félix Mendelssohn
(7) Piano Concerto No. 21, K. 467: Andante = Wolfgang Amadeus Mozart
(8) Of Foreign Lands and People = Robert Schumann
(9) Kinderszenen: Daydream (Traumerei), Op. 15 = Robert Schumann
(10) Lullaby (Berceuse), Op. 57 = Frédéric Chopin
(11) Lullaby (Wiegenlied) = Franz Schubert
(12) Flute and Harp Concerto, K. 299: Andantino = Wolfgang Amadeus Mozart
(13) Songs without Words No. 40, Op. 84, No. 4 = Félix Mendelssohn
(14) Songs without Words No. 19, Op. 53, No. 1 = Félix Mendelssohn
(15) Serenade, Op. 6: Adagio = Josef Suk
(16) Suite for Lady Radnor, Minuet Slow (Lady Radnor's Suite, Slow Minuet) = Hubert Parry (This track also appears on the list of Delta brainwaves on the research of Dr. Jeffrey Thompson)

List of classical music and its effects on different states and physical conditions

Classical music that relieves hypertension:
Four Seasons by Vivaldi.
Serenade No. 13 in G Major by Mozart.
Aquatic Music by Handel
Violin Concerto by Beethoven
Symphony No. 8 by Dvorak

Classical music that relieves insomnia:
Nocturnes (Op. 9, No. 3), (op. 15, No. 2), (op. 9 No. 2) by Chopin
Prelude to the Afternoon of a Faun by Debussy.
Canon in D by Pachelbel.

Classical music that relieves anxiety:
Concierto en Aranjuez by Joaquín Rodrigo.
Four Seasons by Vivaldi.
The Linz Symphony, K425 by Mozart.
Violin Concerto by Beethoven.
Symphony No. 8 by Dvorak.

Classical music that soothes headaches:
Dream of Love by Liszt.
Serenade by Schubert.
Hymn to the Sun by Rimsky-Korsakov.

Classical music that relieves stomach pain:
Musique de Table by Telemann
Harp Concerto by Handel.
Oboe Concerto by Vivaldi.

Classical music that stimulates good energy:
The Karalia Suite by Sibelius.
String Serenade (Op. 48) by Tschaikowsky.
William Tell Overture by Rossini.

Classical music that stimulates healing and harmony in your home:
All symphonic works of Wolfgang Amadeus Mozart.

The effects of Baroque music

The effects of sound are evident in our daily lives. For example, Baroque music has been tested by Bulgarian psychiatrist Georgi Lozanov. Dr. Lozanov was able to demonstrate greater learning capacity and retention in people who listened to Baroque music (Bach 1700, Vivaldi, Telemann, Handel.) He instructed his students to breathe to the rhythm of music. His experiments can illustrate that sound and music can have a profound effect on our physical, mental and emotional health and well-being.

Our health and mood can be affected by music, tone, rhythm and singing. We know that the sound of a person's voice changes if the person is ill or in a negative emotional state; or when suffering from depression, anxiety, fear, stress, etc. You can hear the difference in the person's tone of voice compared to when he or she was healthy or in a better emotional state.

49

Gregorian Chants

Gregorian chants stimulate good energy and healing.

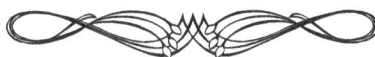

Gregorian chants originated from the monastic life in medieval times and were used in the early days of the Christian liturgical music. They are the roots of Western classical music. The Gregorian chants are usually sung in unison, without accompaniment, and they are generally sung by small choral groups.

The musical scale of **old solfeggio** has been used by the monks in their Gregorian chants. The intonation of this music was originally established at a frequency of **432 Hz**. The music in pitch of **432 Hz** contributes to higher consciousness.

Gregorian chants were sung in Catholic Masses during special festivities and their lyrics were written in **Latin**.

Over the centuries these songs have been heard by millions, causing a feeling of relaxation and peace that calms the spirit and helps us to live in harmony with our world and with others.

According to scientific studies; these songs stimulate **Delta and Alpha** brain waves that induce relaxation, rejuvenation and healing. The intention of the monks when singing this music is to convey messages that generate frequencies of harmonic sounds, which help to create a world of peace and tranquility.

The unique sounds and vibrations of the Gregorian chants have also been integrated in some classics such as Handel's Messiah, the Ave Maria by Schubert and Gounod.

In the late 60s, Alfred Tomatis, a French physician and specialist in human hearing, conducted an experiment in a Benedictine monastery where monks were suffering from fatigue and depression. Tomatis discovered that their fatigue and depression was due to a change in their usual routine. They stopped singing their songs from six to eight hours. Tomatis suggested to them to practice their singing every day. When the monks began to do so, they recovered quickly and were able to resume their demanding schedule of work and prayer. Tomatis concluded that the songs actually stimulate the bones of humans at approximately 2,000 Hz.

"The sound can really change our immune system," explains Dr. Mitchell Gaynor, "Our Interluken -1 level, which is an index of our immune system, **rises between 12½ and 15% after listening to Gregorian chants or some kind of harmonic music**. After listening to this music for 20 minutes, our levels of immunoglobulins in the blood are significantly increased."

According to Dr. Gaynor, therapeutic sound affects our body at the cellular and subcellular level. "There is no organ or system in the body that is not affected by the sound, music and vibrations. The harmonic and melodic sound can help people with cancer and many other diseases."

Recordings of Gregorian chants that stimulate relaxation, alleviate stress and uplift the spirits:

The CD recordings containing the Gregorian chants from the **Benedictine Monks of Santo Domingo de Silos, from the monastery of Burgos in Spain**, has a repertoire of songs that are very effective to relieve stress, stimulate the mental state of Alfa and uplift the spirit. That recording was titled **CANTO (CHANT)** and was recorded in 1970. In 1994, it was released by the record label Angel as an antidote to the stresses of modern life and has sold over three million copies worldwide.

The themes of the Gregorian chants from the **Benedictine Monks of Santo Domingo de Silos from the Monastery of Burgos in Spain** are:

1) "Puer Natus Est Nobis" Introit (Mode VII) - 3:36
2) "I Iusti": Gradual (Mode I) - 2:49
3) "Christus Est Factus Pro Nobis": Gradual (Mode V) - 2:39
4) "Mandatum Novum Do Vobis" Antiphonal And Psalm 132 (Mode III) - 1:41
5) "Media Vita In Morte Sumus" Responsorio (Mode IV) - 6:11

6) "Alleluia, Beatus Vir Qui Suffert" Alleluia (Mode I) - 3:10

7) "Spiritus Domini" Introit (Mode VIII) - 3:46

8) "Improperium" Offertorio (Mode VIII) - 2:36

9) "Laetatus Sum": Gradual (Mode VII) - 2:17

10) "Kyrie XI A": Kyrie (Mode I) - 1:06

11) "Puer Natus In Bethlehem": Rhythm (Mode I) - 1:58

12) "Jacta cogitatum Tuum": Gradual (Mode VII) - 3:34

13) "Verbum Caro Factum Est": Responsorio (Mode VII) - 4:04

14) "Genuit puerperal Regem" Antiphonal And Psalm 99 (Mode II) - 2:56

15) "Occuli Omnium": Gradual (Mode VII) - 3:21

16) "Ave Mundi Spes Maria" Sequenza (Mode I) - 4:18

17) "Kyrie Fons bonitatis" Trope (Mode III) - 4:00

18) "Veni Sancte Spiritus" Sequenza (Mode I) - 2:42

19) "Hosanna Filio David": Antiphonal (Mode VII) - 0:42

The monks from the Monastery of Christ in the desert of Abiquiu, New Mexico, work and study in silence. They pass their daily hours in prayer for world peace. They have recorded a CD titled **"Blessings, Peace and Harmony"** containing selections of harmonic Gregorian chants that stimulate physical, mental relaxation and spiritual uplifting.

The Gregorian chants from the CD recordings of the **monks from the Monastery of Christ in the desert of Abiquiu in New Mexico** are:

1. Alma Redemptoris - Desert Monks 2:21

2. Salve Regina - Desert Monks 2:42

3. Salve Mater - Desert Monks 3:56

4. Ave mundi spes Maria - Desert Monks 4:20

5. Stabat Mater - Desert Monks 5:10

6. Kyrie IV - Desert Monks 1:42

7. Gloria IX - Desert Monks 3:14

8. Sanctus IV - Desert Monks 1:26

9. Agnus Dei IV - Desert Monks 1:05

10. Rorate Caeli - Desert Monks 4:42

11. Puer Natus - The Monks of the Desert 6:03

12. Parce, Domine - Desert Monks 3:54

13. Alleluia, O filii et filiae - Desert Monks 2:58

14. Salve festa dies - Desert Monks 5:18

15. Kyrie III - Desert Monks 3:07
16. Gloria III - Desert Monks 3:17
17. Sanctus III - Desert Monks 1:38
18. Agnus Dei III - Desert Monks 1:54
19. Alleluia, Confitemini - Desert Monks 2:57
20. Alleluia, Vir Dei - Desert Monks 3:25
21. Alleluia, Lustus Germinabit - Desert Monks 3:01
22. Alleluia, De Profundis - Desert Monks 3:02
23. Alleluia, Paratum Cor Meum - Desert Monks 3:22

There are other groups with very good recordings of Gregorian chants. Among them is the community of **Monserrat in Barcelona, Spain, along with the communities of the Miracle and San Miguel of Cuxa**, which consists of about seventy monks governed by the rules of San Benito. As in all Benedictine monasteries, the monks of Montserrat devote their lives to prayer and work. **The Angel Choir of the Abbey of Montserrat** has recordings of Gregorian chants that were produced by RCA Victor. They have an extensive repertoire of Gregorian chants that also have very favorable effects by activating relaxation and spiritual uplifting.

50

The Influence of Music on Animals

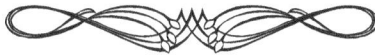

The Influence of Classical Music on Cows

Daniel McElmurray, a 10-year old student at the Goshen Elementary School in Augusta, Georgia, in the United States, was helping his father milk 300 cows at his ranch. His father, Mr. Earl, complained because he was not happy with the cows' milk production.

Daniel noticed that his father liked listening to music while milking the cows, but he did not have a wide selection. Daniel surprised his father by helping him to solve the problem of the cows' low milk production. He tested the effects of classical music, country music and rock music on the cows.

When the cows were exposed to classical music, their milk production increased 1,000 pounds above what they produced when they were exposed to rock or country music.

On March 15, 2003, Daniel McElmurray was awarded first prize at the Regional Science Fair in Hepzibach, Georgia, in the United States, for his project about the effects of classical music on milk production in cows.

A similar experiment was performed in Villanueva del Pardillo, Spain, at Priegola, a dairy farm owned by Mr. Hans Pieter Sieber. The secret of his success is not due to trendy technology or special machinery.

Sieber exposed his herd of 700 heifers to crescendo chords and cadences of the famous Austrian composer Wolfgang Amadeus Mozart.

The dairy cows, which are treated by animal psychologists, listen to classical music, sleep in comfortable areas and take relaxing showers.

Incredibly, when the heifers were being milked, the researchers played the *flute and harp concerto in R Major* by Mozart and there was a dramatic change in their behavior.

The heifers were lining up by themselves to be milked, and each produced 1-6 liters more per day. Mozart's music relaxes the heifers and also keeps them active. Hans Pieter Sieber claims that if comfort is offered to cows, they are more willing to cooperate.

Since early 1990, Dr. Gordon Shaw and Dr. Francis Raucher presented the theory that when babies listen to Mozart's music, their intelligence quotient (IQ) increases. Listening to Mozart's music also helped adults to become more creative and intelligent. This is known as **"The Mozart Effect"** and has influenced the study of sound therapy or **music therapy**, but only recently have researchers used animals to test this theory.

According to investigators, Mozart's gentle harmonies, and combination of sustained flats and allegros stimulate the brain and help muscles in humans and bovine relax and activate their power.

The cows' owners reaped unexpected rewards due to this experiment. Classical music, especially Mozart's, stimulates levels of relaxation in cows and makes them feel comfortable. Not only do the cows produce more milk, but the milk is sweeter, and has higher levels of protein and healthy fat.

Classical Music Helps to Calm Elephants, Gorillas and Dogs

Classical music by Elgar, Puccini and Beethoven has been shown to reduce elephants' abnormal behavior of balancing their bodies and shaking their trunks. Researchers have not indicated that elephants have a favorite composer; however, melancholic tones from the aria Nessun Dorma and the eight notes of the opening allegro brio of Beethoven's Fifth Symphony seem to soothe elephants.

Dr. Deborah Wells, from Queen's University Belfast, and other experts that have been studying elephants, have observed that elephants face difficulties when in captivity, due to their natural instinct to roam great distances. The core of the study is to try to improve the elephants' welfare and to observe their behavior patterns while living in captivity.

The team of researchers working for Dr. Wells recorded the behavior of four female Asian elephants for four hours a day for three periods of five days. They recorded everything that the elephants did during the time they were observed.

During the first five days, the elephants were not exposed to any kind of music. In the next five days, the researchers played classical music by Mozart, Elgar, Handel and Beethoven. During the last five days the speaker was off.

Dr. Wells and her group of researchers wrote a report in the Animal Welfare journal which stated that abnormal behavior was drastically reduced while elephants were exposed to classical music.

Mr. David Field, director of the Whipsnade Zoo in London, said that elephants are very sensitive animals. They have the ability to hear sounds that go far beyond human beings' auditory perception. Elephants communicate through deep infrasonic vibrations.

Dr. Deborah Wells has also researched the effects of music on dogs and gorillas. She concluded that classical music produces the best effects in these animals. Heavy metal music had very negative effects on dogs. Due to the results of studying the effect of music on animals, dog shelters are playing classical music to keep them calm.

51

DNA Sound Repair

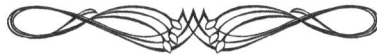

Sounds that can help repair DNA, and release energy blockages and negative beliefs

Scientific studies around the world have accumulated information on the power of intention. Language - the spoken word, with precise terminology along with the power of intention and thought, is a key to healing. Russian geneticists and linguistic scientists Fosar and Bludorf give credence to the concept that verbal mantras, self-talk, clairvoyance, spontaneous and remote healing acts are ways in which the human body communicates with itself and the world around it to heal.

Only ten percent (10%) of DNA in the human genome is used to build proteins and control physiology. This portion of DNA (codons) is what Western medicine has been studying in hopes of eradicating disease. The remaining ninety percent is considered **"junk DNA."** But Russian researchers rejected this notion of **"junk"** and found in their experiments that DNA is not only responsible for body building, but that it also has a communication function and a date storage function. **They found that DNA follows the same rules as all human languages.** By comparing the rules of syntax (the way words combine to form sentences), semantics (the study of meaning in the forms of language) and the basic rules of grammar, they found that the base pairs of DNA have established rules similar to those seen in language. Thus, human language can be a reflection of the inherent structure of our DNA.

Even more astounding, when exploring the vibrational behavior of DNA, the Russian researchers could modulate certain frequency patterns on laser ray and influence DNA frequency, and its genetic information. Since the basic structure of DNA base pairs and language have the same structure, no decoding is necessary - **one can simply use the words of human language to effect changes in DNA.**

The human mind has the ability to produce changes in matter, among other scientific investigations. Dr. Masaru Emoto, in his scientific studies and book **"Messages in Water,"** presented evidence about how our mind energy and words can affect the atomic structure of water (H2O). Positive thoughts, words and harmonic music can activate beautiful pentagonal and hexagonal geometrically shaped water crystals when water is frozen and photographed using an electronic microscope. One example is the one presented in this book about the photographs that Dr. Emoto took of the CD Music **"The Healing Forces of Harmonic Sounds and Vibrations."** When water is exposed to disharmonic music and negative thoughts the water formation is deformed and ugly. **Collective mind consciousness can have a powerful effect on matter.** Dr. Emoto gathered a large group of people and led them in reciting positive affirmations and prayers, and singing harmonic sounds in polluted bodies of water. When the water was tested afterward, Dr. Emoto observed beautiful hexagonal crystals. Many of the bodies of water were almost completely cleared after they repeated the same practice in several sections.

Everything in the universe is connected. Each person's thought has a powerful influence on the collective consciousness, that is, on the collective matrix. Each sub-atom, atom, molecule and cell is in a constant state of vibration, producing frequencies of sound, and is affected by the power of our minds. We live in an ocean of energy, frequencies and vibrations and when we learn to express our thoughts and words creatively, positively and with the intention of healing and doing good, we can transmit powerful vibrational frequencies that can regenerate and heal our DNA. We may also be able to help sick people, animals, and plants and contribute to heal the planet. Our planet can benefit from environmental healing, to help eliminate carbon and nuclear waste and to remedy the deforestation of jungles and forests that is causing ecological contamination in the oceans, in the atmosphere and climate changes.

When a group of people come together to pray, recite mantras, and affirmations, sing healing music, and meditate for **world peace and planetary healing,** a powerful vibratory frequency is activated in the atmosphere. This can open portals so more light can enter the planet, and help manifest peace and harmony on Earth. Scientific evidence supports the effectiveness of these practices. Humans must unify their minds in prayers, mantras, harmonic healing sounds, creative visualization and affirmations with the intention for global peace and to heal and regenerate our beautiful planet **Mother Earth (Gaia.)**

At the National Library of Argonne (Chicago), there are writings about the practice of using **"sound waves to levitate pharmaceuticals;"** and **"this practice increases** the longevity and effectiveness of products". Dr. Richard Goodbar wrote the book "Vibrational Medicine", in which presents a new branch of medical science on "how sound interacts with molecular structures and how this interaction results in a healing medicine." Dr. Barkaran Palua used PHONEMES in an experiment to help individuals reprogram their habits, behaviors, and balance their general emotions. Within these experiments, emphasis was placed on the individual "search" and the "location of the destructive negative emotion used unconsciously" and replaced with "positive, creative and prosperous words and phrases."

My dear friend and colleague, Clinical Psychologist, Dr. Estela Laufer, taught me the **Emotional Freedom Technique (E.F.T.)** I have been using this powerful practice for many years to help my friends and myself liberate negative energy, fears, emotional blockages, and to recuperate from allergies and other conditions. **E.F.T.** works by repeating creative and positive words and affirmations, and gently tapping the fingers in different areas of the body. This practice can remove negative and emotional blockages from tissues, organs, the sub-conscious and conscious mind. It is like a self-touch acupuncture with the hands, using vocal sounds and affirmations to erase negative emotions, traumas and thoughts. It has helped people to liberate emotional blockages, recover from many conditions, and accelerate the body's natural healing process.

In my experiments, I place a pyramid with a triangular face correctly oriented towards the North Polar and the opposite triangular face of the pyramid towards the South Polar. On the square surface of the pyramid I place a sacro-geometrical mandala and a sound speaker with the sounds of the **CD "The Healing Forces of Harmonic Sounds and Vibrations",** and I place herbal supplements, essential oils, water, and minerals to expose them to the frequencies of harmonic sounds for several hours. When I do a kinesiology test for those items placed in the pyramid, they are highly potentiated and energized. When I use these products, I can feel the difference compared to those that have not been energized. I have also used the sounds of Vedic Mantras, Tibetans, Hebrews and Gregorian Chants to energize herbal supplements, essential oils, water and minerals. The results have been very favorable. Most elements, herbal, water, minerals and oils have the peculiarity that they can store frequencies of sounds and those frequencies are recorded on these items, similar to recording music on tape or CD.

A study entitled **"Rapid changes in Histone Deacetylase and the expression of inflammatory Gene-Expression in Expert Meditators"** was carried out by Russian biophysicists and molecular biologists. In it, they questioned the validity of the scientific assumption that humans only use **10% of their DNA that contains all the information,** the information that dictates our genetic development and our ultimate behavior. In attempting to understand **90% of our unused DNA,** they concluded that the so-called **"worthless DNA"** was actually a **"productive DNA,"** a **truly useful DNA reservoir.**

In an investigation of the power of sounds and the effects associated with words, they came to the conclusion that there are basic words that, when repeated, release energy blocks related to negative beliefs, and also help release blockades, and can help manifest prosperity and abundance. These words represent a type of vortex or door that could be used by the individual according to his or her **"free will".** According to the Hindu Philosophy these words are: **Hum, Gum, Shreem, Lakshmi Yei, Narma and Maha** (the Hindu mantra for the Lashmi deity believed to provide abundance, prosperity and beauty), there are also other powerful basic words from Hindu Mantras like the **"Gayatri Mantra", Om, Bhur, Bhuvah, Swaha, Tath, Savithur, Varenyam, Bhargo, Desvasya, Dheemahi, Dhiyo, Yo, Nah, Prachodayath,** also the words from the **Maha Mrityumjaya Mantra, Om, Tryam-Bhakam Yaja-Maje, Sugan-Dhim Pushtivar-Dhanam, Urvaru-Kamiva Ban-Dhanan, Mrityour Mukshiya Maamritat",** and **Om-Na-Mah-Shi-Va-Ya.** According to Jewish Mysticism, other words such as **"Kodoish, Kodoish, Kodoish, Adonai, Tsebayoth, Yud-Hed-Waw-Hed", "Baruch Hashem", "Zohar Hadash" "Shalom" and " Amen", Ya and Ma.** According to the Tibetan Mysticism, other words such as **"Om-Mani-Pad-Me-Hum", "Oum-Aah-Hum", "Oum-Tare-tu-Tare-Ture-Soha".** The sounds produced when reciting these words and mantras are considered to have positive frequencies that resonate with DNA and the subconscious mind. The meaning of these mantras is described in more detail in the chapter on the scientific healing power of mantras and prayers in this book.

In my personal experience when reciting the Bijas Vedic words or the vowel sounds that resonate with each chakra, such as **Lam (U,U,U) Root Chakra, Vam (O,O,O) Reproductive Chakra, Ram (O,O,O) Solar Plexus Chakra, Yam (A,A,A), Heart Chakra, Ham (Ei,Ei,Ei) Throat Chakra, Sham (I,I,I) Third Eye Chakra, OUM (I,I,I) Crown Chakra** used in the same context produce considerable benefits. There are **"Sacred Mystical laws"** that control all levels and aspects of reality and these laws can be harnessed to achieve what might be considered **"supra-human or superhuman"** levels and elevated states of consciousness. The individual's experience is above what is considered normal. **The sounds of these mantras have a strong resonance with the structure of DNA and in turn influence the personality and experience of the person.** In this sense, singing harmonic vowel sounds, Vedic sounds, reciting mantras, praying, doing affirmations and meditating can help repair and heal DNA.

The **Bijas Vedic words or mantras Ham, Yam, Ram, Vam and Lam** represent the five elements: **Ether, Air, Fire, Water, and Earth.** When these Bijas Mantra or words are chanted aloud or in your mind, they activate energy and balance in the chakras, purify and heal the mind and body. According to the Bindu philosophy, if one recites or chants the Bijas Mantras every day, then one can experience divine energy flowing through the body, mind and spirit. **The sounds of the Bijas Mantras or words resonate with DNA.** Bindu spiritual practice states that the sound of these words helps to divert the negative energies around the person, attract positive energy and will help the person attract more successes.

When the mind and body simultaneously reach a state of complete relaxation, and absorb harmonic vowel sounds, mantras, affirmations, prayers, music of the CD **"The Healing Forces of Harmonic Sounds and Vibrations,"** and Gregorian chants, the frequency (528 Hz) releases negative energy. This helps to encode DNA's structure in a positive way. It also acts as glue that cements new words in place and produces a higher state of consciousness. This **"Musical Mathematical Matrix of all Creation"** is characterized by feelings of total euphoria, and is associated with periods of greater awareness of creative expressions. This influences the individual's physical and emotional health in a positive way.

The recoding of DNA cellular memory

In our DNA cellular memory there are accumulated experiences of this life and inheritances from our ancestors. Many times, we have also inherited emotional traumas of our ancestor's. Resentments, insecurities and emotions of fear that are passed down from generation to generation are recorded in the memory of our DNA. These memories are usually stored in our DNA at an unconscious level and can interfere with our evolutionary development.

The emotional traumas and fears that have accumulated in the DNA's memory according to their nature can affect organs, meridians, tissues of the body and can also affect the natural functions of some of the chakras.

For something to be manifest itself on the physical level, first it is created on the energetic level in our mind, heart and through the power of sound and the word activates the energetic frequency that has the power to alter the atomic structure of matter. The manifestation of everything that is created or manifested takes place first from the energy level to the physical level.

Through the infinite power of our mind, the heart, the power of intention, the power of the word and through the power of affirmations, creative visualization, mantras, prayers, healing harmonic sounds and meditation, we can release the stagnating energy in the cellular DNA memory and change the state of the vibrational frequency of our records at the cellular level.

This practice helps to **recode DNA** with positive energy that replaces the memories of the past, frees fears, insecurities and traumas, and helps the person to achieve a productive and creative life, with good health and vitality.

"The Healing Forces of Harmonic Sounds and Vibrations", the power of words and creative affirmations in combination with the stimulation of the vibrational effect of the spectrum of colored lights and sacred geometry (mandalas) also offers very good benefits for **recoding DNA** with creative energy, with good health and vitality.

The use of symbols

Symbolism has been used to communicate ideas, thoughts and intentions for many ancient civilizations such as the Egyptians, Sumerians, Mesopotamian, Tibetans, Hindu, Arabia Islamic, Japanese and Chinese dynasties. Hieroglyphs and other symbols were a means of communication. Aborigines from Australia are registered as one of the first pre-industrialized groups to use symbolism to record, maintain, and transmit relevant information about the origins of their group. The Caribbean Indians from the Caribbean Islands and Pre-Colombian Cultures, the Mayan, Aztecs, Olmec, Toltec's from Mesoamerica, Mexico and Guatemala, the Chavin and Incas Pre-Colombian Culture from Peru, Ecuador and Chile (South America), and the Native American Indians all of these cultures utilized specific symbolisms to communicate their cultural and mystical ideas. The species and its cultural and religious histories are associated with interactions with nature.

Most religions and secret societies use symbolism including the cross, pentagon, flower of life, seven-point star, David star, spiral symbol, kabbalah, Fourth Moon, Scale and a variety of other physical symbolisms. The ancient "seers" and "shamans" used various symbols to educate, inspire and influence others. The Hindus and Buddhists of Tibet use mandalas. Mandalas are spiritual and ritual symbols used to support meditation and help them elevate their mental state of consciousnes. Large companies have experimented with using symbols to convey the effectiveness of their products, such as the use of national, sporting and corporate symbols. However, they may use such symbols to control and manipulate people to consume their products, even when they are aware that their products are not of good quality.

52

The Power of Affirmations and Creative Visualization

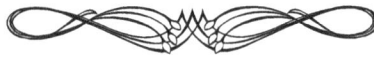

Affirmations penetrate your awareness. Affirmations help liberate mental blockages related to negative energies and help manifest positive changes. Affirmations are important tools, which work subliminally and they are more powerful and effective when recited in loud voice. It has been scientifically proven that affirmations generate positive frequencies that have resonance with DNA and with the subconscious mind. Allow the affirmations to go deep into your consciousness. The mind will soon develop an automatic reaction to the affirmations. If you practice affirmations, it will deeply penetrate your awareness, it will help you to recode the structure of your DNA and create many positives results in your life.

Each of the trillion of cells that form our bodies has a memory and an amazing faculty to respond to the messages that are generated by our thoughts. Send messages of love, harmony, peace, divine order and light to every sub-atom, atom, molecule, cell, tissue and organs that forms your microcosmic universe, the Divine Temple of your Soul, your amazing body.

Thoughts are the essence of human creation, so it would seem that thoughts are a medium of travel, manifesting and healing. One thought can be as powerful as the whole universe. One thought, one mind, unify consciousness. One thought can manifest into an illness or disease. Another thought can erase it. The power of your mind knows no limit. Thoughts produce words and sounds with a tremendous vibratory force that can mold man's body and affairs. **Good will produces a great aura of protection around those who send it, and there will be peace, love, harmony and prosperity for those who send good will to others. Love is a cosmic phenomenon. Real love is selfless and free from fear. Love is God in manifestation and the strongest magnetic force in the universe.**

Statement of Intention

In the name of the **"I am that I am..."**

I choose to be aligned with and to serve the highest consciousness of God/goddess/All that is, the Divine One who is the source of all love.

I choose to allow myself to faithfully serve my own highest good, allowing others to do the same.

I choose to allow myself to consistently emit the purest vibration of who I am, allowing others to do the same.

I choose to allow myself to experience unconditional love in this and all of my multidimensional existences.

I choose to communicate with, and be guided by, the most evolved beings of the highest orders of consciousness who choose to faithfully serve my highest good with truth, love, wisdom and compassion.

In all spaces and times, dimensions and planes, I choose unconditional love. On the Earth plane, I choose to manifest love, peace, harmony, bliss, laughter, abundance, prosperity, good health, happiness, wisdom, creative energy, divine order and light. I choose truth and integrity in all my dealings. I choose peace and harmony with myself and others. In total safety and in total health, I choose to be a divine human of love and light, prepared and evolved for Ascension.

I am the master of my own light.
I am the truth of my own love.
I am eternal...
This shall remain so.

So be it...

I am that I am = It means = God is where you are. As God is in heaven, so God is in Earth within me. Right where I stand God is. I am here below that which I am above... Gods love, wisdom, compassion & light is in every sub-atom, atom, molecule and all the trillions of cells of my divine temple, my divine body, spirit and soul…The divine presence goes before me and prepares my way…and that is the way it is, Amen, Amen, Amen…Oum, Oum, Oum…

Affirmation Experiment

Here is an experiment that can be highly revealing. Sit down comfortably somewhere, say the following statement out loud, close your eyes after you finish, and go into a meditation state for at least 15 minutes.

"Everything is going well for me, I am successful, prosperous and happy. Every day I'm better, better and better."

Many people find it difficult to say those words. They don't feel as if everything is going well for them. They certainly don't feel successful, prosperous or even particularly happy. Think about the words and what they mean. **Your subconscious mind accepts, and acts upon, the suggestions given to it.** When you say: **"Everything is going well for me, I am successful, prosperous and happy, every day I'm better, better and better."** your subconscious mind is not going to argue. Your conscious mind might disagree, but your subconscious mind accepts good thoughts that are presented to it. It then acts on them, and makes them happen. Consequently, if you say: **"Everything is going well for me, I am successful, prosperous and happy, every day I'm better, better and better."** often enough for the thought to become lodged deeply into your subconscious mind, it will become a fact in your life.

Creative Visualization

Visualization is pictures in our mind to train the mind and manifest any kind of goals. Visualizing specific moments, images, pictures, performance and techniques endeavor to create patterns in the brain. The more we visualize the more ingrained these neutral patterns become. When we recite affirmations loudly, along with visualization, the message goes to the subconscious mind which conveys it to the super-conscious, which enables us to reach any heights if done correctly.

The affirmations and visualizations must be done with strong power of intention and the objective desire will materialize and the goal desire will manifest.

The most powerful formula is: Intention+Visualization+Affirmation = Manifestation (You most have a clear mental picture of the objective or goal desire, and believe deeply in your heart and mind that is already manifested. It is not in the future, **it is already manifested in the present moment,** you must see it in your mind, and feel it and it will manifest.)

Wealth and Success: "I have a desire to be wealthy and I become wealthy. My creative thinking opens the door of the monastery of abundance. What I imagine is, what I create. I am persistent, ambitious and determined."

Health and Healing: "Day by day in very way I am becoming healthier and healthier. My immune system functions at optimum efficiency and keeps me in good health. I choose perfect health and use the unlimited power of my mind to heal myself."

Brain Power: "Day by day my mind is becoming agile and alert. My learning abilities and performance increase daily. I think more clearly and creatively."

To have a Positive Attitude: "I am self-reliant, self-controlled, and filled with independence and determination. I have great inner courage and project a positive self-image. I am confident, optimistic and enthusiastic and look forward to new challenges and emerge as a winner."

Accelerate Learning: "I have the ability to focus my energy concentration to accelerate healing and learn new concepts. I am developing a photographic memory and remember what I learn. I remain alert and focused and can instantly compare data."

Self-Discipline: "I have the self-discipline to accomplish personal and professional goals. I direct my time and energy to manifest my desires and increase my self-discipline. I am taking control of my life and am committed to my goals."

Self-Esteem: "I am self-confident. I believe in my abilities and enjoy high self-esteem. My positive self-image generates success and happiness. I am proud of myself and do things that make me proud."

Goal Accomplishment: "I have the power to do more things in less time. I am increasing my speed and productivity. My time is valuable and I use it efficiently to accomplish my goals fully."

Addictions Removal: "I have the will-power and discipline to do anything I desire. I ignore all craving and insecurity. I am letting go of the past, freeing myself and enjoy a deep inner peace and love for myself." "I do not live in the past or in the future, I live in the present time and my mind is in the present."

Enhance Creativity: "Day by day I am becoming more and more creative. I draw creative inspiration from the universe and release the unlimited power of my creative ability and so I am creative and happy."

Inner Peace: "I am at peace with myself and the world and everyone in it. My mind is like calm water and that's all I need. I now feel peaceful, balanced and harmonious, and experience tranquility, love and joy. Use peace, balance, and harmony as trigger words."

Creative Visualization: "I am visualizing what I want. I see it in my mind and set it to manifest. I can visualize my dreams into reality. I hold a clear picture in my mind and combine it with emotional desire."

Daily Affirmation

There is only one mind and life, and that is the reality of being. It is whole, in perfect balance and harmonious. It is the structure of existence, and it is the basis for my personal existence and experience right now.

I express the beauty, order, symmetry of the spirit. It appears in my health as increased vigor, well-being and clear thinking. In my financial supply, it manifests as increasing abundance. In every relationship, it expresses as deepened understanding and harmonious relationships. As a creative being my insight are stimulated by the spiritual ideas that always project through me.

I am in state of serenity. My life is in order. I express only the beautiful, the good and the true. I am fulfilled and content. All things are joyous in my world.

My eyes are open, now I see, fullness of truth revealed to me. My heart now holds the wonderful key. That open my mind and makes me free. Joyously now love works for me. Ready my God, my good to be. My eyes are open, now I see Spirit Divine…

347

Daily Affirmation to Attract Abundance and Prosperity

Be it known that _____(write your name here)_____has all necessary qualifications to demonstrate unlimited abundance, and I am now certified to practice the millionaire's consciousness.

Divine order is established and maintained in my financial affairs now. I am rich, well, and happy in every phase of my life now. Everybody and everything prospers me now. I am a money magnet. I create beauty, joy, health, happiness, inspiration to humanity with my creative talents and works. I inspire humanity with peace, love, harmony my creative works and with the divine light that is within myself. I create more money with my money and help others and myself to have a more creative, productive, prosperous and inspiring life. I work for the mission of Divine Light in order to awaking the Buddhist and Christ consciousness of love, peace, harmony, abundance, divine wisdom, prosperity, divine protection, good will and divine order in this dimension and all dimensions. I also do work for the protection and preservation of the ecology of our natural space ship our beautiful planet Mother Earth (Gaia). Every dollar that I spend, comes back to me multiplied. I deserve to be wealthy and guided by the divine knowledge, wisdom and the protections of the Universal Creator, The Holy Spirit, Christ & Buddha's consciousness of light, the Deities, Angels of the divine mission of love, peace, harmony and light. The divine presence goes before me and prepares my way, and that is the way it is… Amen, Amen, Amen.

Affirmation to liberate unwanted energy from the past

Life give me the right to choose, and I always select the best. Unhappy memories of the past are now erase from my consciousness, as I accept this unique moment of thinking. All patterns of limitations are gone. I envision a new life of freedom and easy. Mind's provision is an eternal good. I am not a repetition of old concepts. I am an expression of a fuller and more creative experience. This is my divine right. I live in a moment of change. My vision is clear, my sights are high, the expanded reach of my mind has made all things new. I am part of the creative spirit. The Infinite Power, the one presence and life divine. I know the Divine Presence goes before me and prepares my way. I know the Divine Presence goes before me and prepares my way. I know the Divine Presence goes before me and prepares my way and that is the way it is… Amen, Amen, Amen…

53

Vocalization Exercises for Good Health Maintenance

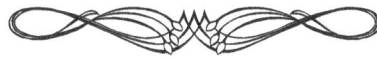

The voice is the most powerful instrument of all instruments and can generate a wide variety of sounds, words, buzzing, the sound of mantras and songs that help balance the chakras and which in turn stimulate the natural healing process in all systems of the body at the cellular level. When I studied **"Vocal Techniques & Music,"** at the Pablo Casals Music Conservatory in Puerto Rico, I remember that in my private singing lessons with my teacher Raquel Gandia, she used the Italian Bel Canto technique, and a vocal method used by famous Spanish singers. She said, to warm the voice, relax the vocal muscles and make them more flexible, we had to start the exercises by making vocalizations with the **vowels A, E, I, O, U.** She used the piano and covered an average of two scales of 8th musical notes on the piano, during the vocalization. The vocalization exercise starts by pronouncing each vowel for 4 to 5 seconds. Then the lips are joined and the vowel sound joins with the sound of the consonant **M,M,M** and continues to vibrate and create a humming sound for about 8 to 10 seconds for each vowel. Vocalizations are as follows:

1st section of vocalization exercises:

A,A,A-AM-M,M,   E,E,E-EM,M,M   I,I,I-IM,M,M,   O,O,O-OM,M,M,M   U,U,U-UM,M,M

Do these exercises for about 3 to 4 minutes, moving up through the 7-note musical scale and 5 semi-notes of the piano keyboard, starting at the central piano **C** and traveling on the 12-note scale with the repetition of the vowel exercise towards the **C sharp** and from the **C sharp** towards the **C Central** of the **Piano.** As you continue to do these exercises your vocal range will become more flexible and begin to expand. With practice, you could continue to do these vocalization exercises, covering two sets of 12-notes of the piano keyboard scales, going up and down. In other words, you can cover vocalizations of two 8vas of the piano keyboard, but this is achieved by practicing these exercises every day. Be sure to keep your pitch and vocal tone very natural without shouting or putting pressure on the vocal cords, and make sure is pleasing to the ear, and similar to the tone of the musical note of the piano keyboard or instrument that you use to vocalize.

2nd Section of vocalization exercises:

Repeat the same routine, with the same vowels and the same format, but starting with the **M** for about 3 to 4 minutes).

MA,A,A-M,M,M, ME,E,E-M,M,M, MI,I,I-M,M,M, MO,O,O-M,M,M, MU,U,U-M,M,M.

This vocalization exercise is performed with the throat and tongue relaxed. Visualize a pear (the pear fruit). The large round part of the pear is displayed behind the throat and the tip of the pear is displayed on the front of the mouth and lips. It's like yawning, but with an inner smile, keeping the back of the throat open and relaxed with an inner smile and an external smile on the lips. After four seconds of pronouncing the sound of each vowel (**A, E, I, O, U**) the lips are joined, the mouth closes gently without pressure, and the sound continues in the form of an internal humming with the consonant **M, M, M.** The sound must be heard and felt as an internal vibration. No pressure should be placed on the vocal cords. The vocal cords should be very relaxed during the performance of this exercise. Do not put pressure on your tongue or jaw. The facial muscles, throat and chest cavity should remain very relaxed during these exercises. It is important to breathe deeply, very relaxed and maintain the support of the sound from the diaphragm.

The chest cavity is kept expanded, relaxed, and the body and arms must be very relaxed. The only thing that moves, dilates and contracts is the diaphragm by means of controlled or rhythmic breathing. In other words, the diaphragm expands and moves when we inhale and contract when we exhale, making sure that the rib cage does not move up or down. Only the diaphragm moves, which is the area that supports the sound, and the rib cage remains dilated and relaxed with no motion during this exercise. The Thoracic Cage is the sound box that amplifies the sound in conjunction with the facial muscles. The rib cage can be compared to the case of a guitar or violin whose function is to amplify the sound generated by the strings of those instruments.

Proper Breathing: Make sure your breathing is correct and that you are not putting tension in your throat, or movement in the chest cavity, and that the sound is sustained all the time through the diaphragm. Lie on the floor or on a bed for a few minutes and place a book on your abdomen or diaphragmatic area, and observe that when you breathe normally only the book that is on the diaphragm moves and the rest of the body remains relaxed and not moving. This type of breathing is very effective in the vocalization exercises to get the sounds done correctly.

Visualize that the sound you generate comes from your third eye, between the eyebrows and the frontal top that connects the nose to the eyebrows. Another way for you to feel the vibrational frequency and mentally program it is to visualize the sound coming out of your third eye. Place the fingers of your two hands forming a triangle, and as if it were a pyramid, and place your hands with the base of the triangular position between the top of the nose and between the eyebrows. The tip of your fingers should point to the sky or above the crown chakra. Once you place your hands with the triangular shape on your forehead, begin the **vocalization exercises and visualize** that the sound comes out from that region **(the third eye)** and not from the throat. This will help you not to put pressure on the vocal cords. If you do this exercise correctly you will feel a powerful vibration in the bones of your face, head, chest cavity and throughout your body.

3rd section of vocalization exercises:

This new vocalization routine includes the consonants and vowels in the order that they resonate with the chakras and the **N** and **M** consonants are used. The exercises are performed as follows:

Do these exercises for about 3 to 4 minutes, climbing through the 7-note scale and 5 cemi-notes of the piano keyboard, starting at the **central C** of the piano and covering the **12-note scale** with repetition of the vocal exercises from the **central C** upward to the **acute C** and from the **acute C** down to the **central C.** When doing these sounds, touch the tip of your tongue to the top front or top of the teeth, without putting pressure, and very relaxed. Visualize that the sound comes from the third eye. This exercise produces very powerful sounds that resonate with the chakras and removes the blocks in those centers.

Niii-UUU-MMM, Niii-OOO-MMM, Niii-OOO-MMM, Niii-AAA-MMM, Niii-EEE-MMM, Niii-III-MMM, Niii-III-MMM

Once you have made the sounds in the musical scale up in the order indicated, covering the 7 combinations of sounds, in the 12 notes of the musical scale of the piano keyboard, make the combinations of the 7 sounds starting with the last combination of vowels, going down on the piano keyboard of 12 musical notes. Vocalizations are as follows:

Niii-III-MMM, Niii-III-MMM, Niii-EEE-MMM, Niii-AAA-MMM, Niii-OOO-MMM, Niii-OOO-MMM, Niii-UUU-MMM

Vowel Sounds and consonants that resonate with the Chakras:

Niii-UUU-MMM = Has resonance with the **Root Chakra.**
Niii-OOO-MMM = Has resonance with the **Reproductive Chakra.**
Niii-OOO-MMM = Has resonance with the **Solar Plexus Chakra.**
Niii-AAA-MMM = Has resonance with the **Heart and Thymus Chakra.**
Niii-EEE-MMM = Has resonance with the **Throat and Cerebellum Chakra.**
Niii-III-MMM = Has resonance with the **Third Eye Chakra.**
Niii-III-MMM = Has resonance with the **Crown Chakra.**

Once you learn to do these exercises correctly and master your execution more safely, you can use the rotational movement of your hands, moving the hands toward clockwise direction in front of your body, and within six inches distance from each chakra. Visualize that there is an energy moving out from your hands to the physical level and harmonizing your body. The rotational movement of your hands in conjunction with the power of sound that is generated by your voice will resonate with the chakras. This exercise will help release blockages, negative emotions, conditions and diseases that may be stoked in the chakras. Make sure that when you do the rotational movement with your hands, that the fingers of the hands remain separated and the palms of the hands move at least 6 inches from the front of the body. Through this exercise, you will be regenerating and harmonizing your chakras, organs and systems of the body from the energy level, to the physical level. It is one of the Qigong systems that I have created, incorporating harmonic vocal sounds and consonants in combination with the rotational movement of the hands to connect with the Ki or Chi energy coming from

Earth and the Universe, and to help release blockages at the physical level. This will accelerate the regenerative energy systems of the body.

When doing this vocalization exercise in conjunction with the clockwise movement of the hands, it connects the person with negative ions coming from Earth's surface, connects with the positive ions coming from the atmosphere, and activates the Ki or Chi Life energy. The electric plant of the human body is located at the Dantien (reproductive and solar plexus area) and from the Dantien the Ki or Chi energy of life expands throughout the body creating a very powerful toroidal field of energy around the body.

Continue the vocalization exercises and the rotational movement of your hands in conjunction with the corresponding vocal sound for each chakra, and raising the energy up above the crown chakra. Visualize that energy blockages, conditions, negative emotions and illnesses leave your body and point your hands and fingers above your head straight towards the universe. Visualize that you are connecting with the golden, silver, white and violet rays of light coming from the universe and any de-harmonizing energy or disease is disintegrated. Continue the rotational movement of the hands down bringing the golden, silver, white and violet light that comes from the center of the universe and activating the healing energy of love, light and divine order in each chakra of your divine temple or body. Continue moving that energy below your feet towards the center of mother Earth. When doing this exercise, visualize that from the soles of your feet, roots come out and connect with the heart center of Mother Earth (Gaia) and the golden, silver, white and blue rays coming from the center of the earth move upwards toward your body, through each of your chakras and you connect Earth's energy with the rays coming from the Universe. When we do this exercise correctly we stimulate the natural healing process of all our bodies; the energy, physical, mental, emotional and spiritual body harmonizes, and contributes to harmonize and heal Mother Earth. Many people who I've taught these exercises have had excellent results in improving their emotional balance, mental health, and many other conditions, including good health maintenance.

4th section of vocalization exercises:

This new vocalization routine includes the vowels in the order they resonate with the chakras and begins with the pronunciation of each vowel with the **G.** The exercises are performed as follows:

Do these exercises for about 3 to 4 minutes, climbing through the 7-note scale and 5 semi-notes of the piano keyboard, starting at the **central C-C** of the piano and covering the **12-note scale** with repetition of the exercises of vowels from the central **C upwards to the C sharp C** and from the **C sharp C down to the C Central C**. This is the **guttural sound** and when making the **guttural sounds** visualize that the sound is generated on the top behind your throat or pharynx, without putting pressure, and very relaxed. Also, see that the sound connects with the third eye and the center of the head. This exercise produces a very powerful **guttural sound** and vibration that vibrates the whole head, stimulates the pituitary gland and the pineal gland. These guttural sounds also resonate with the chakras and remove the blocks in these centers.

GUUU-MMM, GOO-MMM, GOO-MMM, GAAA-MMM, GEEE-MMM, GIII-MMM, GIII-MMM

Once you have made the sounds in the musical scale moving up in the order indicated, covering the 7 combinations of sounds, in the 12 notes of the musical scale of the piano keyboard, make the combinations of 7 sounds starting with the last combination of vowels, going down on the piano keyboard of 12 musical notes. Vocalizations are as follows:

GIII-MMM, GIII-MMM, GEEE-MMM, GAAA-MMM, GOOO-MMM, GOOO-MMM, GUUU-MMM

5th section of vocalization exercises:

This new vocalization routine includes the vowels in the order they resonate with the chakras and begins with the pronunciation of each vowel with the R, R, R. The exercises are performed as follows:

Do these exercises for about 3 to 4 minutes, climbing through the 7-note scale and 5 cemi-notes of the piano keyboard, beginning at the **central C of the piano** and covering the **12-note scale** with repetition of the exercises of vowels from the **central C upwards to the C sharp** and from the **C sharp down to the Central C**. This is the sound of **R, R, R,** and to make this sound place the tip of the tongue touching and vibrating with the top and front part of the teeth. Do not put pressure on the vocal cords and stay very relaxed. This sound connects with the third eye chakra and the center of the head. This exercise produces a very powerful sound that vibrates the whole head, the brain, stimulates the pituitary and pineal gland, and the whole body. This sound of **R, R, R** could be compared to the sound produced by the engine of an automobile.

RRR-UUU-MMM, RRR-OOO-MMM, RRR-OOO-MMM, RRR-AAA-MMM, RRR-EEE-MMM, RRRIII-MMM, RRRIII-MMM

Once you have made the sounds in the musical scale up in the order indicated, covering the 7 combinations of sounds, in the 12 notes of the musical scale of the piano keyboard, make the combinations of the 7 sounds starting with the last combination of vowels, going down on the piano keyboard of 12 musical notes. Vocalizations are as follows:

RRR-III-MMM, RRR-III-MMM, RRR-EEE-MMM, RRR-AAA-MMM, RRR-OOO-MMM, RRR-OOO-MMM, RRR-UUU-MMM

6th section of vocalization exercises:

The previous vocalization exercises are related to **Vedic sounds,** which resonate with the chakras. In my technique of **"Harmonic Healing Sounds Qigong"** I incorporate the Vedic sounds in conjunction with the coordinated movement of the hands facing the chakras. I recommend that you follow the instructions given in previous exercises, but in this exercise, apply the Vedic sound corresponding to each chakra, moving the hands in the direction of the clock and the coordinated movement of the hands from below the body upwards of the body and vice versa. When making the vowel sounds be sure to hold the sound of the M, M, M for about 4 to 5 seconds.

Do these exercises with the rotational movement of the hands in the direction of the clock, moving the hands from the **Root chakra, up towards the crown chakra** and continue to move the hands above the head and point the two hands towards the sky to connect with the energy of the universe. Do this exercise on various musical scales of the piano or with any instrument you select.

LAAA-MMM, VAAA-MMM, RAAA-MMM, YAAA-MMM, HAAA-MMM, SHAAA-MMM, OOO-UUU-MMM

Once you have done the exercises to get above the crown chakra, repeat the rotational movement of the hands with the same routine descending and using the Vedic sound corresponding to each chakra. When reaching the Root Chakra point your hands and fingers down to connect with the energy of Mother Earth (Gaia.)The exercise is listed below:

OOO-UUU-MMM, SHAAA-MMM, HAAA-MMM, YAAA-MMM, RAAA-MMM, VAAA-MMM, LAAA-MMM

Do these exercises at your own pace. Be sure to master an exercise correctly, before doing the next exercises outlined in this chapter. Do not rush, or try to do too many vocal exercises in a single day. Spend at least 15 to 20 minutes a day practicing these exercises, and gradually increase to 30 minutes or whatever time is most conducive to you. The exercises are easy to do and safe for all people. **However, for the person who has disability, back pain or any physical disorder it is recommended that you consult your doctor or therapist before attempting any form of exercise.** After completing the vocalization exercises it is also very effective to rest and meditate for about 10 to 20 minutes so that the sounds and exercises that have been performed have a better effect by activating harmonization of the charkas, relaxing the mind and body.

Additional Recommendations: Have a good sense of humor and be patient with yourself. All movements and sounds generated by your voice should be free of tension, fluids and using natural rhythmic breathing. Wear loose and comfortable clothing and if possible made of natural cotton and linen fibers, and wear comfortable shoes, sneakers, or sandals. It is even more effective to do the exercises barefoot. If possible, record each section and hear and compare each day, to see if there is improvement in your vocal range and the sounds you produce. As you continue to do these exercises in combination with meditation, you will notice that your mental abilities will become sharper, you will feel more focused, and happy with more energy and vitality. Harmonic sound vocalizations are the best natural medicine to influence the body and mind, and provides excellent therapeutic benefits.

54

Light and Chromotherapy

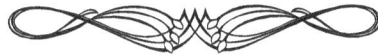

Light is energy that moves in tiny particles known as photons. **Light waves are very similar to sound waves, but can move much faster. Sound travels at about 1090 feet per second or 330 meters per second, while light travels at 186,000 miles per second or 299792.458 kilometers per second.** In equations, the speed of light is often written as the letter **C.** Another difference between light and sound waves is that while sound must have some form of matter in which to travel, such as air or water, light can travel through the vacuum of space. That is how light from the sun gets to us and how we can see the light from distant stars.

Visible light moves at a certain wavelength. If each wavelength was laid out on a chart, it would create what is called the **electromagnetic spectrum.** The shorter waves would be on one end and the longer ones would be on the other. In the middle, would be where visible light would end up. That is because it moves at just the right wavelength for our eyes to see it.

Each wavelength is **perceived** by our eyes as a different color. The **shorter wavelengths of visible light are violet** - we might call them **purple.** Then **as the wavelengths get longer and longer,** the visible **light changes in color to blue, green, yellow, orange,** and **finally the longest is red.**

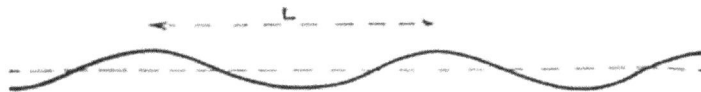

Illustration of a wavelength

The visible spectrum of light is often mixed together in what is called **white light.** We do not see each of the colors when they're mixed together. For that to happen, something must separate the wavelengths into their various colors. **This can happen in a rainbow.** When light passes through certain materials such as water droplets from a storm or a sprinkler, **the light can bend.** If it bends just right each of the different wavelengths can be seen. The colors in a rainbow appear to be **red** on the top and progress down through **orange, yellow, green, blue, indigo and violet.**

Color plays a major role in setting up a particular state of mind. **Colors affect and influence feelings, moods, and emotions.**

Visible light is the small part within the electromagnetic spectrum that human eyes are sensitive to and can detect. Visible light waves consist of different wavelengths of electro-magnetic energy. The colors of visible light depend on its wavelength. These wavelengths range from **700 nm** at the **red** end of the spectrum to **400 nm** at the **violet** end. **Prisms** are another way that light can be bent. Prisms are a specially cut piece of glass or other clear material. If placed just right in a stream of white light, they can separate the light into its various colors.

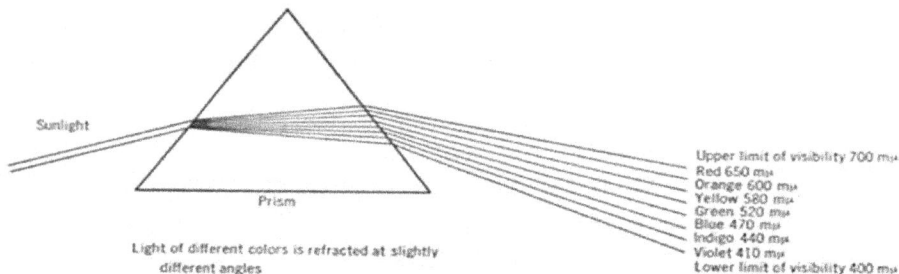

Illustration of white light passing through a prism crystal glass and reflecting the 7 colors spectrum.

White light is made of all the colors of the rainbow because it **contains all wavelengths,** and it is described as **polychromatic light.** The sun light is a good example of this.

Objects appear different colors because they absorb some colors (wavelengths) and reflect other colors. The colors we see are the wavelengths of the visible spectrum that are reflected or transmitted back by an object. White objects appear white because they reflect all colors. Black objects absorb all colors but no light is reflected.

There are three **primary colors - red, yellow and blue -** that are used in television to create all the colors that you see. If you were to mix any two of these colors, you would get the **secondary colors - orange, purple, and green.** These six colors are known as the basic color wheel. Artists, photographers, interior designers, exterior designers, and architects use these colors in their work to give rooms, buildings and spaces a pleasant and harmonious atmosphere.

How the Eyes Perceive Colors

There are three types of cones in the human eye nerves that are sensitive to short (**S**), medium (**M**) and long (**L**) wavelengths of light in the visible spectrum. (These cones have traditionally been known as blue-sensitive, green-sensitive and red-sensitive, but as each cone is responsive to a range of wavelengths, the **S, M and L** labels are more accepted now.)

These three types of color receptors allow the brain to perceive signals from the retina as different colors. Some estimate that humans can distinguish about 10 million colors.

Some animals can see wavelengths of light that humans cannot. Those wavelengths would be just outside the edges of human visible light. For example, insects can see ultraviolet waves - waves just before purple on the electromagnetic spectrum. But we are not able to see these. At the same time, there are colors of red that insects are unable to see, but that humans can.

Healing with light

Color healing, known as **Chromotherapy**, can be implemented in several ways. The ancient's civilizations built great chambers and halls painted with different colors for healing purposes. When people entered those chambers or halls they were immediately bathed with the color vibrations that were activated with the light.

Colors have strong effects on people's moods, feelings, emotions and states of mind. Ancient engineers, architects and artists knew about the effect of colors, and interior designers of this time also used colors to create different moods in different rooms, to inspire, energize, and soothe. The color we wear in our outfits also has a strong effect on our state of mind, on our physical and energetic field, and the way people see us. We should also use colors on bed sheets when we sleep, with a specific color that helps activate frequencies that relax us and that at the same time stimulate the natural healing process of mind, body and spirit.

The listing of colors and healing effects

Red: stimulates the root chakra and the adrenal glands to release adrenalin and activate strength. Brings warmth, energy, and stimulation; energizes heart and blood circulation; builds up the blood and raises a low blood pressure. Energizes all organs and the senses of hearing, smell, taste, vision, and touch. Increases sexual desire and activity. Red causes hemoglobin to multiply, thus increasing energy and raising body temperature. It is excellent for anemia and blood-related conditions. It loosens clogs, releases inflammation, stiffness and constrictions. **Do not apply red light color directly in areas affected by cancer.** The color red stimulates cell growth.

Orange: stimulates the reproductive or sacral chakra. It is warm, cheery and has a liberating action on the body and the mind, relieving the repressions. Open new possibilities and options in life. Stimulates creativity, new ideas, and sexual expressions. It stimulates lungs, digestive, and respiratory systems. Stimulate thyroid functions, alleviated muscles spasms, and cramps.

Yellow: stimulates the solar plexus and the psychic center. Yellow color stimulates the mind, the nerves and inspiration. It helps harmonize the nervous system and alleviate nervous conditions. It invigorates the muscles. Dark yellow soothes nerve pain. The yellow color can be effective to help harmonize liver, intestines and stomach conditions. It helps the digestive process, assimilation and elimination. It also offers healing benefits to the skin pores and for scar tissue. It activates and encourages depressed and melancholy people.

Green: stimulates the heart chakra. It is the color of vegetation, nature and the green grass on earth. It balances and sooths body and mind. It is often used for healing physical, mental, emotional and psychological imbalances. It has energizing and soothing effects. It helps regulate blood pressure, heart functions and hormonal metabolism. It can activate growth hormones and rejuvenation. It is effective against bacteria and germs. It stimulates healing effects on the digestive system, liver, gallbladder, kidneys. It helps fortify the nervous system and the immune system. Stimulates muscle, bones and tissue development. It helps to activate inner peace.

Blue: stimulates the throat chakra, the center of expression, communication and speech. It is cooling, electric and an excellent astringent. It helps cool down inflammation, fever, rheumatoid arthritis. It helps balance high blood pressure, headaches and stop bleedings. Soothes the nervous system, activates tranquility, alleviate stress, anger, aggression and hysteria. Blue color offers powerful antiseptic properties, anti-irritation and anti-itching healing effects. It helps to alleviate skin redness and irritations. The color blue like the color of the mineral **lapis lazuli** offer excellent healing effects for larynx inflammation, for speech ailments, hoarse voice, for communications or for any throat imbalances.

Indigo Blue: stimulates the third eye chakra and the pineal gland. It is cooling and electric. It activates physical and spiritual perception. It helps to harmonize the mind. It is an excellent purifying agent that stimulates blood purification. It can be of great assistance stimulating the healing process of the eyes and ears.

Violet/Purple: stimulates the crown chakra, the center of devotion, trust, inspiration, happiness and positivity. It is the center for deeper spiritual connection with ourselves and a peeper connection with the force of life that is greater than ourselves. These are colors of transformation, meditation, mysticism, contemplation, spirituality. They assist healing delusions, melancholy, hysteria, alcohol addiction and help to slow down an over-active heart. These colors also stimulate the immune system, white blood cells, the spleen, soothe mental and emotional conditions, help people with overactive sexual activities to decrease the need for obsessive sex. It helps people suffering from sleeping disorders, unhealthy sleep habits or insomnia to sleep better. These colors stimulate detoxification and help in decreasing the sensitivity to pain. These are the colors of sensitive people with paranormal abilities and with well-developed psychic faculties.

White: is the color for perfect balance, peace and harmony. It is associated with light (Divine light). It is the color of perfection, for the awakened spirit, for high cosmic consciousness. This color elevates the vibrational frequency of mind, body and spirit and helps to activate harmony and good energy. The color white and white light is often utilized for healing, for purification, for cleanliness and for protection. Qigong master and Pranic healers send white healing light with Ki or Chi energy to the affected area of the person that needs healing assistance and for also healing their aura or energy field. They know that everything comes from the energy field level to the physical level, and when you heal the energy field of a person, it will effectively heal the physical body. White is used by doctors, therapists and healers. It raises the vibrational frequency of the person and activates peace, trust and spiritual enlightenment. White means safety and protection against negative energy. The white light is often used to cover the energy field, and physical body of a persons creating an oval of a white light protective energy field, which neutralize any type of mental or spiritual negative or disharmonic energy invasion.

Magenta: represents universal love at its highest level. It promotes compassion, cooperation and kindness. Strengthens contact with your life purpose. It is the color of magnetism, to speed or attract desired goals. This color stimulates the heart and the adrenal glands. It encourages a sense of self-respect and contentment in those who use it. It is the color that imparts extra power for immediate action in one's life purpose and path. It is the color of strong passions and emotions for the realization of new ideas and goals but controlled. It is the color for activity, focused, great energy and for self-realization.

Pink: is the color of universal love of oneself and others. It is a delicate color that means tenderness, softness, romance, nurturing, caring, innocence, charming, feminine, sweetness. It is also related to peace, friendship, children, youth, femininity, emotional healing and love. This color vibration helps to restore youthfulness, heals sadness, grief and brings the person more in contact with his or her own feelings.

Turquoise: is associated with meanings of refreshing, feminine, calming, sophisticated, energy, wisdom, serenity, wholeness, creativity, emotional balance, good luck, spiritual grounding, friendship, love, joy, tranquility, patience, intuition, and loyalty. This color increases intuition and sensitivity. It works as an antiseptic and disinfectant. It helps in the regeneration of the skin and also assists in relaxing stress sensations. It is the color for intellectual and intuitive insights, for renewal, originality, for brotherhood and humanism. **To the Native Americans, the color turquoise represents life.** Native Americans believe that the earth is alive and that all things, no matter how small or apparently inanimate, are precious. Their medicine men use the turquoise color and the turquoise stones and keeps them in their sacred bundles because they believe that it possesses great healing powers.

Brown: is the color of earth, wood, stone, wholesomeness, reliability, elegance, security, grounding, foundation, stability, conservation, warmth and honesty. It is the color associated with the seasons of fall and winter. It is warm and stimulates appetite. It imparts protection of household, family and friend. It is the color of many materials utilized for constructions. It is used for healing animals, for making relationships solid, for concentration and for attracting help in financial crisis.

Gray: is a cool, neutral, and balanced color. The color gray is an emotionless, moody color that is typically associated with meanings of dull, dirty, and dingy, as well as formal, conservative, and sophisticated. It is a timeless and practical, often associated with loss or depression. It helps to neutralize negative influences, erasing or cancelling situations.

Black: is associated with power, elegance, formality, mystery. Denotes strength and authority and it is a very formal, elegant and prestigious color. It helps to banish evil and negativity. It is good for protection, opens deep unconscious levels and good for deep meditation. This color helps people to liberate bad habits and additions. It also symbolizes darkness, seriousness, depression, death, mourning, secrecy, underground, underworld, things that must remain hidden. It is the color of the extremes-ties, everything or nothing. It also represents standing apart or revolting against something or from provocation. People with high and strong self-confidence use black.

Gold: is associated with illumination, love compassion, courage, passion, magic power and wisdom. Gold is a precious metal that is associated with wealth, authority, grandeur, and prosperity, power, financial riches, luxury, investments, creativity, confidence as well as sparkle, glitz, and glamour. **It is the color that represents solar energy, perfection,** male energy and the winners. It helps heal people from addictions, and bad habits. It is often associated with success, achievements and triumphs.

Silver: is associated with wealth, prestige, glamour, graceful, sophisticated and elegant. It is also associated with industrial, sleek, high-tech and modernity, as well as ornate. Silver is a precious metal and like gold symbolizes riches, wealth and prosperity. It a color related to female energy, the cycle of rebirth and reincarnation. It restores equilibrium, intuition, emotional stability and stability to both feminine power and spiritual energy. It assists in healing hormonal imbalances. It helps remove and neutralize negative energy. It is the color that stimulates psychic abilities and dreams.

Copper: represents wealth, but cooper is less valuable than gold and silver. It is the color of conduction, and it is the best conductor of electricity after silver. Cooper is recognized as the father of the modern techniques. It represents love and passion, positive relationships in love, friendship, business, career opportunities, promotions and negotiations.

Color Light Therapy

Color light therapy also known as photodynamic has been used by dermatologists and therapists for skin rejuvenation, to activate cell energy, and for skin whitening. It has anti-inflammatory and sterilizing effects that help inhibit the production of acne, slows aging, strengthens and reaffirms the facial muscles of the skin, eliminates fatigue and relieves inflammation of tissues and nerves.

LED light is one of the forms used for photodynamic color therapy. Scientific research has found that LED light can enhance the energy potential of skin cells. It acts directly on the cell mitochondria, which is the cell's energy production center and activates enough energy to promote aerobic respiration of the skin, stimulates the removal of freckles, repairs the skin and delays senescence.

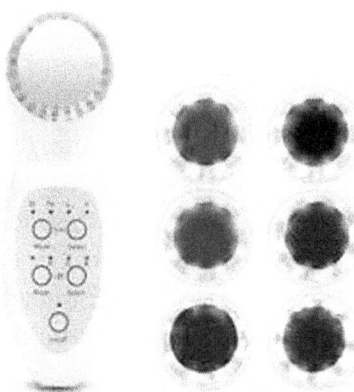

Illustration of LED light photodynamic color therapy for the skin facial and body.

Photodynamic skin therapy effects

Red Photodynamic skin therapy: with wave **640nm** (Penetrate the skin 1-6mm) Red color has the most penetrating power of all the colors, promoting cell's recycling, increases the oxygen content in the blood and helps to activate cells vitality. It promotes the skin production of collagen, make the skin more translucent, white and thus reducing fine lines and wrinkles. Red light is one of the most anti-aging light color therapies that activates deep skin absorption of nutrients, creams and oils. Tightens pores, improves overall skin color and brightness, leaving the skin smooth and elastic. Fades freckles and redness, promotes facial blood circulation, moisture skin. It is very effective in reducing skin and joint swelling and pain. It is also very effective for therapeutic treatments of dermatitis allergy conditions. It helps reduce scars, acne and activates skin relaxation.

Yellow photodynamic skin therapy: with wave **583nm,** (penetrates the skin 1-2mm) improves cell's oxygen absorption, strengthens muscles and stimulates the immune system, relaxes and restores the balance of sensitive skin, improves microcirculation and circulation deficiencies, regulates cell activity and gradually fades freckles and skin pigmentation. Improve skin dullness and relaxation. Helps to cure skin roughness, and red spots. Relieves erythema and lymphatic swelling.

Green light photodynamic skin therapy: with wave from **532nm to 640nm,** (Penetrate the skin 0.5-2mm) Effective helping to reduce melanin cell production, decreased pigment formation, adjustment skin gland function and help reduce glands grease production. When green and blue lights are combined, they can assist improving oily skin and black pigmentations. They are also effective for acne treatment. It also promotes the synthesis of protein, collagen and for skin contraction.

Blue light photodynamic skin therapy: with waves from **423nm to 480nm** can help with vasoconstriction, strengthen the protein fiber tissue, penetrate the skin and kill bacteria, activates injury recovery, shrink pores, suitable for aging skin, ease skin wrinkles, relieve a symptom such as edema, promote the synthesis of protein and collagen, activate cleansing and recovery of skin cells, activate the relaxation of skin contraction and has a calming effect on sensitive skin.

Purple light photodynamic skin therapy: with wave **640nm.** The **purple** light results from the combination of **red** and **blue,** it can help strengthen protein fiber tissue, shrink pores, eliminate face yellowing (a yellow face), decrease wrinkles and assist in the treatment of premature acne. It stimulates blood circulation and activates skin tissues vitality.

White light photodynamic skin therapy: with wave at **510nm** can calm, sooth, prevent allergies, and so on.

Infrared Red-light heat wand massager therapy

Infrared red-light heat wand massagers are well known to penetrate below the skin to stimulate blood flow, relax muscles and helps speed healing, reduce joint stiffness, relieve and relax muscles pain. It is very effective for the spine, neck, shoulder, arms, and feet therapy, relieving aches, strains and cramped muscles. The heat produced by the red-light infrared heat process is much the same as the feeling of warmth produced by the sunrays, but without the danger of the ultraviolet and radiation damaging effects.

Colors clothing's mental, psychological and physical effects

Red color clothing: Red **empowers and draws attention** toward the wearer. It's also strongly associated with **romance and passion,** making it a perfect date and night color. But be careful - it's also been said that red stimulates the appetite and makes us hungry for junk food, so wear with caution if you're trying to eat healthier.

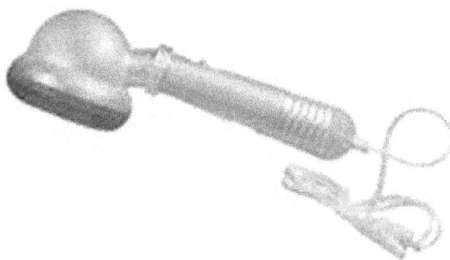

Illustration of the red light infrared heat wand massager

Orange color clothing: Like red, orange draws attention and energy, but unlike intense red, it's a little more soothing. While **orange is a difficult color for some skin tones to pull off,** if you have the coloring to make it work, orange will help put you in a positive, energetic mood.

Yellow color clothing: Sunny shades of yellow are the perfect thing to cheer you up on a bad day, so if you're feeling down, wearing yellow could help perk you back up. Yellow is also associated with **intelligence and inspiration,** so wearing something yellow on the day of your big final exam might help you come up with some extra answers.

Green color clothing: Shades of green are **calm and soothing,** as well as associated with nature and the outdoors. That's why green is one of spring's most popular shades. Green is also refreshing and has been found to **reduce stress** in those who look at it. If you're feeling really overwhelmed during finals week, add green to your outfit and you might **feel more relaxed.**

Blue color clothing: Blue is a color that can be both **peaceful and calming** as well as cold and standoffish. If you're feeling really stressed out, blue can help you feel more relaxed. If you're sad, however, you might want to steer away - blue can subconsciously make you feel more "blue." Studies also show that blue **can make you more creative,** so if you want to channel some genius for your art project, wearing blue might be able to help.

Purple color clothing: Regal and sophisticated, purple is associated with **creativity and luxury.** Like red, purple is a very **stimulating color which can boost your energy level** when you see it. It's also a color that's sometimes **associated with spirituality and intuition,** so if you're having trouble making a decision, wear lavender and see what comes to you.

Pink color clothing: Pink is the favorite color for females, but it's also associated with **romance and happiness.** Pink is very **soothing, calming, soft and deep,** so don't wear it if you need tons of energy. Because of its romance association, pink is a good choice for a date. You can also wear it anytime you're a little bummed out for a boost. Of course, if you personally don't like pink, then (obviously) this won't work for you.

White color clothing: The white color is used in the four seasons of the year but it is used more frequently during summer and spring. It **reflects light** and reminds us of sunnier days. It is the purest color of all colors and induce **protection, peace and harmony.** It is also **associated with peace, innocence, simplicity, and cleanliness,** although in Japan, white carnations mean death - who knew? **Wear white when you want to bring out any other colors you're wearing** - it enlivens anything you pair with it.

Black color clothing: If you're going for a promotion at work or interviewing for a new job, you might want to wear black - it signifies **power, seriousness, authority, and responsibility,** all qualities your boss is likely looking for. The black color is associated with **elegance** and **conservative** people who have authority. Outside the office, black is also a color that will give you some rocker-chick edge. If you're shy and want to feel like a badass one day, some black studded ankle boots should do the trick!

Color psychological effects in your home, business and healing areas.

Color is a nonverbal universal language that generates a powerful vibrational frequency that has profound effect on the emotional well-being of people. The colors you use in the walls of your house, business or public places activate an intuitive emotional and behavior response on the people that are observing or exposed to the colors. When painting a wall of a room with a color, you should first consider the primary function of the room that you are going to paint.

There are rooms painted with colors that offer a relaxing and calming experience and other rooms that can irritate a person and make them un-comfortable. The colors should be used to create a healthy emotional response and comfortable environment for the people that are going to be impacted by the vibrational frequency of the color in a specific room. There are professional color consultants that can be contacted to help best select the proper color for a specific room or area. It has been scientifically proven that some colors work better than others at encouraging certain activities. The right color can help create the right energy frequency for the most important rooms and to help activate the right environment in your home, office and businesses. **The surrounding colors in a room have strong influencing emotional and mental response in people.**

Colors for a living room or foyer: Warm tones like **reds, yellows** and **oranges** or **earth tones** like **browns** are often used in these rooms because they stimulate **conversation and interaction.** These are colors that encourage people to sit around and talk. These colors make people feel warmth and activate the desire to connect with other people.

Color for kitchen and restaurants: In the restaurant industry, many of them have some walls painted in a **red color** décor because it has long been recognized that the red color is an appetite-stimulating color. If you wish to maintain good weight maintenance and good health **do not use red in the kitchen or dining room** in your house. **Yellows in combination with some walls in white or bone white can be a good color** for the kitchen and the dining room since is a warm color that stimulate conversation and interaction and encourage people to talk.

Bedrooms and high-traffic rooms: Blue colors are suggested for high-traffic rooms and for areas where people spend a significant amount of time. In a bedroom it is good to combine some walls in **soft blue and white,** or **mint blue and bone white** or **lavender and white** or **light mint green and white or soft turquoise and white.** Using two colors for the bedrooms walls, two walls painted in one color and the other two in any white. The combination of these colors is relaxing, calming and activate a serene environment. It's said that they harmonize respiration and lower blood pressure. It is important to only use in the bedroom one of the colors recommended in combination with white. Do not use more than two colors in a bedroom since it can alter the relaxation state.

Business office or home office: Light purple is said to result in a peaceful surrounding and relieve tension. Purple utilizes **red and blue color** which provides a nice balance between stimulation and serenity that is supposed to encourage creativity. A **light purple color** is good for a business office since it stimulate harmonious conversation and effective interaction in a relaxing environment.

Healing space or therapy room: 1st. Combination of one wall in **turquoise,** one wall in **lavender** and the other two walls in **white** color, **2nd.** Combination of one wall in **Light Blue,** two walls in **white** and one wall in **indigo blue** color, **3rd.** one wall in **mint green,** one wall in **turquoise** and two walls in white colors, and **4th.** Two walls in **light turquoise** and two walls in **white.** The turquoise, lavender, mint green, light blue and white colors stablish positive calm emotions, peace, harmony, serenity, and happiness in an environment where people are looking to receive healing energy, therapies or treatments.

Light: It is also very important for the illumination of these rooms, with natural spectrum light bulbs that project the light similar to the light from the sunrays. **Neon fluorescent light do not generate healthy frequencies** and should not be used in the office, home and never in rooms for healing or that will be used for healing therapies. The color perception inside a room change as per the lighting variations. It is recommended to illuminate a room with natural spectrum light bulbs that resembles the light from the sun, and that will enhance the colors utilized for a specific environment in a room.

In conclusion: the light and colors generate powerful frequencies of vibrations that have **strong effects on people's moods, feelings, emotions and state of mind. Light, colors as well as sound frequencies** should be implemented in a way that can stimulate the natural healing process of the mind, body and spirit.

Testimonial Letters

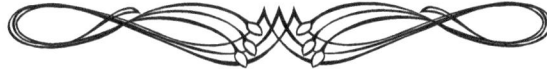

Dra. Raquel Liberman
Psychotherapy Specialist
Playa Mirador 427, CP 08830, México, D.F.
Tel: 011-52-55-5634-5969
Tel: 011-52-55-24-4848
Email: Raquel_Liberman@yahoo.com
Webpage: metatron-galactron.com

The Healing Forces of Harmonic Sounds and Vibrations and Magnetic Harmonic Vibrational Therapy.

In 2010 I met Jay Emmanuel Morales, who has values and spiritual virtues like no one else I ever encountered. Balance, harmony, congruence, service and love are the virtues that characterize Jay.

Throughout my professional life as a specialist in psychotherapy, as well as in my spiritual learning path, I have rarely received information that integrates learning through sensitivity, creativity and free expression, as well as its counterpart, the structure given by accurate and well-informed theoretical information.

The workshops I have taken with Jay Emmanuel display these principles so I do not doubt that his book will display the same powerful wisdom and concepts. "The Healing Forces of Harmonic Sounds and Vibrations and the Healing Power of the Human Voice and the Mind" contains the keys needed for achieving integral health. In his work, Jay Emmanuel displays love and dedication to humanity with a base of extensive studies and scientific evidence.

February 4, 2014

Raquel Liberman

—————————————
Raquel Liberman
Professor and Psychotherapy Specialist

Estela Laufer
Clinical Psychologist, Holistic Psychotherapist, Reiki Master
E-mail: elauferhipnoterapia@yahoo.com
Tel: (347) 599-7594

"The Healing Forces of Harmonic Sounds and Vibrations & Healing Through the Power of the Voice and the Mind."

Dear Readers:

This book is an invitation to activate the natural healing process in all bodies of our Divine Being by simply applying the VIBRATIONAL MEDICINE teachings which Dr. Jay Emmanuel Morales has masterfully put together in his book and based in his deep investigations about ancestral wisdom. He presents very powerful information about his professional holistic practice, healing through harmonic sounds and vibrations, kinesiology, homeopathy, ayurvedic medicine and most of all his love and the dedication that hi puts into his work.

Thank you Jay for the amazing legacy that you are giving to humanity, without a doubt, his book is a great tool for our evolution, and it will contribute to improve the quality of life of all the people that have the opportunity to read it. May the Divinity bless and expand this wonderful teachings and scientific message.

I use the CD **"THE HEALING FORCES OF HARMONIC SOUNDS AND VIBRATIONS"**, in my personal meditations and in my professional practice with my patients to contribute to the integral energy balance with excellent results, to achieve a state of relaxation, to harmonize and to help to improve the immune system. The sounds of this masterful CD generate an atmosphere of peace that expands to the environment and at the same time it contributes accelerating the natural healing process in all its listeners.

The book **"THE HEALING FORCES OF HARMONIC SOUNDS AND VIBRATION"** & **"HEALING THROUGH THE POWER OF THE VOICE AND THE MIND"** offers us a guide to improve the quality of life do to the great diversity of ancient knowledge and techniques that has been presented in this book. Healing through the power of specific harmonic sounds, the voice and the mind has also already been wisely supported scientifically and it is a great toll for spiritual evolution.

The CD and the book Dr. Jay Emmanuel Morales leaves to humanity are a legacy of wisdom, love and light that will contribute activating evolutionary transformation in the people who put these teachings into practice. You will find an immense variety of natural methods that will help you in your quest to maintain the integral balance of the mind, body and spirit.

February 10, 2014.

Estela Laufer

Estela Laufer
Clinical Psychologist, Holistic Psychotherapist,
Hipnoterapist, Reiki Master,
Emotional Freedom Theraphy Specialist (EFT) and
Regression Therapy

Marisol Carrere

85-05 85 Road
Woodhaven, N.Y. 11421
Carrere Films International, L.L.C.
E-mail: **Marisolcarrere@gmail.com**
Tel: (646) 229-6022

The Healing Forces of Harmonic Sound and Vibrations

"The Healing Forces of Harmonic Sounds and Vibrations" CD by Dr. Jay Emmanuel Morales is powerful and uplifting. I listen to it during my morning and evening meditations. I am so grateful for this compilation of powerful harmonic sounds because along with positive affirmations, it helped me go through the healing process of surviving cancer. Jay Emmanuel Morales sincerely helped me transform my life through his process of healing and natural holistic recommendations. In addition, listening to **"The Healing Forces of Harmonic Sound and Vibrations"** It takes me to a creative heightened state as I continue to develop my film scripts and other artistic projects. Thank you so much for your amazing work, your wisdom and dedication!

January 15, 2014

Marisol Carrere

_____

Marisol Carrere
Actress, writer and producer,
"I am Julia" & "The I Am Peace Project"
http://www.iamjuliamovie.com

Anita Velez Mitchell
171 West 57th Street, Apt. 9-A
New York, N.Y. 10019
Tel: (212) 246-3631
E-mail: **avelezmitchell@yahoo.com**

"The Healing Forces of Harmonic Sounds and Vibrations" & "Magnetic Harmonic Vibrational Therapy"

Dear Jay,

Your CD is divine!

The frequency of vibrations. The harmony tones such deep, rich and colorful tones possesses one. I began to feel levitation and vibrations through the energy center of my body, from the first day I submitted to your therapy.

I remember when I would come to you for consultation. How I came out dancing...singing... such a joy! And you said to me: "Your etheric body is pleasurably lifting you up." My aura became visible and my sensitivity was heightened, since that moment, I could see other people's auras.

Once, immediately after receiving your therapy, I went to a singing class, and about to start it, I could see the aura of my teacher. I gasped. She understood what I saw. I stood by the piano, determined to sing. I was amazed to see her bathed in colors. "What colors do you see, Anita?" My teacher asked me. As I said it, she got up from the piano and said, "I cannot give you the class. Those are the colors of death!" And so, it was; a week later she was dead.

I want to thank you, Jay, for helping me refine and raise the level of my consciousness. This is already evident in my poetry and other creative works. It adds contentment and harmony with everything that surrounds me. Now, thanks to you, I am much more aware of my inner attunement and my chakra vibrations. I am glad to acknowledge publicly how you have enriched my life.

Gratefully,

February 4, 2014

Anita Vélez Rieckehoff

—————————————————————
Anita Vélez Rieckehoff Vda. de Mitchell
Poet, Drama Director, Theater Director, Actress,
Singer, Dancer and Cultural Themes Columnist

The infinite evolutionary process of existence

... In the sacred temple of my body, in the inner biological sanctuary,
Invisible and silent to the outside world,
today, in a very accelerated way, a reconstruction and re-structuring of my body
is happening, produced by the extraordinary alchemy knowledge of Jay Emmanuel
Morales, his knowledge in the culinary arts and his use of pyramidal energy, the
holistic machines hi utilize in his practice, his crystal quartz and Tibetan bowls music,
his mighty mantras chanting, his songs and of course, his powerful and vibrant voice
energy, his alchemy knowledge and above all, "the purity of his healing intention."

I am writing memories of this special visit that has healed me physically
and spiritually.

This morning, before dawn, Jay and I were walking through the streets of New York
City, lugging large suitcases to the Port Authority bus station that took us to the
airport, where we boarded the plane that took us on a twenty-two days unforgettable
spiritual and mystical pilgrimage to Japan And Thailand.

Jay walks in New York City daily to many places and he does it always with great
speed. In the three days of my visit we walked many streets. "It's good exercise," he
explains.

I followed him almost running, blocks and blocks. Sometimes Jay stop to wait for
me with a childlike smile, and he would move his hands sending messages with the
physical language to encouraged me to continue walking, and before crossing an
avenue ... he said to me "Walk a little faster" ..., "Look" He demonstrated to me, Walk
with your chest open, happy, with a nice smile in your lips and against the wind." I
smiled. He is 15 years younger than me and in perfect physical shape, like that of a
young athlete,
I notice that I am not.

On that morning, there were hardly any people in the streets; The city was full of black
plastic trash bags, tied up and piled with discipline, a well-organized work done at
night. New York City "The Big Apple" is like that, the big city must be cleaned daily
...The same apply to our human life, we need to cleanse our mind,
our soul and our physical body daily.

Jay Emmanuel teaches us to use the sacred healing power of our voice and mind,
through specific harmonic sounds and creative visualization, we can cleanse our
hearts and minds, and we can stimulate and accelerate the natural regenerative healing

power of all our body systems, our divine physical temple.
Before arriving at the bus stop we saw three homeless asleep on the sidewalk. People that do not have a place to live. Anonymous, shipwrecked in life.
Internally we bless them with our love.

At the airport, we kept walking and walking at high speed through long corridors. People, many people from all over the world. How interesting are the airports! A great analogy of life. "We are all travelers," always moving like the stars in the universe towards new paths and dimensions in the infinite evolutionary process of existence ...

Pilar Alvear Farnsworth,
February 2014
Founder of the Natural Birth Movement
http://www.farnsworthproductions.com/PilarDeLaLuz/

Acknowledgements

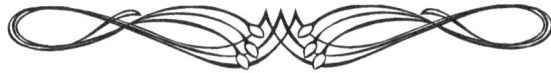

My deepest thanks to all those who have participated in this project, and especially for their support which helped me launch this book and present it to the world.

Teodorico Enrique Ampudia, for helping me with the book's original concept and edition, graphic designs, photographs, promotion, website, translation from Spanish to English, and for his continuous support throughout this extensive project and for the fraternal and family support that he and his distinguished sister **Juana Isabel Ampudia** have offered me over the years.

Carlos Alberto Quintero, for his creative and innovative artistic expression, his great talent which has been expressed through his designs of the book's front and back covers, and for being an honorable representative of spiritual arts through his transcendental paintings that activate frequencies and expand evolutionary consciousness towards infinite cosmic spaces. www.xcreativegroup.com/alberto

Pilar Alvear Fansworth, for helping me with the pre-edition of the book, for her recommendations, prologue redaction, and her spiritual support and benevolent affection. For presenting me at events that she coordinates and directs, such as "The One Human Race Festival" in Washington, D.C. and Pagosa Spring, Colorado. For her participation in several of the mystical and educational trips I organized to Egypt, the Riviera Maya in Yucatan Mexico, Mexico City, D.F., Thailand, Japan and Ecuador.

Dr. Estela Laufer for her support during the verification and grammatical corrections for many versions of the book, for her spiritual support, for her presence at my conferences, workshops, activations and concerts, and for her affection as family and as a sister. I thank her for sharing her knowledge on her therapy practice Emotional Freedom Technique (E.F.T.), regressive therapy for mental reprogramming; and for her participation in one of my mystical and educational journeys to Egypt. And primarily for her fervent dedication to helping humanity through her practice as a psychologist and clinical hypnotherapist.

Thomas Aksness, scientific director of Health Tech Sciences in Norway, for submitting my CD **"The Healing Forces of Harmonic Sounds and Vibrations: Healing Through**

the Power of the Voice and the Mind" to scientific examinations through the Aquera Voice Analysis system, and for concluding that my CD is effective in improving blockages and imbalances of the chakras. I am infinitely grateful to Thomas and his organization for the scientific analysis of the CD and for recommending my work to the scientific community and the general public, and for defining my work as "**an effective sound therapy to improve the chakras.**" Thank you for all your support and friendship.

Dr. Masaru Emoto, for his November 5, 2004 submission of my CD "**The Healing Forces of Harmonic Sounds and Vibrations**" to examination tests in his laboratory in Japan which resulted in photographs of 24 beautiful hexagonal patterns created by my CD and the harmonic sound frequencies. Infinite thanks for his valuable scientific report and for the fascinating work he presented in his book "**The Hidden Messages of Water.**"

Dr. Premala E. Brewster Wilson, PhD, CCH, CNS, LN, founder of the Institute of Preventive Medicine, Homeopathy and Nutrition in Silver Spring, Maryland, USA, for recognizing the therapeutic value of my CD "**The Healing Forces of Harmonic Sounds and Vibrations**" and for recommending it to her patients as an important part of their health protocol. My most sincere gratitude for also recommending my practice and work "**Magnetic Harmonic Vibrational Therapy,**" for her family's support and hospitality, especially her distinguished husband, Theodore D. Wilson, Indiana State Attorney Assistant, Colonel and Judge of the Army of the United States, and her late brother, Dr. Seth J. Edwards, who was a professor at the University of El Paso, Texas.

Dr. Leonel Eduardo Lechuga, inventor, architect, professor and founder of the Metatron Center in Mexico for recommending my work and my book to help activate the natural healing process, and for giving me the opportunity and the honor of successfully presenting my workshops, thesis, conferences and sound healing activations through his organization in Mexico. For his continued brotherly support and knowledge in sacred geometry, design and architecture, and for the knowledge he provides to mankind through his organization "Espacio Metatrón de México."

Dr. Raquel Liberman, Teacher and Specialist in Psychotherapy for the Metatron Center of Mexico for recommending my work, and expressing that this book has been presented with great wisdom, sensitivity, accurate and well-researched information. I also express to Raquel and her distinguished husband Dr. Leonel Eduardo Lechuga my most sincere thanks for giving me the opportunity and honor to successfully present my Vibrational Medicine workshops and conferences in Mexico. For her dedication and mission to help humanity as a teacher and specialist in psychotherapy and constellations workshops.

Dr. Paul T. Sprieser, DC, DIBAK, Director of the Institute of Kinesiology Studies, Pine Brook, N.J. For the knowledge I obtained from him in the area of Applied Kinesiology, which is a powerful science that has the ability of being used as a tool for diagnosis. My infinite thanks to Paul and his distinguished wife, Priscilla Sprieser for their family support and affection over the years.

Dr. Bruno Casatelli, for his support throughout my singing career and as a Vibrational Medicine Therapist, and for opening the doors for my kinesiology studies through his friend Dr. Paul T. Sprieser. But the most important thing was the encounter I had with Bruno in Egypt more than 16 years ago, on my first trip to Egypt, where I was able to find the brother I had from many past lives. In the temple of the Cosmic Mother Isis, at Philae in Aswan, during a powerful meditation, where all people present felt the immense frequency of love and light of Mother Isis, we meet again at this powerful sacred temple. The greatest gift that transformed my life was when Bruno made arrangements with his contacts and Egyptian friend Fergany Al Komaty, for a friend and I to climb to the top of the Great Pyramid of Cheops. On the return from Luxor to Cairo, at 1:00 a.m. we started to climb to the top of the pyramid. We were at the top of the pyramid of Cheops for 5 hours where I could feel Mother Earth's powerful frequency as a deep hum that came from Earth's center and was similar to the sound AUM. That subtle sound, similar to ultrasound, vibrated all the fibers of my being and I felt the light energy of the stars descend from the center of the universe to us at the center of the pyramid. Later I learned about the power of the pyramid and that from its center the Tachyon Energy connects the pyramid with the center of the universe. Tachyon Energy moves much faster than the speed of light. There are no words that can express what I perceived. The powerful energy at the top of the pyramid had an amazing impact on me. I felt that from then on my powers of perception were sharpened. I felt a strong motivation to help humanity, especially through my humble mission and message **"The Healing Forces of Harmonic Sounds and Vibrations and The Healing Power of the Voice and the Mind."** Thank you Bruno for being such a benevolent being, for your light and for being my eternal brother.

Dr. Rubén Ong, Oncologist, for all the knowledge he has shared with me about the nature of cancer, the sophisticated mechanism of the body's healing systems and the direct relationship they have with the emotions and mental energy in that process. For supporting my studies, research, experiment and work in the area of **"Vibrational Medicine and Healing Through the Power of the Voice and the Mind."** For his suggestions, recommendations and articles that he sends to me so I can be aware of the latest therapeutic systems and perfect my practice. Thank you Rubén for your brotherly and benevolent friendship.

Jesús Gutiérrez, for his benevolent energy, support and talent creating the musical arrangements, the sound engineering, and the creative ideas that contributed to the successful recording of the CD **"The Healing Forces of Harmonic Sounds and Vibrations"** at his recording studio "Jesús Gutiérrez At TV Music Recording Studios" in New York City.

Palmira Ubiñas, President and Founder of the International Association of Hispanic Art and Culture (AIPEH) in Orlando, Florida, and New York, for her recommendations, preparation and writing of the editorial note, and for all spiritual and benevolent support and her sisterly affection. For presenting and introducing my work at the AIPEH organization and for coordinating my presentations and lectures through her organization and different institutions in Orlando, Florida.

Susana Bastarrica, president and founder of The Vigil for World Peace. For giving me the honor of presenting my thesis on **"The Healing Forces of Harmonic Sounds and Vibrations: Healing Through the Power of the Voice and the Mind"** in several conferences at the United Nations. For granting me the honor of participating, singing and activating the harmonic sounds with my voice and the alchemy crystal singing bowls in the vigil of peace in New York's Central Park for the International Week of Peace Celebration. For her benevolent friendship, her support in my creative works, her interest in presenting my scientific research, and especially for everything she does to bring the message of peace and harmony to humanity.

William Jones (Lupito) & Paul Utz, the founders of Crystal Tones, owners and distributors of alchemy crystals of precious and semi-precious stones, located in Salt Lake City, Utah. For giving me the honor of being an exponent of the healing power of crystal singing bowls and harmonious sound by appearing at their shows during The New Life Expos in New York City, Florida, Arizona, and Colorado. For being the carriers and facilitators of The Pure Quartz Crystals and Alchemy Singing Bowls, which stimulate people's natural healing process. For their benevolent, fraternal affection and support, and for their extensive mission to bring the music of the spheres to humanity through the powerful instruments that they distribute.

Dr. Gloria Godinez, M.A.Sc., N.D., H.M.D., O.M.D. President, Founder and Director of the Institute of Energetic and Biological Medicine SC. For her support in my research and Vibrational Medicine works, and honoring me with her distinguished presence at my workshops in Mexico, and for recommending my work and practice to her friends in Mexico. For her presence at the sound activations and meditations that I have performed at The Pocito's Church in México D.F., which is the sacred place where the Cosmic Mother Guadalupe made her appearances, also at The Pyramid of the Sun in Teotihuacán, The Astronomical Chamber of the Acropolis in Xochicalco Morelos, and at the energy vortex of the Grand Canyon of Colorado and Canyons in Sedona, Arizona. What strikes me most about Gloria is the unconditional love she radiates, and her dedication and interest in helping humanity through her extensive knowledge of biological nanotechnology, Energy and Vibrational Medicine. Thank you Gloria for being so special, for your beautiful friendship, for your affection and unconditional love.

Lama Thupten Kunkhyer, from the monastery of Tibetan monks of Sera Je in Mysore, Karnatak state in India. For teaching me how to sing and vocalize Tibetan mantras, and anchor and activate my internal energy so I could help others activate their chakras to accelerate the natural healing process through the singing practice of mantras and meditation. For the mystical teachings he and his brother monks shared with me, for continually including me in their prayers, for being my brothers, for their mystical wisdom, compassion for humanity and constant communication with me from the Tibetan region of India to New York.

Anita Vélez Mitchell, poet, playwright, theater director, actress, singer, dancer and cultural topics columnist. Anita was born on February 21, 1916, in Vieques, Puerto Rico. She lived for almost a century. I knew her for 32 years, to be more specific, since I came to New York. Her mind and creative energy was very sharp, and radiated a light that inspired deep appreciation for life. She was very talented, sensitive, creative, and intelligent, and receptive to the practice of Vibrational Medicine. She gave me the honor of being able to assist her through **"The Healing Forces of Harmonic Sounds and Vibrations," The Magnetic Harmonic Vibrational Therapy, and Biomagnetism Therapy.** Anita honored me with her words when she said that the frequencies of the vibrations and tones I use in my activations and treatments with sounds "are so deep, rich and colorful that they possessed her," she continues, "I left, dancing, singing and with great joy. " Her evaluation of my work inspires me to continue to do my utmost to strive and to help humanity through my scientific research and work in the area of vibrational medicine.

In one of the many interesting conversations I had with Anita through the years that I knew her, she mentioned to me that in the mid-1950s she was married to Mr. Mitchell and they wanted a baby. However, Anita was active in her artistic career which involved a lot of physical dance activity, and could not conceive. Her husband knew the scientist Royal Raymond Rife, who had a "Vibrational Medicine" laboratory in New York City, and he told him about Anita's problem. Rife at that time was confined in a prison. Rife told Anita's husband to speak to his assistant, who was running his Vibrational Medicine Laboratory in New York, that Anita should have three treatments with his "Rife Machine." She went for the treatments and a few weeks after Anita finished Rife's third treatment, she became pregnant with her daughter Jane Vélez Mitchell (Jane is moderator of TV news). Anita is a source of inspiration for our generation and will be for many generations to come. Thank you Anita for your wisdom, for loving life, for your creative work and for the love you always gave to me.

Antonio Kabral, television producer and programming director. For his support and direction during my presentations and interviews with Omar Cabrera, moderator of the TV show "Crecer" with TV Azteca. For presenting my thesis of **"The Healing Forces of Harmonic Sounds and Vibrations and The Healing Power Through the Voice and the Mind"** in his conference cycles at the Elmhurst Hospital Theater in Queens, New York. For his fraternal and benevolent friendship and interest in helping humanity through all his informative events.

Marisol Carrere, actress, writer and producer. For granting me the honor of assisting her with my therapies through **"The Healing Forces of Harmonic Sounds and Vibrations," "Magnetic Harmonic Vibrational Therapy, Biomagnetism and Nutrition Therapy."** Marisol honored me when she said that my Vibrational Medicine CD, Nutrition and Bio-Magnetism Therapy and positive affirmations helped her survive cancer. For her beautiful and benevolent friendship, and her desire to promote my Vibrational Medicine work. For creating and directing theater and film projects that enhance the quality of life and for her recent short film "I Am Julia & I Am The Peace Project."

Linda Russo, for her recommendations and legal advice. For her intensive and amazing support during the English editing of this book. For being my sister, friend and family since I arrived in New York City 33 years ago, and specially for her benevolent interest to help people through her talents and profession.

Laurisa Brandekam, for her support during the verification and grammatical corrections in Spanish for some of the chapters of this book, for her recommendations, spiritual support, and for her presence at my conferences, workshops, activations and concerts. Mainly for her affection as a sister and friend. For sharing her knowledge with me and for her desire to help humanity through her Mayan Shamanic Mystical practices.

Nilda M. Tapia is a writer from Buenos Aires, Argentina who has been a journalist since the end of the 60's. She has maintained columns in several Spanish-language publications in New York and is dedicated to collaborate in the editing of literary works of new writers in Spanish. Nilda has collaborated in the final corrections in Spanish of the second edition of this book. We know each other since 1997 when she worked as a publisher for the magazines Canales and Temas which gave me the cover and published very interesting articles titled **"The Spiritual World of Jay Emmanuel."** That occurred when I released an album and performed pop Latin music. In 1997 Nilda was in my home and I offered her as a gift, an activation through **"The Healing Forces of Harmonic Sounds and Vibrations"** and using my voice in combination with the Pure Quartz Crystals Singing Bowls. At the end of the session she said to me "This vibrational therapy has activated a powerful healing energy and frequency in me. I feel that it will help me greatly." Thank you Nilda for your help, sensitivity, receptivity and appreciation for the healing forces of harmonic sounds (Vibrational Medicine,) and for your friendship.

I am deeply grateful to all the teachers with whom I studied singing voice techniques, breathing support techniques and voice projection to sing professionally and for better musical performance. **Rafael Elvira,** musical director from Puerto Rico, **Raquel Gandía,** voice teacher at the Conservatory of Music of Puerto Rico, **Puli Toro,** mezzo-soprano and voice teacher in New York City, **Ted Taylor,** musical director, voice coach and teacher, **Sigmund Jasinski**, tenor, voice coach and teacher.

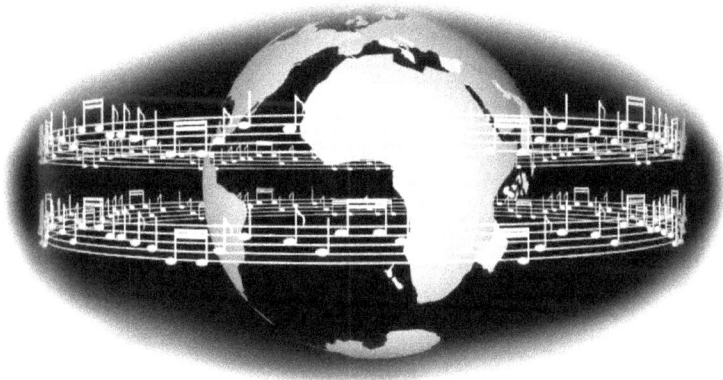

"Our Planet, Mother Earth (Gaia),
is a gigantic symphonic orchestra,
incessantly in concert, generating
sounds and vibrations naturally."
- J.E.M.

About Jay Emmanuel Morales

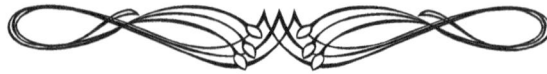

Jay Emmanuel Morales, A.K., V.M. (Kinesiologist, Vibrational Medicine Therapist.) Mr. Morales uses many techniques to help individuals maintain good physical, mental and spiritual health. Mr. Morales works with Qigong and Pranic Healing Energy, Reiki, Hatha Yoga, Kundalini Yoga, and meditation. He works and experiments with the acoustic effects of specific harmonic sound frequencies in chambers and pyramids and their therapeutical effects on people, animals and plants. He teaches healing techniques using the power of the voice, mind and specific vowel sounds that resonate with the organs and chakras of the human body. Mr. Morale's purpose is to awaken the consciousness in people so that they realize that **"The power is within each one of us,"** and when we learn to cultivate our natural faculties, we raise the mind and spirit to higher levels of consciousness. Jay Emmanuel bases his work on historical and scientific evidence from ancient civilizations that have used these techniques for thousands of years as preventive and self-healing remedies.

Jay Emmanuel developed a powerful Qigong technique called **"Harmonic Healing Sounds Qigong."** He bases his technique on the use of specific vocal sounds, different coordinated movements of the hands and body, breathing techniques and meditation. The purpose is to harmonize the chakras, and eliminate blockages of the meridians so the energy of live (Ki or Chi) flows freely without obstacles and can effectively energize and revitalize body meridians, tissues and organs. This practice contributes to strength, flexibility, balance, greater resistance to injuries, recovery from stress, and mental and physical well-being.

Jay Emmanuel is the founder of the **"Power of Harmony Organization, Health and Global Wellness Network."** His organization focuses on educating the community with information about alternative health methods that incorporate organic natural nutrition, herbology, harmonic sounds and vibrations, music therapy, creative visualization, mental power, affirmations, mantras, prayers, meditation, yoga, qi gong and other methods. The purpose of these practices is to help people achieve good health by stimulating the natural healing process of the mind, body and spirit. Jay has given several presentations without charge, as a service to the community.

Jay Emmanuel is an ambassador of peace and has appeared in countless conferences to present his thesis **"The Healing Forces of Harmonic Sounds and Vibrations and Healing Through the Power of the Voice and the Mind."** Venues include the United Nations, the Universal Fraternity of Master Serge Reynaud de la Ferriere, and New Life Expos in New York, Florida and Colorado. He has given lectures and workshops for the One Human Race Festival in Washington, D.C. and Pagosa Springs, Colorado. He has been invited on three different occasions to lecture at La Serenísima Masonic Grand Lodge of the Spanish Language for the United States of America, in New York City. He has brought his expertise in music therapy, the healing power of the voice, mind, music and specific harmonic sounds to public school students in the Bronx, New York. He has also presented workshops at Metatron Space in Mexico, and at many organizations in Spain, Egypt, Israel, Russia, Ecuador, Colombia, Puerto Rico, Japan and other countries.

On September 27, 1997, the Governor of New York, the Honorable George E. Pataki, granted Jay Emmanuel a letter of acknowledgment for his participation in the celebration of Culture and Hispanic Educational Month. Governor Pataki expressed in his message "I applaud his dedication and talent and thank him for his contribution. His music and talent enriched our program and augured the success of our ceremony."

On September 27, 1998, the Puerto Rican Institute of Culture in New York awarded Jay Emmanuel Morales with the "Art of Music Award" for his excellent work and willingness to serve the community. On Wednesday, February 17, 1999, Jay Emmanuel was a special guest for the tribute offered to Puerto Rican poet, playwright and singer Anita Vélez Mitchell at Merkin Concert Hall in New York's Lincoln Center, where Jay Emmanuel was accompanied by the Pan American Symphony Orchestra, under the direction of maestro Joseph Lliso.

On Monday, February 22, 1999, Jay Emmanuel was a special guest for the event "Knowing and Loving Puerto Rico, USA" a multicultural concert at Dag Hammarskjold auditorium at the United Nations, organized by diplomat Ms. Nilda Luz Rexach.

Jay Emmanuel performed as lead singer in the production of **"The New Age Musical Ballet," "King David"** in Moscow, Russia in 2003, written, choreographed and directed by Yuly Zorov. He co-acted with dancers of the Bolshoi Ballet of Moscow. Jay Emmanuel gave a wonderful performance, with his extraordinary scenic presence and with a masterful command showing different shades of his powerful voice. Jay Emmanuel sang all songs with light and strong versatility, demonstrating the talented agility of his extensive vocal record. People from different parts of the world have witnessed his performance on YouTube and on social networks. (Gail M. Carrillo, Impacto Latino News.)

In 2002, Jay Emmanuel gave a lecture on **"The Healing Forces Sounds and Harmonic Vibrations"** at the **"One Human Race Festival"**, followed by a concert, and several harmonic sound activations. The festival was held in Washington DC and Pagosa Springs, Colorado, and was coordinated by Ms. Pilar Alvear.

Jay Emmanuel has a powerful voice and extensive and melodic musical range. He has been working and experimenting for more than 30 years with **"The Healing Forces of Harmonic Sounds and Vibrations"** to develop his **Magnetic Harmonic Vibrational Therapy Technique.** He defines his practice basically as the technique used to heal the body, mind and spirit through specific sounds, musical tones and frequencies that produce vibrations that restore the harmony of the chakras. Since each energy center of the body better know as the chakras vibrate in a specific musical note, "The Magnetic Harmony Vibrational Therapy" contributes to the harmonization of the vital energy of the etheric body, the auric body and the physical body.

Jay Emmanuel is an initiate in Egyptian mystic teachings and has coordinated innumerable educational and metaphysical journeys to Egypt for more than 16 years. In his lectures he shares his knowledge of Egyptian antiquity so each participant might experience a positive transformation in his or her life. He uses specific harmonic sounds in ancient solfegus chords in his lectures to help the participants to activate their own natural healing force.

Jay Emmanuel has performed studies, sound acoustic experiments and recordings using his voice and pure quartz alchemy crystal singing bowls in the King and Queen Chambers of the Great Pyramid of Cheops, the Temple of the Hathors in Dendera and the Temple of the goddess Isis in Philae in Egypt.

In October 2004 Jay Emmanuel and Dr. Masaru Emoto participated in a conference at the Dag Hammarskjold auditorium in the United Nations, organized by Reverend Susana Bastarrica, of the Department of cultural activities of Feng Shui at the U.N. Dr. Emoto subsequently analyzed Jay Emmanuel's CD; his findings are on the website healingpowerofharmony.com, in the section "Analysis of Sounds".

In June 2012, on the summer solstice, six months before the end of the 25,900 year cycle of the Mayan calendar, Jay Emmanuel coordinated an educational and metaphysical trip to the Mayan Riviera. He experimented with acoustic healing sounds using his voice, quartz crystal singing bowls and Tibetan bowls at historical and sacred places including the pyramid of Chichén Itzá, the pyramid of Uxmal and other Mayan pyramids, and the Cenote EkBalam Au in Yucatán, Mexico. Jay presented "The Healing Forces of Harmonic Sounds and Vibrations" in three conferences at the Okaan Hotel, in the Mayan plateau.

To celebrate the closing of the 25,900-year Mayan calendar cycle that took place on December 21, 2012, in Cuernavaca, Mexico, Dr. Leonel Eduardo Lechuga and his wife Dr. Raquel Liberman invited Jay Emmanuel to participate in an event they coordinated, **"The Closing of the Mayan Cycle and the Trajectory Towards a New Era,"** where the Shamanas Julia Nava and Lulu López Garay were present. Here, Jay gave two lectures on **"The Healing Forces of Harmonic Sounds and Vibrations and Healing Through the Power of the Voice and the Mind."**

On December 23, 2012, two days after the beginning of the new era according to the Mayan calendar, Jay Emmanuel was led by the shamans Julia Nava and Lulu Lopez Garay to the Capilla del Pocito to the Sanctuary of the Cosmic Mother of Guadalupe, where he sang with the alchemy crystal singing bowls Franz Schubert and Charles Gounod the "Ave Maria" to a large audience.

For the past eight years, Jay Emmanuel has been a guest of honor at "The Vigil of World Peace" which takes place every year on September 21st in New York's Central Park to celebrate the International Day of Peace.

To celebrate the solstice twice a year and under the new moon or full moon lunar cycle, Jay Emmanuel organizes largely attended meditation and outdoor concerts at Cleopatra's Obelisk in New York's Central Park.

Jay Emmanuel has toured internationally and appeared in national television programs including "Diálogo de Costa a Costa" hosted by Malin Falu, and "Crecer" with the Argentinean moderator Omar Cabrera, TV Azteca.

Jay Emmanuel masterfully mixes voice, colors lights, sounds and alchemy crystal singing bowls to offer his patients and audiences harmonic sound vibrational frequencies capable of elevating them to an incomparable healing journey.

Jay Emmanuel tells us in his composition:

The healing power is within each of us…

Open your heart to the power of vibrations,
Open your mind to the power of harmonic sounds,
Everything in the universe is in a state of vibration,
Reflection of light, consciousness of God…

Open your heart to the power of divine light,
Open your mind to the power of creative thoughts,
Every thought your mind creates,
Is in a state of vibration,
Reflection of light, consciousness of your soul,

Harmonic frequencies turn into light,
And seven colors the rainbow form,
And all the spaces are filled with love,
The strongest force in the Universe,

Harmonic Frequencies manifest transformational changes,
That ignite healing energy in all systems, atoms and cells,
Within the heart and in all fibers of our being…

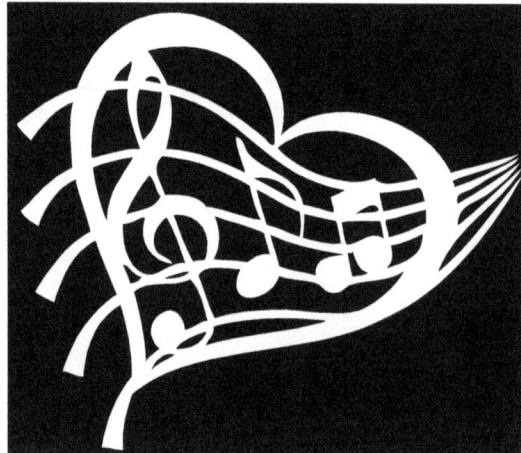

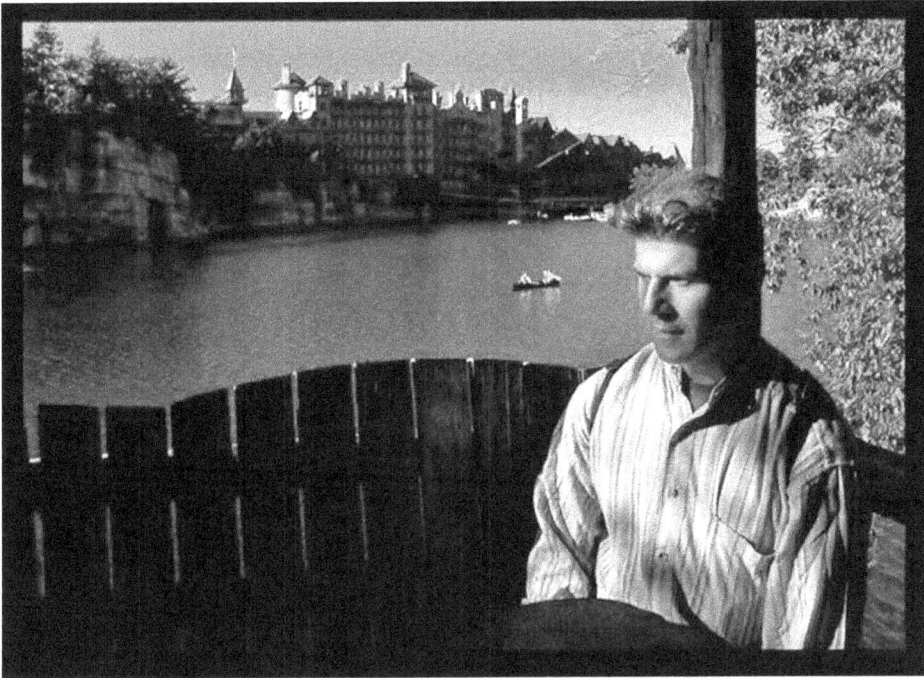

"Contemplation Journey"

Traveling in the infinite space of our sacred inner universe, opens the doors that connect our divine being with the universal light and consciousness of creation. It's transcending beyond space and time, a state of stillness and serenity, where the inner sound of silence, makes us levitate in the frequency of peace, harmony and love. It's the unification of the spirit with the Universal Creative Intelligence ... "Oum, this must be Nirvana" ... J.E.M.

(Nirvana in Buddhism = a transcendent state in which there is neither suffering, desire, nor sense of self or ego. It is the state of perfect happiness.)

"Meditation"

Meditating on the peak of the mountain, feeling the strength and sound of the wind, the heat of the sun's rays, Earth's magnetic force, and the fresh scent of vegetation. Listening to the symphony of Mother Nature, the melodic serenade of birds, insects and elements, elevating my senses, and my spirit is traveling in a different dimension, unified with the magnificent spirit and force of creation ...J.E.M.

<u>Harmonic sounds, mantras and meditation</u>

Harmonic vocal sounds and mantras,
Activate the sublime silence of meditation,
Sounds echoes make our whole being vibrate,
Turning up the light that connect spirit with the universe.

The music and harmonic chants,
The mantras and meditations,
They make the spirit dance,
In the spiral orbits of the universe,
Unifying hearts and consciousness,
With the immense cosmic creation.

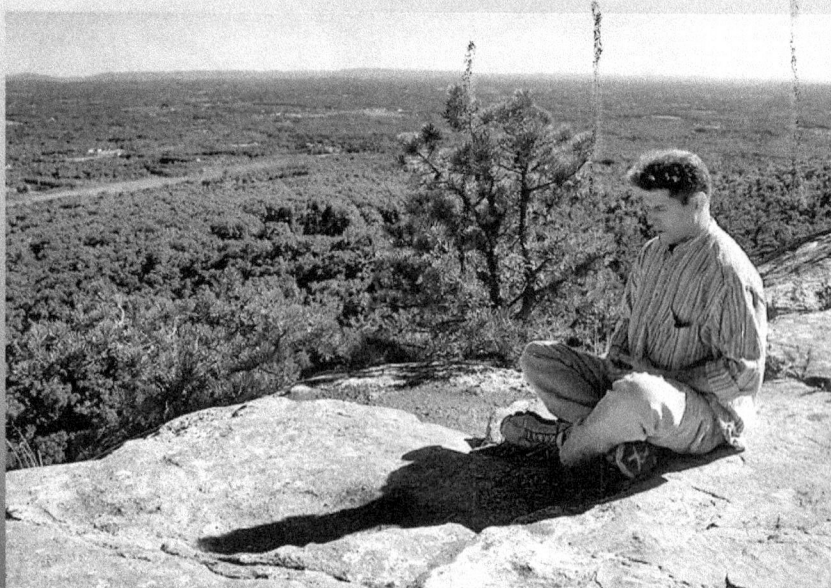

The whole universal creation is in motion,
Everything that exists, atoms,
celestial bodies are spinning,
Living things vibrate in an infinite revolution,
All of them particles
of the symphonic music of the spheres.

Harmonic sounds, mantras and meditation,
Connecting the mind with the collective consciousness of creation,
Lighting flames in the spirit
with the unconditional love force of the heart.

Let your life be the musical note of the immense universal pentagram,
bringing peace, harmony, wisdom, creative energy and enlightenment to the world.

Sincerely, in the power of harmony and light,

- Jay Emmanuel Morales

www.ingramcontent.com/pod-product-compliance
Lightning Source LLC
Chambersburg PA
CBHW081644280326
41928CB00069B/2915

9 780991 623716